Register Now for Online Access to Your Book!

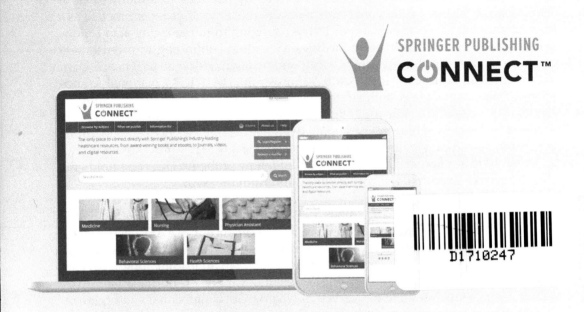

SPRINGER PUBLISHING
C⭘NNECT™

D1710247

Your print purchase of *The Health Services Executive (HSE*™*)* **includes online access to the contents of your book**—increasing accessibility, portability, and searchability!

Access today at:
http://connect.springerpub.com/content/book/978-0-8261-7733-9
or scan the QR code at the right with your smartphone
and enter the access code below.

B2UL2ETY

*Scan here for
quick access.*

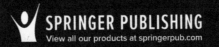
SPRINGER PUBLISHING
View all our products at springerpub.com

Keith R. Knapp, PhD, MHA, HSE, CFACHCA, currently serves as associate professor in the Department of Health Management and Policy at the University of Kentucky's College of Public Health and as Senior Advisor on Adult Programs for the Secretary of the Cabinet for Health and Family Services, Commonwealth of Kentucky. His current professional endeavors are rooted in 37 years of practice as a licensed nursing home administrator (NHA), ranging from managing stand-alone skilled nursing and rehabilitation facilities to leading continuing care retirement communities and a multi-site senior living organization. He is the past board chair of the American College of Health Care Administrators (ACHCA), National Association of Long Term Care Administrator Boards (NAB) and its affiliated foundation, Kentucky Board of Licensure for Long-Term Care Administrators, and Leading Age (Kentucky). He earned his undergraduate degree in arts and sciences and doctorate in gerontology from the University of Kentucky and his MHA from Xavier (Ohio) University. He is a licensed NHA and certified fellow of the ACHCA and holds the Health Services Executive (HSE™) qualification from the NAB.

Douglas M. Olson, PhD, MBA, LNHA, FACHCA, is the director of the Center for Health Administration and Aging Services Excellence (CHAASE) and professor of health administration at the University of Wisconsin–Eau Claire (UWEC). Prior to his academic career, Dr. Olson devoted 12 years to leading long-term care communities. Dr. Olson has been published in a variety of journals, has given numerous presentations, and has served on a variety of professional and organizational boards. His current research about advocacy for the profession has sparked a national collaboration among senior living organizations, academic programs, trade and professional associations, consumers, and regulatory agencies to mount a concerted, intentional, and coordinated effort to properly prepare enough future leaders in this field to meet the anticipated demand—known as Vision 2025. He earned his BS in healthcare administration from UWEC, MBA from the University of St. Thomas, and PhD in health services administration, research, and policy from the University of Minnesota. He is a licensed NHA and fellow of the American College of Health Care Administrators (ACHCA).

The Health Services Executive (HSE™)

Tools for Leading Long-Term Care and Senior Living Organizations

Keith R. Knapp, PhD, MHA, HSE, CFACHCA

Douglas M. Olson, PhD, MBA, LNHA, FACHCA

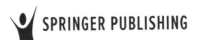 SPRINGER PUBLISHING

Springer Publishing Company, LLC
11 West 42nd Street, New York, NY 10036
www.springerpub.com
connect.springerpub.com/

Acquisitions Editor: David D'Addona
Compositor: Amnet Systems

ISBN: 978-0-8261-7732-2
ebook ISBN: 978-0-8261-7733-9
DOI: 10.1891/9780826177339

Qualified instructors may request supplements by emailing textbook@springerpub.com

Instructor's Manual ISBN: 978-0-8261-7734-6
Instructor's Test Bank ISBN: 978-0-8261-7736-0
Instructor's PowerPoints ISBN: 978-0-8261-7735-3

20 21 22 23 24 / 5 4 3 2 1

The author and the publisher of this Work have made every effort to use sources believed to be reliable to provide information that is accurate and compatible with the standards generally accepted at the time of publication. The author and publisher shall not be liable for any special, consequential, or exemplary damages resulting, in whole or in part, from the readers' use of, or reliance on, the information contained in this book. The publisher has no responsibility for the persistence or accuracy of URLs for external or third-party Internet websites referred to in this publication and does not guarantee that any content on such websites is, or will remain, accurate or appropriate.

Library of Congress Cataloging-in-Publication Data

Names: Knapp, Keith R., author. | Olson, Douglas M., author.
Title: The health services executive (HSE) : tools for leading long-term
  care and senior living organizations / Keith R. Knapp, Douglas M. Olson.
Description: First Springer Publishing edition. | New York, NY : Springer
  Publishing Company, 2021 | Includes bibliographical references and
  index. |
Identifiers: LCCN 2020016878 (print) | LCCN 2020016879 (ebook) | ISBN
  9780826177322 (paperback) | ISBN 9780826177339 (ebook) | ISBN
  9780826177346 (instructor's manual) | ISBN 9780826177360 (test bank) |
  ISBN 9780826177353 (powerpoints)
Subjects: MESH: Health Facility Administrators | Long-Term
  Care—organization & administration | Leadership | Homes for the
  Aged—organization & administration | Assisted Living
  Facilities—organization & administration | Health Services for the
  Aged—organization & administration
Classification: LCC RA999.A35 (print) | LCC RA999.A35 (ebook) | NLM WX
  155 | DDC 362.1606—dc23
LC record available at https://lccn.loc.gov/2020016878
LC ebook record available at https://lccn.loc.gov/2020016879

Contact us to receive discount rates on bulk purchases.
We can also customize our books to meet your needs.
For more information please contact: sales@springerpub.com

Publisher's Note: New and used products purchased from third-party sellers are not guaranteed for quality, authenticity, or access to any included digital components.

Printed in the United States of America.

I dedicate my contributions to this text to my lovely wife, Jane, without whose love, support, encouragement, and patience throughout the writing and editing process I would have faltered; to my family—parents, siblings, children, and grandchildren—who inspired my drive to share valuable lived experiences with the next generations; and to the nation's senior living organizations, their consumers, staff members, and families of both.

—K²

I dedicate my contributions to this text to my son, Lukas, who tolerated evenings when his dad was on his computer rather than playing another game of one-on-one hoops in the driveway; to my mom whose quiet selfless devotion to her family and long-term care nursing career taught me how to balance the best of both; to my immediate and extended family who always valued the wisdom of elders and the joy of young ones; and to the colleagues I have been blessed to get to know and be inspired by over the years.

—DO

Contents

Foreword

Our long-term care administrative profession has not received the attention it requires to train future leaders for what likely lies ahead, and that needs to change. The scope of practice has broadened considerably since the days when an administrator managed a nursing home and for good reason. In the next 10 years, the 75+ population is expected to grow by almost 40% as the boomer generation ages, and this growth is highest among adults 80 to 84, which is expected to grow by 55% from nearly 6 million today to over 9 million in 2030. Many of these elders will need services, and our current capacity and service mix will not meet that need. Responding to anticipated demand and the changing interests of consumers, existing services have evolved, and more lines of service have emerged to support older and disabled people, forming a more seamless *continuum* of care with varying funding streams, regulatory requirements, and opportunities for person-centered coordination. Sound leadership in our profession is one informed by these developments, working knowledge of their common denominators and differences, and nimble adaptability to this constantly evolving environment. Our noble profession, which is critically important to our aging country, deserves the same level of educational materials that other, more academically mainstream disciplines have today. This book is a big step forward for us.

We have the honor of leading the two largest national associations that defend and fight for providers across the continuum of aging services. It is a challenging but worthwhile battle. In that capacity we have seen firsthand the changing landscape of how and what services are paid for, public policies that support or inhibit good care and support, innovative models and approaches, the evolving role of technology, and a host of new stakeholders interested in our field. Services and supports vary greatly in whom they serve, how well and for how long they serve, and how they are structured at the organizational level. Many are excellent and provide care that we can all be proud of. But some are not, and often the gap comes down to knowledge and leadership. To address this divide, the authors have produced a comprehensive textbook that not only provides the how-to information concerning the profession but also provides the leadership lessons needed to succeed. At this moment in time, our sector really needs this.

The authors address both knowledge and leadership in this important text and are uniquely suited to do so. Their careers are rich and varied. But there is one step along their path that really stands out. Each has been a certified nurse aide (CNA). CNAs are in the forefront of everything that we do. They are underpaid, overworked, and underappreciated. But the work they do is heroic, inspiring, and skilled. It is what we are all about. For Keith and Doug, that practical experience is an incredible foundation for everything else to which they have devoted themselves. Each has been a licensed nursing home administrator (LNHA), each has had multiple leadership positions, and each now holds a PhD. For them, this is not theoretical. They have walked the walk.

The book comes at a critical moment. Demographics are changing rapidly. Millions of Americans are turning 75 years old every year, and many will need our care, services, and supports. And at the very time that we are needed, the profession is changing. Long gone are the care homes of the past. Skilled nursing facilities have become small hospitals. Assisted living communities are offering services more like the nursing homes of the past. The multitude of community and home-based services has grown exponentially, making it possible for older adults to remain in their homes longer. As such, we need sophisticated operations and talented, well-prepared leaders.

This book will help in both categories. It provides the historical context for our profession and the lessons needed for success today and tomorrow. Equally important, it teaches the value of leadership and leadership training. Facts and processes alone are of little value, but when combined with motivated leaders, they become powerful tools.

Undoubtedly, this is an important book at an important time. We have an incredible opportunity in this profession: We have the honor of supporting millions of people who desperately need our care and services. Our decisions and actions determine whether and how the final years of their lives will be spent in dignity and with purpose and value. We have the chance to change lives for the better. It is a huge responsibility but an incredibly rewarding career path. As you work with this book, we hope you will make the choice that we have. We have chosen a career in this profession and hope that you get to feel the same privilege and satisfaction every day that we do when we are making a positive difference in someone's life.

Katie Smith Sloan
President and CEO of LeadingAge and Executive Director of
the Global Ageing Network

The Honorable Mark Parkinson
President and CEO of the American Health Care Association and
National Center for Assisted Living

Preface

As an aging America seems certain to drive up demand for services, consumer expectations for more service options, choices, and flexibility are growing and affecting strategies among long-term care facilities and service lines. Regulations are in constant flux, and the rules surrounding their enforcement are not only inconsistently interpreted, they are sometimes even in conflict with one another. Reimbursement rates—publicly or privately funded—fall increasingly short of the true cost of providing quality care and services. Competition for hiring and then retaining qualified and motivated care and service staff presents challenges in a period of anticipated growth.

Why would anyone consider walking into such an apparent firestorm as a potential career path? The answer lies in the list of rewards—both professional and personal—of leading an organization charged with protecting, serving, and enhancing the lives of our nation's elders, rewards that are matched by so few other career options. It is not for the fainthearted or anyone who relies on predictability or routine for life satisfaction. However, there are plenty of opportunities for filling one's cup to serve those in need, to aspire to make a meaningful difference in the lives of others, to effectively overcome seemingly insurmountable odds, and to experience firsthand the living history of those an organization serves.

The field of senior living is not "Grandma's nursing home" anymore. It continues to expand in scope and complexity, with borders among service lines becoming increasingly vague or overlapping. The combination of skills and knowledge required of tomorrow's leaders in this profession will be broader and demand ongoing refinement after entry to practice. Preparation for a meaningful and successful career in senior living leadership is the warm-up for a journey—not an event. The journey is less likely to include a few successive stops with employers offering the same set of services than either (a) adapting—at any one site—to expanding or modified service lines or (b) adjusting to new environments with different blends of service lines.

Understanding the differences and similarities among senior living lines of service will not adequately equip tomorrow's executive leaders in this field to succeed. Having command of the applicable terminology, familiarity with the relevant regulations, and grasping the fundamentals of financial and human resources management will fall short; they are merely tools in the tool chest. Building or repairing something with those tools takes critical thinking, team building, creativity, flexibility, compassion, and courage—*leadership*. This book provides basic tools for successfully leading senior living organizations, as the title suggests, with a purposeful emphasis on the importance of exercising sound executive judgment and using the right tools for the job.

The National Association of Long Term Care Administrator Boards (NAB) periodically performs a professional practice analysis to determine the knowledge and skills a person should possess to assume the chief leadership position in a long-term care organization, referred to as its Domains of Practice. All states license nursing home administrators, and many are beginning to also license or consider licensing administrators of residential care/assisted living (RC/AL) facilities and some home- and community-based services (HCBS). The NAB commissioned a study that suggested four out of five of the skills and knowledge areas included in its established domains were comparable across multiple lines of service. That served as the basis for the NAB's development of the Health Services Executive (HSE™) qualification, which is discussed in more detail in this text. The authors also reviewed the work of the Senior Living Certification Commission that developed an assisted living director certification program sponsored by Argentum.

Textbooks on this subject published prior to the implementation of the HSE™ qualification model provide useful information for those preparing to become licensed administrators or credentialed assisted living managers. However, they tend to concentrate on managing the daily operation of institutional provider organizations, particularly skilled nursing facilities (SNFs) or assisted living facilities (ALFs), and not across multiple lines of senior living services. Fewer provide helpful discussions about the aging services continuum of care, and for those that do, it may be only from a social policy or broad conceptual perspective.

This book follows the NAB's current approach in describing the knowledge and skills covered. There are "core" competencies that apply to leading organizations across the senior living continuum and others that have unique, service line–specific qualities because of variances in regulations, reimbursement, or other practical considerations.

This text is divided into three sections. Section I provides an overview of the senior living field today. Chapter 1 offers a brief history of elder care in the United States, including changes in society's expectations and political initiatives responding to shifting demographics. Chapter 2 addresses the first of the NAB's Domains of Practice: customer care, supports, and services. How we develop and deliver truly person-centered care—starting with what we even call the customer—in such different settings is one of the key challenges for an HSE™. The relationship between monitoring clinical care metrics and quantifying the consumer experience is shifting in ways that add autonomy and power to care recipients and their families.

Section II addresses the nuts and bolts of operating the nonclinical support systems. Chapter 3 discusses the operating elements of human resources management—the NAB's second domain—from regulatory compliance issues to practical aspects of recruiting, screening, hiring, training, scheduling, evaluating, and retaining qualified, engaged staff members. Chapter 4, dealing with the NAB's third domain, covers providing leadership for the financial performance of the organization, from preparing budgets, monitoring cash flow, and managing other fiscal outcomes to risk management and capital financing. The NAB's fourth domain is featured in Chapter 5, leading the organization's efforts to exercise responsible stewardship in maintaining its physical plant and related assets; protecting the safety, dignity, and comfort of its customers, employees, and visitors; and aligning with regulatory compliance. This chapter also discusses various forms of organizational governance, their respective advantages and limitations, and an HSE™'s roles in interacting with a governing board.

Section III spreads the final NAB domain across five of the next seven chapters, tying together theory and practical application with an intentional emphasis on leadership. Chapters 6, 7, and 8 provide context for leadership while pulling together the other four domains, leveraging them to enhance the strategic and marketing direction of the organization. Chapter 9 addresses effective implementation of the strategic plan and adjusting to changing environments. Chapter 10 emphasizes the importance of valuing people as a critical asset. The uniqueness of senior living when it comes to customer service and its complex array of customers and stakeholders are at center stage in Chapter 11. Chapter 12 is devoted to the importance of continually developing the person in the mirror—professionally and personally—through acting on one's commitment to lifelong learning.

During the final stages of preparing this book, the world unexpectedly encountered an assault of unprecedented scale by the novel coronavirus, or COVID-19. In recognition of the pandemic's implications for both emergency disaster preparedness and customer care, service, and supports, we have added an afterword sharing important lessons learned from the early stages of this horrifying series of events.

Inserted throughout the chapters are relevant insights and recommendations shared by many of the profession's most highly respected and accomplished leaders. The appendix offers a robust, annotated glossary of acronyms and selected terms that commonly appear in the realm of senior living leadership.

At the end of each chapter appear the following:

- *Key Points* summarizing the "take-home" facts and concepts covered
- *Leadership Role(s)* related to that chapter's content
- *High-Impact Practices* of innovative senior living organizations
- *Questions for Discussion* to facilitate group interactions among students
- *Case Problems* providing fictional—but realistic—scenarios that invite exercising discernment and executive judgment
- *NAB Domains of Practice* highlighting specific sections directly related to that chapter's content
- *References* and *Additional Resources* including references plus suggested resources for further information about selected topics

At least four potential groups of readers will likely find this book useful:

1. **Instructors:** Faculty of an undergraduate or graduate course on long-term or postacute care administration can adopt this book as the course text or as a resource for specific content. (Recommended course prerequisites for consideration: basic math, financial accounting, medical terminology, psychology, and any introductory health systems or management courses.)

2. **Administrators-in-Training (AITs):** A non–academic degree track candidate for state licensure in the management of nursing homes, ALFs, or HCBS may find this book informative while framing their AIT schedule, during the field experience, or as a resource in preparing for the licensure examination.

3. **Practicing Senior Living Executives:** This book can serve as a reliable desk reference for applying one's knowledge and skills in the NAB domains across the three designated service lines; as a catalyst for inspiring internal leadership team discussions about high-impact practices, critical thinking, and problem-solving; and as a resource when serving as a preceptor for an AIT or student intern.

4. **Public Servants and Consumer Advocates:** The list of stakeholders with a keen interest in the ultimate success of a contemporary HSE™ includes regulators, policy makers, clients, their families, and other consumer advocates.

For an instructor who adopts this book for a course, the ancillary resources are:

- Chapter-summarizing slides in PowerPoint format
- Test Bank: HSE™ core and service line–specific questions (multiple-choice, true-or-false, and short essay questions for each chapter)
- Instructor's Manual: Suggested student activities and test bank with answer key

We welcome your thoughts, comments, and suggestions, which we will gladly consider incorporating into a second edition. You can reach us at HSE.Yodas@gmail.com.

Keith R. Knapp and Douglas M. Olson

Qualified instructors may obtain access to supplements by emailing textbook@springerpub.com

Acknowledgments

Several widely recognized leaders in the field of senior living leadership have offered insightful comments, recommendations, observations, and opinions concerning a host of topics; their names and affiliations appear with their contributions. David D'Addona and Jaclyn Shultz have been extraordinarily helpful in shepherding this project, as have been the editorial and production staff at Springer Publishing. Our colleagues at the University of Kentucky and University of Wisconsin–Eau Claire (UWEC) have consistently provided encouragement and scheduling flexibility throughout the process, affording us the professional space and time to complete it. The classes of UWEC healthcare administration students devoted some of their time to gathering related resources and exploring concepts that helped inform the development of the textbook. Our peers in academe who teach courses regarding senior living leadership and long-term care administration have clamored for a new textbook that truly reflects the current environment and have supported our attempt at producing one that is relevant and rooted in practice. We are extremely grateful to all!

Introduction

THE CHANGING ENVIRONMENT IN SENIOR LIVING: TERMS OF ENDEARMENT

The phrase *long-term care* is used to refer to the services provided by a nursing home. However, the array of service lines that comprise today's senior living sector has expanded to include a much broader range of care options. This evolving continuum of service lines has less well-defined boundaries. Varying regulatory and payment environments exist, sometimes overlapping and occasionally even conflicting. Multifaceted interorganizational relationships continue to emerge between long-term acute care hospitals (LTACHs), in-patient rehabilitation facilities (IRFs), skilled nursing and nursing facilities (SNF/NFs), residential care and assisted living (RC/AL) communities, congregate senior housing, and home- and community-based services (HCBS), such as medical and nonmedical home health agencies, hospices, adult day centers, and providers of transportation and telehealth services. Their interconnections continue to grow in complexity and depth, and the gaps between them have steadily eroded over the past two decades.

Postacute care began gaining popularity as a descriptive term following the enactment of the Patient Protection and Affordable Care Act of 2010 (Ackerly & Grabowski, 2014). It is sometimes shortened to the Affordable Care Act, abbreviated as ACA, or referred to as ObamaCare because President Obama strongly advocated for and signed the enabling legislation into law. The proliferation of this phrase's use seems somewhat ironic for at least two reasons. First, the ACA actually did very little to directly affect the realm of long-term care and related supportive services. Second, people access the service lines included in the continuum described earlier before (pre-), after (post-), and sometimes in lieu of acute care services. Describing this cluster of services as *post*acute care is unnecessarily limiting and technically insufficient. While the authors hold that the field deserves a label that is more descriptive, we acknowledge *postacute care* as a leading one in contemporary use.

Senior living has become an increasingly embraced term of art that encompasses all of the elements mentioned across the postacute, long-term care continuum. We tend to prefer it because it replaces the traditional institutional bias by emphasizing the service *recipients* (rather than service providers) and the overarching goal of them *living* their lives (instead of receiving care). Although the terms appear throughout the text somewhat interchangeably, *senior living* captures the essence of the field better than anything else we have yet seen or heard.

CHIEF CONTRIBUTING INFLUENCES

Demographic shifts toward an increasingly mature American population are profoundly influencing payment models, available resources, and consumer expectations. The underlying population growth trend of an aging citizenry has as its most significant contributor the arrival of the baby boomer generation (born between 1946 and 1964) at the door of retirement age. Nearly 10,000 of them turn 65 every day, a phenomenon that will likely continue for another decade, according to the U.S. Census Bureau (2019). By 2030, we expect one in five Americans to be at least 65 years of age. Accordingly, we can reasonably anticipate an unprecedented level of demand for health and human services aimed at supporting people with needs that typically accompany advanced ages (Colby & Ortman, 2014).

Both government-sponsored systems for financing such services and commercial insurance products are already undergoing significant revisions in order to address actuarial imbalances between the inflow of contributions (tax revenues and premiums, respectively) and outflow of benefit payments. As we enter a new decade, Social Security and Medicare account for over 45% of all federal spending (U.S. Social Security Administration, 2019). The trustees of the Social Security and Medicare Trust Fund predict the combined cost of the Social Security and Medicare programs to rise from its current 8.7% of gross domestic product (GDP) to 11.6% by 2035. Policy options for addressing this before the trust fund empties include raising taxes, reducing benefits, changing eligibility requirements, or some combination of two or more of them. Evolving public payment models receive substantial attention in Chapter 4, Financial Management in Senior Care.

According to the American Association for Long-Term Care Insurance (AALTCI), indemnifying the risk of long-term care expenses with traditional insurance approaches has already become unsustainable. There are fewer commercial carriers offering traditional policies, due either to a business decision to withdraw from that market or to consolidating mergers and acquisitions (Gleckman, 2017). The AALTCI conducted a survey of over 1,000 insurance professionals who had prior experience selling both traditional and contemporary long-term care policies. Nearly one half predicted that their sale of traditional products would drop during the next 5 years and their sale of linked-benefit products would grow; one in 12 predicted that traditional products have a short future. Aimed at improving sales and mitigating actuarial risk, a budding approach by those remaining is linking long-term care benefits with other types of benefit with which the public may be more familiar, such as life insurance or annuities (Gleckman, 2019).

Consumers have also become more aware of and better informed about available senior living options, as well as about what to expect in each setting. Decisions about meeting acute care needs tend to be episodic and time limited, and those needs are often unexpected and/or urgent. Choices about senior living tend to be slower to develop, deliberative, and dynamic. They often involve more people than the actual end user, such as a spouse, adult child, other family member, or friend. Except for the case of needing postacute *rehabilitation* services, there is less likely to be an *event* that inspires one to explore senior living options than either a *series of negative events* or a *steady decline in functional independence* (Kane & Kane, 2001).

LEADERSHIP DEMAND AND SUPPLY

Amid this increasing complexity, one glaring constant persists: Service providers across the continuum of senior living need appropriately prepared, competent, and effective leaders, and they fully expect that they will require even more in the years ahead. Both the U.S. Department of Labor's Bureau of Labor Statistics and the U.S. Health Services and Research Administration's Bureau of Workforce Development produce estimates of workforce demand for most clinical health professions, but not for the field of senior living administration. The anticipated need for administrative leadership shows steady growth, but the projections combine all healthcare service lines (U.S. Bureau of Labor Statistics, 2019; U.S. Health Resources and Services Administration, 2019). Furthermore, the consensus among leaders of the relevant trade associations and professional societies is loud and clear: We need a pipeline providing talented, well-prepared candidates to both replace retiring leaders and expand our services to meet anticipated demand.

Framework: Essential Elements of Senior Living Leadership

The National Association of Long Term Care Administrator Boards (NAB) is widely considered the leading authority on licensing, credentialing, and regulating administrators of organizations along the spectrum of senior living. Its membership includes delegates from regulatory boards and agencies responsible for licensure of long-term care administrators in all 50 states and the District of Columbia. Since its inception in 1971, NAB has embraced its fundamental charge of enhancing the effectiveness of its member boards to fulfill their respective public protection duties. NAB facilitates the sharing of best practices for preparing and qualifying new administrators as well as for enforcing applicable regulations regarding standards of practice, continuing education, and licensure renewal.

NAB periodically conducts a "job analysis" to determine the most relevant knowledge, skills, and tasks of effective postacute care administrators. The results—referred to as the *domains of practice*—serve as the foundation for preparing administrators to enter the profession and to continue their professional development throughout their careers. The domains of practice also help frame curricula for academic programs and administrator-in-training (AIT) programs, the content of valid and reliable licensure examinations, and criteria for evaluating continuing education programs. The five categories of NAB's domains of practice for long-term care administration—key tasks with specific knowledge and skills expected to perform them—include (NAB, 2019a):

10 Customer Care, Supports, and Services: Nineteen key tasks related to planning, implementing, monitoring, and evaluating direct care and services, from compliance with applicable federal and state laws governing care, documentation, records storage, and contract services to fostering person-centered care through the admission process, care planning and delivery, discharge planning, and quality assurance and performance improvement (QAPI)

20 Human Resources: Fifteen key tasks concerning recruiting, hiring, training, motivating, and retaining the organization's most precious resource—its staff

30 Finance: Ten core competencies regarding sound stewardship of financial resources, such as budgeting, managing the revenue cycle and cash flow, monitoring financial performance, securing capital, and risk management

40 Environment: Eleven central tasks related to planning, implementing, monitoring, and evaluating systems that address the physical plant and environment, such as safety and security, sanitation, emergency and disaster

preparedness, preventive maintenance, technology and care recipients' privacy, dignity, and autonomy

50 Leadership and Management: Nineteen essential tasks that foster the successful pursuit of the governing body's approved mission, values, and vision by implementing, monitoring, and evaluating procedures consistent with the governing body's approved policies

The NAB's 2020 Professional Practice Analysis is expected to lead to adjustments in the knowledge and skills that comprise its domains of practice. However, that seems likely to consist more of reallocating relative weights of emphasis among the domains to reflect contemporary practice than making substantive content revisions; more similar to reshuffling a deck of playing cards than adding another number or suit.

Response: Broader Preparation for Senior Living Leaders

Originally focused on administrators of nursing homes, the expansion of the senior living continuum of care prompted NAB to take a wider view of the profession. The association broadened the scope of its 2013 job analysis by commissioning a professional practice analysis (PPA) designed to examine common and specialized tasks, knowledge, and skills required along multiple lines of service. The results demonstrated that a significant common core of them does apply to leading organizations providing any of those services. This finding served as the impetus for establishing a more broadly based approach to training and credentialing senior living leaders going forward.

In 2015, NAB launched an initiative to establish relevant minimum competency standards for administrators across postacute care lines of service. The triple aim of this plan included proactively (a) fostering public protection beyond the nursing home setting, (b) strengthening the cost-effectiveness of pre- and postacute care, and (c) enhancing access to appropriate care by bolstering professional mobility (NAB, 2014). Competent leadership matters for any organization's quality or financial performance. Professional mobility for administrators across the continuum of care, the map, makes opening or expanding services to meet growing community demand more readily achievable.

The new qualification standard introduced by NAB is the Health Services Executive (HSE™). It is intended to recognize a person achieving minimal proficiency in a common core and unique entry-level competencies concerning leadership in each of three lines of postacute care service: skilled nursing care, RC/AL, and HCBS (Figure 1).

According to NAB, successful demonstration of this combination of competencies—as measured by education, experience, and examination—meets or exceeds the current requirements of licensure to practice as a nursing home administrator (NHA), an RC/AL, and administrators practicing in the field of HCBS, in the vast majority of licensing jurisdictions. NAB describes this approach as Licensure by Equivalency. It continues to support examination and licensure of NHA and RC/AL administrators, while adding the option of licensure for HCBS executives.

Although no federal mandate yet exists for licensing administrators in either of the two additional service lines, there appears to be growing interest in this initiative among NAB's member boards, the legislative branches of their respective jurisdictions, providers of multiple service lines and/or multistate operations, and consumers (Lindner, 2019). Given the anticipated growth in the number of elders

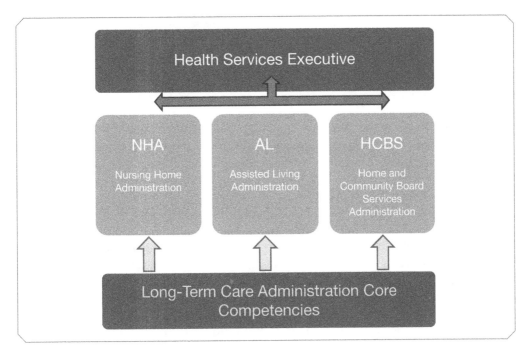

Figure 1 A New Vision for the Profession. Core + Specialized Competencies = HSE™

Source: Reproduced with permission from the National Association of Long Term Care Administrator Boards. (2014). *NAB's professional practice analysis aligns leadership core competencies across expanding continuum of care.* Washington, DC: NAB White Paper.

and disabled adults—and their families—the senior living field expects to serve, as well as the tremendous amount of public and private dollars that will flow through provider organizations, it makes good sense to adopt evidence-based competency standards for the people leading those operations. Why should America wait for a disaster and repeat the unfortunate series of events and subsequent process that led to licensing NHAs four decades ago?

Windshield Versus Rearview Mirror: Watch the Road Ahead

None of the textbooks currently listed on NAB's bibliography for the development of its examinations comprehensively reflect the structure, depth, and breadth of the new HSE™ model (NAB, 2019b). Students and faculty (in either a degree-granting academic program or a state-recognized AIT program), as well as practitioners, point to a dearth of information inside one textbook about gerontology, contemporary views on effective leadership, regulatory compliance, technology, and entry pathways to the profession—as they apply to all three environments.

Our profession also has a storied tradition of relying heavily on the apprenticeship model of learning what truly matters under the guidance of an experienced mentor or preceptor. Although we by no means advocate for the abandonment or erosion of that approach, the framework for *what* an aspiring HSE™ acquires (leadership core and unique service line elements) and from *whom* (possibly more than one mentor) will necessarily need to reflect the increasingly seamless nature of the postacute care continuum. Practicum arrangements will require a parallel reconfiguration so that students have opportunities to learn about multiple service lines from subject matter experts in each of them.

A NEW RESOURCE: *THE HEALTH SERVICES EXECUTIVE* (HSE™)

The current trends in the senior living field drive the direction for preparing its leaders of tomorrow. This text represents the authors' attempt to apply our complementary experiences as leaders of both senior living and human services organizations and academic programs in health and long-term care administration toward charting a new map for that journey with a handy tool chest to go with it. Our chief goal is to provide relevant guidance to both those entering the field and those wishing to strengthen their credentials and career options, to equip them with tools for remaining nimble in a field that is becoming more complex at increasing speed, hence the byline in the text's title: *Tools for Leading Long-Term Care and Senior Living Organizations*.

In anticipation of NAB's success at fostering the adoption of its HSE™ model as the gold standard in the profession, the NAB domains of practice and new exam design (core + service line) serve as the foundation for how we have arranged information. How those domains manifest themselves in each of the three HSE™ service lines receives significant attention through illustrative examples, case studies, and domain-specific discussion questions. Additionally, we include supplemental guidance around key contemporary concepts regarding effective leadership, such as exercising executive judgment and critical thinking, as well as modeling integrity, ethical conduct, accountability, transparency, honesty, confidentiality, and trustworthiness.

The authors intend for this text to serve as much more than a study guide for preparing to pass a licensure examination. We expect the information included will offer relevant and practical assistance—and encouragement—as the senior living field continues to evolve. It is an exciting and challenging time to join this field of endeavor. Welcome to the ranks of those who find it so rewarding and fulfilling.

REFERENCES

Ackerly, D., & Grabowski, D. (2014). Post-acute care *reform—beyond the* ACA. *New England Journal of Medicine, 370*(8), 689–691. Retrieved from https://www.nejm.org/doi/full/10.1056/NEJMp1315350

American Association for Long Term Care Insurance. (2019, May 19). *Long term care insurance trends impact marketplace*. Retrieved from https://www.aaltci.org/news/long-term-care-insurance-news/long-term-care-insurance-trends-impact-marketplace

Colby, S. L., & Ortman, J. M. (2014, May). *The baby boom cohort in the United States: 2012 to 2060*. Current Population Reports, P25-1141. U.S. Department of Commerce, Economics and Statistics Administration, U.S. Census Bureau. Retrieved from https://www.census.gov/prod/2014pubs/p25-1141.pdf

Gleckman, H. (2017, September 8). The traditional long-term care insurance market crumbles. *Forbes*. Retrieved from https://www.forbes.com/sites/howardgleckman/2017/09/08/the-traditional-long-term-care-insurance-market-crumbles/#64c8c8443ec3

Gleckman, H. (2019, April 1). Another shock to the long-term care insurance industry. *Forbes*. Retrieved from https://www.forbes.com/sites/howardgleckman/2019/04/01/another-shock-to-the-long-term-care-insurance-industry/#6473a30e385e

Kane, R., & Kane, R. (2001, November/December). What consumers want from long term care and how they can get it. *Health Affairs, 20,* 6. Retrieved from https://www.healthaffairs.org/doi/full/10.1377/hlthaff.20.6.114

Lindner, R. (2019, November 15). *Author Interview with CEO of NAB.*

National Association of Long Term Care Administrator Boards. (2014). *NAB's professional practice analysis aligns leadership core competencies across expanding continuum of care.* Washington, DC: NAB White Paper.

National Association of Long Term Care Administrator Boards. (2019a). *Annotation of tasks performed and knowledge and skills used across lines of service in long term care.* Retrieved from https://www.nabweb.org/filebin/pdf/Annotation_of_Tasks_Performed_Across_LOS_in_LTC.pdf

National Association of Long Term Care Administrator Boards. (2019b). *Health services executive study resources.* Retrieved from https://www.nabweb.org/hsestudyresources

U.S. Bureau of Labor Statistics. (2019). *Outlook: Medical and health services managers.* Retrieved from https://www.bls.gov/ooh/management/medical-and-health-services-managers.htm

U.S. Health Resources and Services Administration, National Center for Health Workforce Analysis. (2019). *About NCHWA.* Retrieved from https://bhw.hrsa.gov/national-center-health-workforce-analysis

U.S. Social Security Administration. (2019). *2019 social security and Medicare trust fund report.* Retrieved from https://www.ssa.gov/oact/TRSUM/

The Postacute Segment of Healthcare and Human Services

Section I begins with a historical reflection of the field. Chapter 1, The Senior Living Field: Background, History, and Its Current and Future State, takes the reader through the various stages of development of senior living services in the United States. It provides a framework for the context of elder care, its origins, and its status today. The roots of aging services are explored and examined to help future long-term care leaders understand both the positive contributions made by many different stakeholders that have propelled the field forward and some of the challenging times of our field's history.

Chapter 1 also encourages a foundational understanding of the various legislative and policy shifts that have occurred in the United States, underscoring the importance for any health services leader to know why policy matters and how policy impacts each stakeholder and long-term care facility. Being engaged in the conversation is easier for leaders when they have a solid foundation and appreciation of the intended and unintended consequences of both past and current major policy initiatives. Having a clearer picture of the evolving provider landscape also helps both the emerging and practicing leader to consider how the world is changing, how far we have yet to go, and how we may get there with new policies. The proverbial "elephant in the room" is the changing demographic staring in front of us and in the years ahead and drives what may become tomorrow's portfolio of care and services.

In Chapter 2, Customer Care, Supports, and Services, the elements of customer care, supportive factors, and service practices that require a deeper understanding for both the developing and practicing leader serve as an important knowledge platform. The different needs and desires of consumers are explored with a commitment to the person. The true importance of the care and service team is highlighted, including opportunities for improvement through better coordination across disciplines and care settings. Several high-impact practices are described to instill a spirit of optimism that there is always a better way. This reflects the quality philosophy that is introduced in this chapter and embedded throughout the text and the value it brings to all the stakeholders involved in this care and service community—consumers and practitioners.

CHAPTER 1

The Senior Living Field: Background, History, and Its Current and Future State

INTRODUCTION

The field of aging services has evolved tremendously over the years. In 1657, the first almshouses were built in New York (Abramovitz, 1996). Almshouses originally created by the Dutch were also called poor houses or county homes in the United States, which were locally administered public institutions for homeless, aged persons without means. These facilities were often created as extensions of churches or other charitable organizations. The leaders of these settings were typically referred to as wardens or superintendents. More often, during these early years, care and service of elders was still largely dependent on family support.

From the late 17th century until the early 20th century, the so-called poor houses provided by churches or other organizations were the state of elder care facilities in the United States until the government started to play a more significant role during the period of the Great Depression. One of the first notable actions was the passing of the Social Security Act of 1935. Title I of the act forged a partnership between the federal government and states to address, to some degree, the financial challenges of the older population. Additionally, a key element of the Act had both employers and employees make contributions for a supplemental workers' retirement fund. Initially, this social safety net was set at the age of 65, which was based on the life expectancy in the United States at the time (Centers for Disease Control and Prevention [CDC], 2017). Both elements helped provide some modest level of support to elders in their later years.

One of the next significant legislative initiatives was the passing of the Hill–Burton Act in 1946. Although the new law focused on hospital growth, it did serve as a model for some long-term care (LTC) funding. The funding for senior care during this period was largely contributed by nonprofit groups, such as religious-affiliated organizations, and was very limited in scope. There was somewhat of a boom of LTC building growth following the Hill–Burton Act in the 1950s, mostly by for-profit housing and real estate with Federal Housing Authority and Small Business Administration loans being used to finance these projects. One of the characteristics of the funding arrangements that was notable was the significantly financially leveraged funding models that were used by these groups. Due to the limited experience in the provision of care and services for elders, this period of LTC history could be described as one with abundant variation and with little quality control or oversight.

President Lyndon Johnson's efforts in 1965 for comprehensive reform of senior living services launched a much larger role of government in senior care. The Older Americans Act (OAA) was signed into law with many broad aims, including:

- focus on ensuring adequate retirement incomes;
- consideration of both physical and mental health;
- provision of suitable housing;
- good restorative services;
- the pursuit of meaningful activity;
- community services, including access to low-cost transportation;
- supporting demonstration projects and research; and
- enabling individual initiative in planning and managing their own lives.

The driver of these services was mostly through the Administration on Aging (AOA) via matching grants to qualifying states, ranging from community-based planning, demonstration grants, research on aging, and personnel training, to creating recreational facilities and guidance centers. However, funding services for the aging was limited because of other priorities in the country at the time, such as the war in Vietnam (Administration for Community Living, 2019).

The Long-Term Care Ombudsman Program was also authorized under the OAA and administered at the state level. It provides residents of LTC facilities with access to effective advocacy in order to ensure that they receive the quality of care and quality of life they deserve and are entitled to by law.

The year 1965 also saw the passage of Medicare and Medicaid. Medicare was advanced as a health insurance program for the elderly. Medicaid was put into place as a health insurance program for low-income persons in the United States. Both were established as part of the Social Security Act. They embodied a major policy shift for the country in face of greater life expectancy and needed senior services and continue to stand the test of time. Several senior care services, most notably skilled nursing care (or, at the time, nursing home care) and home care, saw tremendous growth and availability for individuals after enaction of the law.

In addition to the growth of senior living services and medical coverage, there was also legislation bringing housing reform with the passage of the Housing and Urban Development Act of 1965. The legislation expanded funding for existing federal housing programs and added new programs that provided rent subsidies for the elderly and disabled; housing rehabilitation grants to poor homeowners; provisions for veterans to make very low down payments to obtain mortgages; new authority for families qualifying for public housing to be placed in empty private housing (along with subsidies to landlords); and matching grants to localities for the construction of water and sewer facilities, construction of community centers in low-income areas, and urban beautification. The Department of Housing and Urban Development (HUD) was also created. In many instances, HUD paved the way for affordable senior housing and LTC facilities' growth across the country, especially in high population urban areas, in the 1960s through the 1980s.

As LTC facilities grew in number, there was a greater call for national standards of quality. The Federal Nursing Home Reform Act, passed in 1987 (also known as OBRA'87), created a set of national minimum set of standards of care and rights for people living in certified nursing facilities. This landmark federal legislation came at a time when many were calling for enhanced quality and service in the nursing home field due to public concerns about some poor living conditions placing frail elders at risk. This legislation had a significant impact on rules and regulations over the next couple of decades.

The American With Disabilities Act (ADA) became law shortly after OBRA in 1990. The ADA, a civil rights law, prohibited discrimination against individuals with disabilities in all areas of public life. The purpose of the law was to make sure that people with disabilities had the same rights and opportunities as everyone else. The ADA gave civil rights protections to individuals with disabilities similar to those provided to individuals on the basis of race, color, sex, national origin, age, and religion. It has guaranteed equal opportunity for individuals with disabilities and is divided into five different sections that relate to different areas of public life (ADA, 2019). As a matter of general knowledge, the ADA applies to all citizens, but LTC facility residents are disproportionately disabled—so they benefit from the protections included in the law.

In the past few decades, there have been several other sections added to shore up legislation and provide more options and better standards to the LTC field.

- In 1997, the Balanced Budget Act was a bipartisan legislation that was an effort to curb Medicare payments. It also launched the creation of Medicare Part C (Medicare Advantage). The legislation also allowed states to advance state Medicaid managed care organization (MCO) programs. It also made enhancements to the State Children's Health Insurance Program (SCHIP) and was initially funded by an increased tobacco tax.

- In 2003, the Medicare Modernization Act (MMA) was passed and created Medicare Part D (prescription drugs), which began in 2006. This law allows individuals to voluntarily enroll in private plans that are approved by the Centers for Medicare & Medicaid Services (CMS) and has helped mitigate the challenges of prescription drug costs for seniors (Kellogg Foundation, 2019).

- Home- and community-based services (HCBS) became even more readily available in 1983, when Congress added section 1915(c) to the Social Security Act, giving states the option to receive a waiver of Medicaid rules governing institutional care. In 2005, HCBS became a formal Medicaid state plan option. Several states include HCBS in their Medicaid state plans. Forty-seven states and DC are operating at least one 1915(c) waiver.

- The Older Americans Act Reauthorization Act of 2016 was passed and signed into law by President Obama. The Act helps older adults age with independence and dignity in their homes and communities and protect elders in LTC facilities and other settings. Reauthorization strengthens and improves this program's effectiveness. It clarifies both organizational and individual conflicts of interest within the program; improves resident access to ombudsmen; better protects the confidentiality of ombudsman information; ensures that state ombudsmen receive ongoing training; and permits ombudsmen, when feasible, to continue to serve residents transitioning from an LTC facility to a home care setting.

THE PATIENT PROTECTION AND AFFORDABLE CARE ACT

The Patient Protection and Affordable Care Act (ACA) was signed into law in 2010 and has three main objectives:

1. To reform the private insurance market—especially for individuals and small-group purchasers—and make affordable health insurance available to more people. The law provides consumers with subsidies ("premium tax credits") that lower costs for households with incomes between 100% and 400% of the federal poverty level.

2. To expand Medicaid to the working poor with income up to 133% of the federal poverty level and expand the Medicaid program to cover all adults with income below 138% of the federal poverty level. (Not all states have expanded their Medicaid programs.)

3. To change the way that medical decisions are made by supporting innovative medical care delivery methods designed to lower the costs of healthcare generally (Healthcare.gov, 2019).

There are also numerous policy advances happening today that are focused on value-based care and services and incentivizing and rewarding efforts to work across the silos of services and settings, including improvements for Medicare Advantage plans and advancing Medicare payment and delivery reforms with accountable care organizations. A few of the other enhancements within the ACA for seniors included providing prescription drug discounts, adding more preventive visits eligibility, and a focus on fraud and abuse within Medicare (see Exhibit 1.1 for more information).

EXHIBIT 1.1 Highlights of the Legislative Initiatives in Senior Care

1935 Social Security Act passed to provide Old Age Assistance and Survivors Insurance.

1946 Hill–Burton Act passed to give hospitals and other health facilities grants and loans for construction and modernization.

1959 Housing Act established Section 202: Supportive Housing for the Elderly as part of the Housing and Urban Development (HUD) program.

1965 Older Americans Act established the Administration on Aging, and Medicare and Medicaid were added to the Social Security Act.

1973 Older Americans Act Comprehensive Services Amendments established Area Agencies on Aging. The amendments added grants for multipurpose senior centers.

1974 Title XX of the Social Security Amendments authorized grants to states for social services.

1975–1981 Older Americans Act amendments authorized coverage of a variety of services for seniors, grants to Indian Tribal Organizations, Congregate Housing Service, and required states to establish a long-term care ombudsman program to cover nursing homes.

1983 Congress added Section 1915(c) to the Social Security Act, allowing home- and community-based services to be more readily available.

1987 Omnibus Budget Reconciliation Act provides for nursing home reform.

1990 Americans with Disabilities Act extended protection to persons with disabilities.

1997 The Balanced Budget Act passed to help curb Medicare payments. It also launched the creation of Medicare Part C (Medicare Advantage). The legislation also allowed states to advance state Medicaid managed care organization (MCO) programs.

2003 Medicare Prescription Drug, Improvement, and Modernization Act enactment, which included the creation of Medicare Part D, a prescription drug benefit, and Medicare Advantage Plans.

2005 Home- and Community-Based Services became a formal Medicaid state plan option based on Section 1915.

2010 The Affordable Care Act was put into place by executive order.

* There have been ongoing amendments to the Older Americans Act focusing on additional protections and expansion of services, particularly in the home- and community-based service arenas with state implementation emphasized.

THE CURRENT STATE AND FUTURE OUTLOOK OF LONG-TERM CARE AND SENIOR SERVICES

Since the Social Security Act of 1935 became law, America has continued to steadily expand the capacity of, elevate the standards for, devote more resources to, and heighten its expectations for senior living care and services. With the senior population expected to grow tremendously in the decades to come and with new preferences emerging for services, there are many opportunities and challenges for the field and for future LTC leaders and administrators. Significant influences on them include various demographic trends, developments in each line of service, and growth in population segments that require specific care and service needs.

Demographic Trends

By 2050, the population of individuals who are 65 and older in the United States is projected to double, growing faster than any other age group. As seniors age, their risk of having chronic diseases or functional limitations increases. According to LeadingAge, a national association that represents non-profit aging service providers, these risks are higher among members of minority groups, who are expected to make up 42% of the senior population in 2050 (LeadingAge, 2019). The risk of having a functional limitation or chronic disease is also higher among those living in poverty, who were 16% of the senior population in 2010 but whose numbers are expected to grow in the future. Many seniors, however, wish to remain in their homes and communities for as long as possible. This presents new challenges for America's senior living field because of its current reliance on institution-based care and the changing demographics of the available workforce (see Exhibit 1.2).

Present-Day Providers and Services

The postacute network of lines of services and settings is robust and ever changing based on the demand and preferences of this aging population. There are some who would say that these lines of service are blurring a bit, yet they do each still have their own distinct set of principles and philosophies of care and service.

Long-term acute care hospitals (LTACHs) are facilities that specialize in the treatment of patients with serious medical conditions that require care on an ongoing basis but no longer require intensive care or extensive diagnostic procedures. A LTACH needs to be designed to deliver more complex clinical care than a skilled

EXHIBIT 1.2 Projected Population of Older Adults by 2035

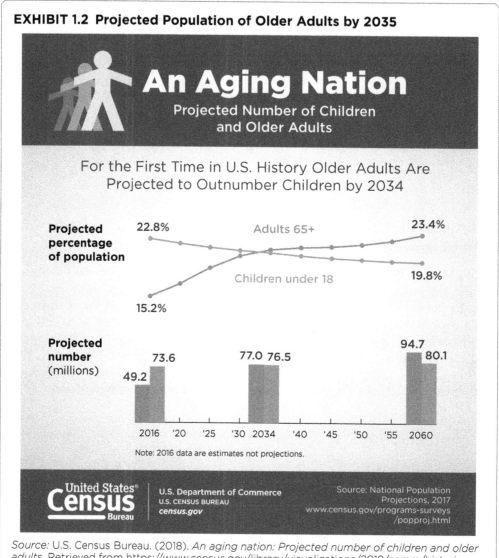

An Aging Nation

Projected Number of Children and Older Adults

For the First Time in U.S. History Older Adults Are Projected to Outnumber Children by 2034

Projected percentage of population

Adults 65+ — 22.8% ... 23.4%

Children under 18 — 15.2% ... 19.8%

Projected number (millions)

2016	'20	'25	'30	2034	'40	'45	'50	'55	2060
49.2	73.6			77.0 76.5					94.7 80.1

Note: 2016 data are estimates not projections.

United States® Census Bureau

U.S. Department of Commerce
U.S. CENSUS BUREAU
census.gov

Source: National Population Projections, 2017
www.census.gov/programs-surveys /popproj.html

Source: U.S. Census Bureau. (2018). *An aging nation: Projected number of children and older adults.* Retrieved from https://www.census.gov/library/visualizations/2018/comm/historic -first.html

nursing facility (SNF), because LTACH residents are in poorer health and less able to care for themselves. Current estimates are that the country has approximately 400 of these operating in the United States.

SNF is an inpatient rehabilitation center staffed with trained medical professionals. Such facilities provide the medically necessary services of nurses, physical and occupational therapists, speech pathologists, and audiologists. There are approximately 15,000 SNFs in the United States. These facilities are still referred to as nursing homes, yet most have moved well past that era. It is true that some residents are still receiving traditional services for a long-term stay; however, many more have shifted their services to much more rehabilitation and specialized services.

Assisted living facility is housing for elderly or disabled people and provides some level of nursing care, housekeeping, social activities, and prepared meals as needed and based on individual preferences. There are more than 28,000 assisted living residences in the United States, housing more than 1 million people, according to the National Center for Assisted Living (NCAL). The "typical" assisted living resident is an 83-year-old woman, and the average age of all assisted living residents is 83. The average female/male ratio in assisted living residences is 3:1. According to the NCAL, the average size of an assisted living residence is 43 units and ranges from 3 units to 200 units. The average number of residents in a facility is 40, with a range of 1 to 175. Residential care is also provided by many states through their Medicaid program with waiver programs and provides a similar level of service than assisted living. Assisted living generally falls into a couple of categories, including either a social model or a medical model. One of the distinct recent areas of development in the more medically oriented sites are facilities that specialize in memory care.

The low-income HUD and its **supportive housing for the elderly program** is an important presence in the field. HUD's Section 202 program helped expand the supply of affordable housing with supportive services for the elderly. It provided direct loans and capital advances from the federal government to support nonprofit entities to build housing for very low-income elderly. Senior housing through Section 202 provided seniors, defined as 62 or older, with options that allow them to live independently but in an environment that provides support activities such as cleaning, cooking, transportation, and others. Although funding has was tightened in 2012, affordable senior housing developments that were built with Section 202 funds continue to provide housing and services to their residents. There are new programs from the Federal Housing Authority that have helped supplement the capital needs of senior housing in recent years.

Independent senior housing in the private market continues to be a viable option for many seniors who explore this option earlier than some of the others. These senior housing properties for those 55-plus years in age often focus on being safe and affordable with convenient amenities. There continues to be tremendous growth in this arena with some recent attention to the middle-income market population (Pearson et al., 2019).

Continuing care retirement communities (CCRC) and life plan communities are retirement communities that include the span of services that offer a continuum of care, including independent living, assisted living, skilled nursing, and home care options. Elderly persons can spend the rest of their life and "age in place" without moving from the community. These settings often require a deposit or an investment as part of entrance fee along with their monthly fees structure.

Group or family care homes are housing settings that include services where seniors or people with disabilities live in the same building; these are sometimes called group homes and are usually smaller in size and often cater to certain populations. For individuals with intellectual and developmental disabilities, a group care home is sometimes an option, although these individuals may also prefer support with home care with their families.

Home- and Community-Based Services

Home health is a range of healthcare services that can be received in the home for an illness or injury. Home health care can be less expensive and more convenient and may be just as effective as care received in another setting. There were approximately 12,200 agencies in the United States in 2016 (CDC, 2019).

Homecare or personal care is also offered in a variety of ways across the country, including covered services for nonmedical or custodial care services. **Homemaker services** are also available for assistance with general household chores that an individual is not able to do at their residence. These services are generally covered under Medicaid depending on the state the person lives in and their waiver program.

Hospice offers four levels of care, two of which happen at home. The four levels are as follows:

- **Routine Home Care:** This is the most common level of hospice care, and this includes nursing and home health aide services.
- **Continuous Home Care:** This is provided when a person needs continuous nursing care during a time of crisis or emergency.
- **General Inpatient Care:** This is short-term care during times when pain and symptoms cannot be managed without a hospital setting.
- **Respite Care:** This is short-term care in a facility during times when the patient's caregiver needs a break in caregiving.

Hospice care differs from palliative care, which serves anyone who is seriously ill, not just those who are dying and no longer seeking a cure (National Hospice and Palliative Care Association, 2018).

Adult day centers provide social and some home health services for seniors. The typical services include social activities, transportation, meals and snacks, personal care, and therapeutic activities. There are approximately 4,600 adult day centers in the United States (National Adult Day Association, 2019).

Multipurpose senior centers serve a wide range of needs both in terms of services and as a connection for other community services. These sites have a variety of funding sources, including a relationship with the OAA with nearly 10,000 centers across the country (National Council on Aging, 2019).

The new Health Service Executive model of licensure for leaders in senior care allows individuals to practice in the broader continuum of senior care services. This model focuses on a critical set of core knowledge and skills required to lead organizations and takes into consideration the ever-changing field of care and service options available to the elders of our country.

Randy Snyder, Executive Director, Minnesota Board of Executives for Long-Term Services and Supports

SPECIAL TARGET POPULATIONS

Memory care is provided in a variety of settings. The most common form is an assisted living–type facility with enhanced safety and security features and generally more staff. The average cost of memory care is about $5,000 a month, but such facilities provide care for those with Alzheimer's or other dementias, with 24-hour supervised care for patients at all stages of the disease (Howley, 2019). There are also options in SNFs with special units designed or adapted for this population. Many individuals also use home health services, especially in the early stages.

Intellectual and developmental disabilities often occur at childhood and are chronic issues that can be cognitive or physical, or even both. For those with developmental disabilities, there may also be related physical issues, as is the case for patients with cerebral palsy. People may also have both physical and cognitive issues in addition to intellectual disability, as is the case with Down syndrome. These populations depend on both Medicare and Medicaid, along with charitable or private resources from the family or caregivers. Typical services and settings vary as much as the individual situation and can include housing, education and employment coordination, and healthcare services.

Older Inmates and Parolees

"Of the 2.3 million adults in state and federal prisons, about 246,000 are 50 or older, according to the National Institute of Corrections. The United States currently spends more than $16 billion annually caring for these aging inmates, and their numbers are projected to grow dramatically in the next 15 years" (Vestal, 2014). Under the 1965 law that created Medicaid, anybody entering a state prison forfeited Medicaid eligibility. An exception to that general rule was created in 1997 when the U.S. Department of Health and Human Services informed states that inmates who leave state or local facilities for care in hospitals or nursing homes can get their bills paid by Medicaid. The federal contribution varies by state for those individuals requiring services. Even in states that have not expanded Medicaid to low-income adults under the ACA, most elderly or disabled prison inmates qualify under existing Medicaid rules if they receive care outside the correctional facility.

LGBTQ Older Population

There are an estimated 3 million LGBTQ seniors over the age of 65 years, and this number is projected to double by 2030. Two common care-related issues are as follows: (a) They have fewer children to support them, and (b) they have discrimination issues that are not protected by federal civil rights laws (National Resource Center for LGBT, 2019). The hope is that the conversation in LTC and senior living facilities about the challenges of discrimination is becoming more frequent and that strides have been gained during the past 10 years with a more public discourse. It is imperative that leaders and administrators are sensitive to the diverse needs of the deserving LGBTQ senior citizens entrusted to our care and service.

Ethnicity and Race

The numbers and corresponding proportions of older people of diverse racial and ethnic origins in the United States are increasing. In 1990, ethnic minorities represented 13% of the population age 65 and older—a percentage that rose to 16% in 2000 and is projected to increase to 23% by 2020 and to 36% by 2050. This increase is projected based on higher birth rates and the immigration numbers among racial and ethnic minority populations. There are several issues about the demographic factors that will impact the care and the delivery of LTC services across all lines of service. Among people over 70 who require care, Whites are most likely to receive help from their spouses, Latinx are most likely to receive help from their children, and African Americans are the most likely to receive help from a nonfamily member (National Academy on an Aging Society, 2000). These likelihoods often impact the types of LTC services a person receives and who provides them.

Immigrant Groups

As of 2017, immigrants accounted for more than 18% of healthcare workers. In nursing homes, nearly one in four workers who directly care for patients are immigrants, as are nearly one in three housekeeping and maintenance workers (Zallman, Finnegan, Himmelstein, Touw, & Woolhandler, 2019). For immigrants who need service, good information is not readily available; however, it is generally believed that they pay for their own care with private funds out of fear and risk of deportation.

Specific Medical Conditions

For many individuals with disease-specific issues, they are likely to select staying at home for as long as they can until care stressors or depletion of financial resources occurs. Patients with greater service needs, such as with multiple sclerosis (MS), for example, which is one of the most common conditions found in skilled nursing care residents, often require some form of residential care. Approximately 20% to 25% of people with MS require some form of HCBS, and another 5% will need residential LTC and often skilled nursing care due to financial funding models. Amyotrophic lateral sclerosis (ALS) is another example of a condition that requires individuals to navigate the use of support and care resources. Often as ALS progresses and financial resources are depleted, a decision is made about the use of home care resources or placement in a residential care setting as the person and family navigate what might be the better option (ALS Association, 2020).

Pediatric LTC

One last service line available in the country is **pediatric LTCFs**, which are defined as LTC, subacute, or rehabilitation facilities. These specialty care settings serve a population of children who have medically complex needs. There are a growing number of patients who require this service. The special care needs of these children are met by the estimated 40 providers across the country who fill this critical niche for these children and their parents (Pediatric Complex Care Association, 2016).

FUTURE FACTORS AFFECTING LONG-TERM CARE AND SENIOR LIVING FACILITIES

So the elephant in the room is clear to most people associated with this field. One of the most significant demographic trends in the United States is that America is graying (see Exhibit 1.3). This presents opportunities and challenges in the years ahead.

EXHIBIT 1.3 Population Changes (by Age) in 1960 Versus 2060

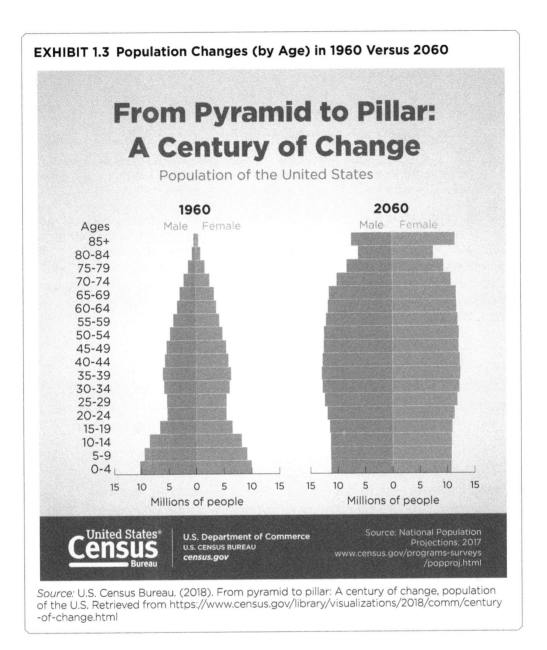

Source: U.S. Census Bureau. (2018). From pyramid to pillar: A century of change, population of the U.S. Retrieved from https://www.census.gov/library/visualizations/2018/comm/century-of-change.html

Based on this huge shift in our population, as well as the changing landscape of public policy and consumer perspectives, there are a few noteworthy issues that require greater awareness for leaders and administrators in the senior living field:

- Consumer expectations of the baby boomers who want good senior care and high-quality services, often in different environments and venues than their parents' generation

- The intersection of customer satisfaction and hospitality models of care and service that are challenging us to reexamine our approach to healthcare services for seniors

- Rising consumer awareness around quality and value that is further heightened with transparency of publicly available quality data

- A variety of workforce development and supply issues, such as addressing the needs and wants of the new millennial workforce or responding to government immigrant policies

- Value-based purchasing being deployed by healthcare organizations and systems with required outcome accountability

- Rural and urban trends with technology driving some of the care and service approaches

- The expanding senior care continuum driving new and more meaningful relationships with both clinics and acute care hospitals

These topics and others will be explored throughout this text in a variety of ways. Determining the future landscape of the field is within the grasp of every individual leader involved and involves adaptation in both micro- and macro-ways.

Steven Chies, an executive who has been deeply entrenched in the development of senior care leaders within the provider, association, and academic worlds, shared some views of aging policy, trends, and the future needs of the profession.

The societal and financial impact of the baby boomer cohort on the United States economy will be felt at multiple levels. This impact will require senior care leaders who are able to meet the complexity of care needs for boomers, the challenging financial issues, and the expectations for control over their living and care settings.

Firstly, with the aging boomer cohort now into their 70s and moving into retirement, having succession plans for senior care organizations should be a key part of their strategic planning. The ability to transfer knowledge from the experiences of boomers who have worked in the "longevity economy" will be of considerable benefit to the organizations as they transition leaders going forward.

Secondly, the boomers will no longer be in the higher tax-paying segment of society but will be using governmental funding resources, including Social Security, Medicare, and probably Medicaid, for their care needs. This will cause serious public policy discussions on the needs versus demands of the boomer cohort to meet their care needs and living expectations.

Thirdly, as the early boomers hit the magical age of 80 in 2026, an age that will peak in the 2032–2033 years, the need for chronic care settings, rehabilitation, and other care requirements will expand to fill the demands.

Finally, current and future senior care leaders will need to expand and broaden their knowledge and skills to avoid becoming narrowly focused in their career decisions. As the National Association of Long Term Care Administrator Boards (NAB) has demonstrated and predicted the need for a broader educational curriculum with their Health Services Executive (HSE™) model, a number of current senior care leaders are seeking to go beyond the care and institutional settings and adopt a more expansive array of skills to lead the future of the sector.

The textbook has been written to provide the starting point for both current and prospective senior care leaders who are charged with leading senior living organizations into the "new normal." The HSE™ credential will allow individuals and organizations to view careers in the "longevity economy" as having expanded options and leadership opportunities across all lines of service and at a national level.

Predicting exactly what the future care and living settings for the boomer cohort is very difficult as consumer expectations and the ability of the aging population to self-fund financial needs will be a key challenge for society. One can look at the demographics and data for each cohort in the United States and see what the growth of a senior care population will be, but how to create, staff, and fund the future for boomers is a challenge for the Health Services Executives going forward.

Steven Chies, Program Director,
St. Joseph's College of Maine

SUMMARY

It is important for the emerging leader to have some context for the landscape of aging services in this country. Understanding the history and development of the field adds depth of perspective to future leaders. A view of the broadening of the landscape of senior services also sets a framework for how this continued evolution of service may evolve to meet both the necessary and desired services delivered and desired by future elders. The changing and diverse populations expected in the decades ahead will also be a key driver that leaders will want to pay attention to as the health and service system responds to these population shifts.

KEY POINTS

1. The history of aging services is a long-standing tradition in society that even predates the United States.

2. Legislative changes are important to understand as is their impact on delivery of services and funding.

3. Providers and services have evolved across the continuum over the years based on needs in the U.S. population.

4. Populations served are diverse and complex with different needs and LTC preferences.

5. Leaders must understand the continuum so they can effectively practice today and position themselves strategically for future changes and challenges.

6. Aging trends should be paid attention to help predict future needs.

LEADERSHIP ROLES

1. Leaders need to be historians.

2. Leaders are responsible for understanding how policy impacts delivery.

3. Leaders need to understand the changing landscape that impacts their services, financials, strategies, personnel decisions, and facilities.

QUESTIONS FOR DISCUSSION

1. Describe the key policy and legislative shifts that influenced senior care delivery.

2. What are some of the unintended consequences of policy changes that have happened over the years?

3. What are some of the major impacts of the baby boomer generation on different lines of service available both today and in the future?

CASE PROBLEM

Consider a specific county in the United States that an individual would like to practice in and explore both the demographic footprint and the current provider availability for the provision of services. You will need to do the research using both public and private databases to get a robust picture of the landscape and the potential opportunities for service needs and supply.

REFERENCES

Abramovitz, M. (1996). *Regulating the lives of women: Social welfare policy from colonial times to the present*. Boston, MA: South End Press.

Administration for Community Living. (2019). *Older Americans Act*. Retrieved from https://acl .gov/about-acl/authorizing-statutes/older-americans-act

ALS Association. (2020). *Paying for home care*. Retrieved from http://www.alsa.org/als-care/ resources/fyi/paying-for-home-care.html

Americans with Disabilities Act. (2019). *An overview of the Americans With Disabilities Act*. Retrieved from https://adata.org/factsheet/ADA-overview

Centers for Disease Control and Prevention. (2017). United States Life Tables, 2013. *National Vital Statistics Reports, 66*(3), 1–63. Retrieved from https://www.cdc.gov/nchs/data/nvsr/ nvsr66/nvsr66_03.pdf

Centers for Disease Control and Prevention. (2019). *Home health care*. Retrieved from https:// www.cdc.gov/nchs/fastats/home-health-care.htm

Healthcare.gov. (2019). *Affordable Care Act (ACA)*. Retrieved from https://www.healthcare.gov/ glossary/affordable-care-act/

Howley, E. (2019). Dementia care in assisted living homes. *U.S. News*. Retrieved from https:// health.usnews.com/best-assisted-living/articles/dementia-care-in-assisted-living-homes

Kellogg Foundation. (2019). *An overview of the Medicare part D prescription drug benefit*. Retrieved from https://www.kff.org/medicare/fact-sheet/an-overview-of-the-medicare-part-d-prescription-drug-benefit/

LeadingAge. (2019). *Why housing plus services*. Retrieved from https://www.leadingage.org/why-housing-plus-services

National Academy on an Aging Society. (2000). *Chronic and disabling conditions: Caregiving*. Washington, DC: The Gerontological Society of America.

National Adult Day Association. (2019). *Overview and facts*. Retrieved from https://www.nadsa.org/consumers/overview-and-facts/

National Council on Aging. (2019). *Senior center facts*. Retrieved from https://www.ncoa.org/news/resources-for-reporters/get-the-facts/senior-center-facts/

National Hospice and Palliative Care Association. (2018). *NHPCO facts and figures*. Retrieved from https://www.nhpco.org/wp-content/uploads/2019/07/2018_NHPCO_Facts_Figures.pdf

National Resource Center for LGBT. (2019). Retrieved from https://www.lgbtagingcenter.org/

Pearson, C., Quinn, C., Loganathan, S., Datta, A., Mace., & Grabowski, D. (2019). The forgotten middle: Many middle-income seniors will have insufficient resources for housing and health care. *Health Affairs, 38*(5). doi:10.1377/hlthaff.2018.05233

Pediatric Complex Care Association. (2016). *2015 clinical pilot benchmark study*. Retrieved from https://pediatriccomplexcare.org/wp-content/uploads/2016/04/PCCA-2015ClinicalBenchmarkPilotExecSum041116LM.pdf

Vestal, C. (2014). For aging inmates, care outside prison walls. *Pew Stateline*. Retrieved from https://www.pewtrusts.org/en/research-and-analysis/blogs/stateline/2014/08/12/for-aging-inmates-care-outside-prison-walls

Zallman, L., Finnegan, K., Himmelstein, D., Touw, S., & Woolhandler, S. (2019). Care for America's elderly and disabled people relies on immigrant labor. *Health Affairs, 38*(6). doi:10.1377/hlthaff.2018.05514

ADDITIONAL RESOURCES

Achenbaum, W. A., & Carr, L. C. (2014). A brief history of aging services. Generations, Summer 2014.

Centers for Medicare & Medicaid Services. (2019). *History*. Retrieved from https://www.cms.gov/About-CMS/Agency-Information/History

Department of Housing and Urban Development. (2019). *Section 202 supportive housing for the elderly program*. Retrieved from https://www.hud.gov/program_offices/housing/mfh/progdesc/eld202

Khan, A., Tavakoli, N., & Stefanacci, G. (2017). Management of medical complications in a long-term care patient with multiple sclerosis. *Annals of Long-Term Care: Clinical Care and Aging, 25*(2), 44–47.

Medicaid.gov. (2019). *Home and community based services authorities*. Retrieved from https://www.medicaid.gov/medicaid/home-community-based-services/home-community-based-services-authorities/index.html

Pandya, S. (2005). *Racial and ethnic differences among older adults in long-term care service use*. AARP Public Policy Institute. Retrieved from https://www.aarp.org/home-garden/livable-communities/info-2005/fs119_ltc.html

Pew Charitable Trusts and MacArthur Foundation. (2014). *State prison health care spending*. Retrieved from https://www.pewtrusts.org/~/media/Assets/2014/07/StatePrisonHealthCareSpendingReport.pdf

U.S. Senate Special Committee on Aging. (2019). *The nursing home reform act turns twenty: What has been accomplished, and what challenges remain*. Retrieved from https://www.aging.senate.gov/hearings/the-nursing-home-reform-act-turns-twenty-what-has-been-accomplished-and-what-challenges-remain

CHAPTER 2

Customer Care, Supports, and Services

INTRODUCTION

People helping people—that is at the very core of what senior living is all about. Whether that takes the form of directly providing a needed service or arranging for it to happen, enabling an older or disabled adult to reach their full potential for functional independence and life satisfaction presents the most challenging—and the most rewarding—aspects of working in this field. As with any enterprise, it is beneficial to know as much as possible about the customers, as well as about the service delivery team and their respective roles, current trends in the field, and key tools available for assessing customers' needs, planning care goals, and monitoring the effectiveness of selected approaches.

GERONTOLOGY BASICS

Not everyone who accesses postacute services is elderly, but the vast majority of them *are* 65 and over. According to the National Center for Health Statistics, they represent over 80% of the care recipients among nursing homes, home health and hospice providers, assisted living and residential care communities, and over 60% for adult day centers (Harris-Kojetin et al., 2019). Accordingly, an effective Health Services Executive (HSE™) becomes knowledgeable (not necessarily an *expert)* about **gerontology**, the study of human aging. If it were not included as part of one's formal preparation, continuing education opportunities are abundant. This should be included in every HSE™'s professional development plan—know as much as possible about the customer.

Physical Well-Being

Physiological changes accompanying advancing age occur gradually and at vastly different rates, making chronological age less reliable as a meaningful determinant of health than we tend to view it. Measures of performance and capacity really make more sense, but a person's age is easier to calculate and remains important in Western culture as a significant marker. Differences in genetic heredity, gender, environment, health behaviors, and income each contribute to the variance observed in how people age.

The greatest decline typically occurs in complex functions involving multiple organ systems, muscles, and nerves. Some form of sensory loss can be expected with advancing age—vision, hearing, taste, smell, and even touch. The risk of acquiring at least one chronic disease rises with age, but most consider their own health as satisfactory. The most prevalent aging-related conditions are diseases of the cardiovascular system. In fact, the leading causes of death among older adults, in descending order, are heart disease, cancer, stroke, and accidents. Some signs of aging are visible, such as changes in hair color, skin texture, posture, or gait. Others are less obvious but profoundly affect a person's life, such as arthritis, adult-onset diabetes mellitus, diverticulitis, or incontinence (Hooyman, Kawamoto, & Liyak, 2015).

Mental and Emotional Health

Cognitive functions and personality can change with advancing age, some of which is normal and some attributed to mental health disorders. Scientists differentiate fluid intelligence—skills such as abstract reasoning, spatial relations, and perceptual speed—from crystalized intelligence—the knowledge we gain through education and experience, such as verbal memory and meaning, social judgment, and numbers skills. The former typically shows more measurable decline with age (Hooyman et al., 2015).

It is difficult to determine the prevalence of abnormal changes in personality and behavior associated with aging because they can also be related to genetic heredity, environmental stresses, or acquired diseases. Depression is the most common mental disorder in old age and the most underdiagnosed condition among cognitively impaired elders (Allan, Valkanova, & Ebmeier, 2014). Outdated cultural norms tend to influence people's expectations about depression, resulting in accepting it as part of normal aging or denying symptoms. Anxiety disorders have been identified as nearly as prevalent as depression among elders, and they often occur together (Darling, 2019). The negative consequences of social isolation—loneliness, helplessness, and boredom—can grow in scope and severity with advancing age due to declining interactions with other people.

A whole chapter could easily be devoted to dementia, both reversible and irreversible types, which can lead to major cognitive impairments, especially declines in short-term memory recall, learning and comprehension, attention span, and orientation to time, person, or place. Regardless of service line, an HSE™ should acquire a fundamental understanding of the causes and characteristics of various forms of dementia, as well as signs and indicators of onset. If leading an organization with specialized services aimed at persons with dementia, an even deeper dive is warranted, including high-impact practices in the field. An HSE™ should become a student—and ultimately, an authority—on this subject.

On the bright side, changes in the aging brain appear to enhance wisdom and creativity. A primary task for older adults is redefining their self-concept as they experience the loss of prior roles in professional, social, family, and community circles. Interventions aimed at assisting elders with coping with those changes, overcoming the associated grief, and embracing new roles typically need to be highly individualized. Positive aging is characterized by avoiding disability and disease, maintaining a high cognitive level, remaining socially engaged with others, and coping effectively with life's events. Resilience and the ability to effectively draw upon both internal strengths and external resources help elders the most in remaining physically, socially, and cognitively active (Hooyman et al., 2015).

Spiritual Wellness

Spirituality sometimes gets included in discussions about a person's mental or emotional health. It is certainly related to both, but it is just enough different to mention here separately. It sometimes is used synonymously with religion or religiosity, but the latter two are more accurately considered possible subsets of the former. What they share is the value people place on faith. How that faith may be practiced varies widely, but the importance that spiritual wellness plays in one's overall well-being tends to increase with age. Some researchers even hold that spiritual wellness contributes significantly to the notion of successful aging. Progressive senior living leaders find creative ways to maintain an organizational culture that nurtures spiritual wellness (Fagin & Pargament, 2011).

Family Dynamics

One of the most unique features about senior living is the challenges surrounding the variations in defining the customer. In most other businesses, the customer is the purchaser or end user of the product or service. In senior living, that is not always the case. It can also mean a patient's advocate, whether a trustee or attorney, physician, clergyperson, neighbor, or family. "Family" is a social construct that has changed dramatically over recent decades, both regarding structure and geographic distribution. We have come a long way from the traditional nuclear family as the predominant model to a much more diverse constellation of interwoven relationships resulting from a variety of social trends.

This complexity makes it imperative for a senior living organization to identify early in the service relationship timeline that one person has the greatest legal authority to represent the interests of the resident. In the absence of a formal guardianship, power of attorney, or healthcare surrogate designation, it may be as simple as having the family stakeholders decide among themselves. The dangers associated with remaining unclear about this can become significant, ranging from staff getting conflicting instructions or guidance from different family members to wondering about whom to call first about a significant change in the resident's condition. Unfortunately, there is not a uniform approach to take in dealing with family dynamics—but one constant is to clearly identify with whom the organization is supposed to communicate.

UNANTICIPATED CLINICAL CHALLENGES: COVID-19 AND PREVENTING COMMUNITY SPREAD

The vast majority of customer needs and preferences are somewhat predictable, based on history and experience, marketing and consumer satisfaction data, and observation. They cover the spectrum of physical, mental, emotional, and spiritual wellness—often overlapping—and family dynamics. Treating people's medical and mental health conditions, providing a safe, secure, dignified, and comfortable environment, honoring their faith traditions and heritages, and empowering their family and community support networks are fundamental charges. Applying contemporary knowledge and skills may demand some tailoring to address varying combinations of needs and preferences, but there is at least an evidence-based, established standard of practice on which to rely.

Rare circumstances occur, which may be unfamiliar to an organization or community. Although there may not be widely accepted response standards, some other providers are likely to have experienced the same or a similar predicament, and they are generally willing to share their insights and lessons learned. Examples range from an infestation by scabies or bedbugs to a pharmaceutical manufacturer's recall of a medication. Outside assistance is typically required in order to swiftly and effectively address such challenges.

Even more infrequently, a new disease or hazard emerges about for which there is very little known about initial defense. When this happens, it is incumbent upon the HSE™ and the leadership team to exercise sound critical thinking skills and executive judgment and to take decisive action based on the best available information. Think of a new strain of flu or airborne pathogen or a large meteor crashing in North America with atomic bomb force and its subsequent radiation release. Although it is impossible to include in an organization's disaster preparedness plan scenarios that either are unpredictable or have an extremely low probability of occurring, it is possible—even necessary—to establish protocols for evaluating them, for deciding a course of action (including contingencies concerning delegation of authority) and monitoring the effectiveness of the response or intervention.

The world's encounter with the unprecedented, rapid, and exponential spread of the COVID-19 virus during 2020 provides a memorable example. The introduction of a highly lethal human pathogen, for which there was no broadly effective antidote or treatment, had the healthcare provider and scientific communities scrambling for answers. Preventing the speed of "community spread" became the primary goal of governments around the globe as the epidemic grew in scope into a pandemic, buying precious time for the development of more permanent solutions. Reducing opportunities for person-to-person contact, either through self-imposed or state-mandated quarantines, became the first line of defense. Following the recommendation from the Centers for Disease Control and Prevention (CDC) of "social distancing"—keeping at least 6 feet between people to reduce the risk of disease transmission—emerged as a new social norm.

At the senior living provider level, leaders dealt innovatively with unforeseen challenges that ranged from implementing more intense infection control practices, procurement of sufficient supplies and personal protective equipment (PPE), and scheduling staff during community-wide quarantines to communicating with residents' families (who were banned from visiting) and managing underlying business operations, such as cash flow, payroll, and billing. Providers fared much better if they had systems in place before the pandemic for engaging those closest to each new challenge and for coordinating their efforts.

TECHNOLOGY'S ROLE: ENHANCING OLDER ADULTS' WELL-BEING

Technological advances occurring in a broad array of related fields hold promising potential to positively impact elders' lives, whether in *applied* technology, for enhancing an older or disabled individual's wellness, comfort, or safety, or in *health information technology* (HIT), for more effectively managing operational information. Expect emerging technologies aimed at doing so to have as their user audiences both consumers and senior service providers. According to the Center for Aging Services Technology (CAST, 2011),

... aging-services technologies can be broadly defined as technologies that can influence the aging experience for seniors, including their quality of life, health outcomes, satisfaction and/or the quality of care they receive. These include technologies that can be used by seniors, caregivers (both professional and informal), health care providers and aging services providers to improve the quality of care, enhance the caregivers' experience, efficiencies and cost-effectiveness. These technologies broadly include assistive, telemonitoring, telehealth, telemedicine, information and communication technologies that intend to improve the aging or care experience. (p. 3)

Many tend to view older adults as technophobic or slow to accept change. However, as members of the generations that witnessed the arrival of radio and television, commercial air travel and GPS, space exploration, personal computers, and the Internet, they have impressive track records of adopting and adapting to technological leaps *throughout* their lives. Tech developers recognize the seniors' segment as one of the most attractive consumer markets on which to focus, partly due to the anticipated growth in the pure size of the group and partly due to its members' affinity for products or services that improve comfort, convenience, safety, efficiency, or any combination of them (Dahlke, Lindeman, & Ory, 2019; Etkin, 2019).

Technology advances for direct consumer use can preserve or restore one's functional independence. They range from artificial limbs, prosthetics, and universal design in homes to hearing aids linked to smart phones, wearable emergency alert devices, and even countertop oral medication dispensers that deliver proper doses on time as prescribed. Incredibly sophisticated devices that rely on user input via voice recognition or eye movement and can control the lived environment (HVAC [heating, ventilation, and air-conditioning], lighting, mobility, communication, and entertainment) add to the tool chest. As capability grows with advances in artificial intelligence technology and robotics, the depth and breadth of self-determined and self-initiated supports seem destined to expand.

HIT is the application of technology—hardware and software—to health data collection, storage and retrieval, interpretation, and operational application. It can help a provider organization internally by facilitating quality assurance and performance improvement (QAPI), operating efficiency, and speed of business. Examples of clinical applications include evaluating residents, care planning, recordkeeping, safety, and monitoring both quality and regulatory compliance. Administrative applications range from managing financial operations (accounting and reporting) to organizing staffing schedules and personnel records, menus and food production, purchasing and inventory control, preventive maintenance, and climate controls.

External applications for effectively managing information with technology focus mainly on the capture, retrieval, sharing, and use of personal health information (PHI), regulatory compliance, and reimbursement. The Health Insurance Portability and Accountability Act of 1996 (HIPAA) contained provisions to protect the confidentiality of any person's healthcare information without handicapping the flow of information that was required to provide treatment, regulatory compliance, or payment for services. The chief technological challenge to that end has been achieving higher levels of interoperability among the various information operating system platforms of providers, regulators, and payers while protecting the confidentiality of that information (HIPAA-Journal.com, 2017).

The Centers for Medicare & Medicaid Services (CMS) and the Office of the National Coordinator for Health IT jointly proposed describing the effective electronic exchange of health information as the "meaningful use" of interoperable electronic health records throughout the U.S. healthcare delivery system as a critical national public health priority. In 2009, Congress moved in that direction with the passage of the Health Information Technology for Economic and Clinical Health (HITECH) Act, with concurrent goals that included (a) improving quality, safety, efficiency, and care coordination, (b) reducing health disparities, and (c) ensuring adequate privacy and security protection for PHI (HIPAA-Journal.com, 2017).

Interoperabilty—the ability of different computer platforms and programs to effectively use shared information—has been steadily but slowly progressing. The chore is somewhat like getting people who speak different Romance languages (Spanish, Italian, French, and Portuguese) to clearly and precisely understand one another. The most widely recognized standards for measuring the *degree* of meaningful use achieved come mainly from a not-for-profit organization called Health Level Seven International (HL7). According to its website, HL7's mission is to provide "a comprehensive framework and related standards for the exchange, integration, sharing, and retrieval of electronic health information that supports clinical practice and the management, delivery and evaluation of health services" (HL7, 2019). Its corporate vision: "A world in which everyone can securely access and use the right health data when and where they need it." HL7 has more than 1,600 members from over 50 countries representing healthcare providers, government agencies, payers, vendors, and suppliers.

INTERDISCIPLINARY TEAM

Senior living involves caregivers from many different fields—commonly referred to as "disciplines." Because of the wide variation in individuals' lived experience with aging, engaging people from a blend of professions in assessing, care planning, and service delivery improves a provider's probability of success. Other terms occasionally used to describe this idea include "multidisciplinary" or "transdisciplinary" teams. While they both portray involvement in a work group by more than one profession, neither calls for team member cooperation and coordination of effort as strongly as *interdisciplinary* team (IDT).

The two main categories of IDTs are clinical services and support services. They can overlap, depending on the situation or the resident's current needs. The HSE™ should develop a fundamental understanding of each discipline and foster a customer-centric organizational culture that values and utilizes interdisciplinary collaboration. The old adage "Two heads are better than one" applies to our field incredibly well. The key to success is working together effectively by (a) sharing relevant information in a timely fashion, (b) clearly assigning roles and expectations, (c) holding one another accountable for performing agreed-upon approaches and interventions, and (d) objectively evaluating results.

Interdisciplinary Teams: Clinical Services

Clinical services are typically led by a licensed physician, regardless of service line, working with a team of healthcare and human services professionals. In an institutional setting, that might include some combination of members from the disciplines of nursing, rehabilitation therapies (physical, occupational, speech and hearing, and others), dining services, social services, chaplaincy, and recreational activities. Depending on the needs of the residents, the IDT might also include additional health professionals either as consultants, such as a registered pharmacist or licensed dietitian, or as preferred direct care providers, such as a podiatrist, ophthalmologist or optometrist, dentist, or even beautician.

The value of sharing client information and coordinating care planning and service delivery remains constant across the service line continuum. However, which disciplines engage in the process and the mechanisms for fostering effective communication among them vary. In a congregate living setting, such as a skilled nursing facility (SNF) or residential care/assisted living (RC/AL), the IDT is more likely to meet in person than it might in a home health agency (HHA), but the composition of the team is shaped in either environment by the customer profile. The service line with the most variance concerning its IDT's composition and information sharing model may be the adult day center. It has a *location*, like an institutional setting, which makes it possible for the IDT to meet regularly in person, but its participants do not *reside* there 24-7, which presents unique challenges concerning service coordination and follow-through because the support persons change between day and night and weekdays and weekends.

Medical Care

In most jurisdictions, a physician's order is required for admission to an inpatient rehabilitation facility (IRF) or SNF, as well as to receive many home- and community-based services (HCBS). Most commercial long-term care insurance carriers also expect a physician's involvement in directing a person's care in order to approve claims for benefits. For either purpose, this generally means a physician who is licensed by the state in which services are rendered as either an MD or a DO.

The medical professional who directly manages the care of a person as their patient is called the "attending physician." It is common—in many instances *required*—for a senior living organization to have policies and procedures addressing the qualifications of an attending physician, such as having a license in good standing or without disciplinary sanctions from the state board of licensure for the past 3 years. Some senior living providers even go so far as to develop medical staff credentialing rules patterned after the medical staff standards that hospitals must meet for accreditation by The Joint Commission on Accreditation of Healthcare Organizations (JCAHO, 2019a, 2019b).

Senior living providers with service lines that participate in Medicare or Medicaid are expected to contract with a physician to serve as "medical director." In addition to fulfilling the administrative role of overseeing the development and implementation of medical care policies and procedures, the medical director might also serve as an "attending physician" for residents. The medical director's role is discussed in more detail later in this section.

Physician Assistant

Initially popularized in rural areas where doctors were few and far between, physician assistants (PAs) have become more prevalent in the senior living arena in rural, urban, and suburban communities. They must work under the supervision of a licensed physician but generally have a broad spectrum of clinical practice, including authority to diagnose and to prescribe medications, approve plans of care and treatment approaches, and document progress. PAs earn a master's degree, and then they are nationally certified by examination through the National Council of Certification of Physician Assistants (NCCPA) and licensed by each state (NCCPA, 2019).

Nursing

The discipline of nursing covers a lot of waterfront, from licensed personnel with extensive training to paraprofessional caregivers with modest formal preparation. Senior living relies on them all, in various combinations. Generally, the higher the acuity level of the patients, the more highly trained and credentialed the nursing staff.

An **RN** in most jurisdictions can hold an academic nursing credential—RN diploma, associate's, bachelor's graduate degree in nursing—from a program accredited by an agency recognized by the Council for Higher Education Accreditation and pass an examination (RegisteredNursing.org, 2019). The test, called the National Council Licensure Examination-Registered Nurse (NCLEX-RN®), is designed to measure a person's command of appropriate professional nursing knowledge and skills for state licensure as an RN (National Council of State Boards of Nursing [NCSBN], 2019a). State boards of nursing typically administer the exam. An RN may also complete further clinical training that results in additional credentials reflecting their advanced proficiency, such as an advanced practice registered nurse (APRN) or gerontological nurse practitioner (GNP), according to GraduateNursing-Edu.org (2019). Nurse practitioners are being increasingly used in skilled nursing environments in consultation with the Medical Director and other physicians. Other members of the nursing department might include the following:

- **Licensed Practical Nurse (LPN) or Licensed Vocational Nurse (LVN):** Upon completion of an accredited course of study, someone who passes the National Council Licensure Examination-Practical Nurse (NCLEX-PN®) exam becomes an LPN or LVN, a term used only in California and Texas (NursingLicensure.org, 2019b). Some states have separate boards of licensure for RNs and LPNs. The scope of practice for an RN versus an LPN varies by state—sometimes considerably. The training required to become an LPN/LVN is 1 to 2 years and emphasizes performance of practical tasks. They report observed changes in a patient's condition to an RN or other medical professional for further assessment (NursingLicensure.org, 2019a).

  - *Note*: According to the NCSBN, over two thirds of the states participate in the Nurse Licensure Compact (NLC), which enables nurses—RNs and LPNs/LVNs—to practice in other NLC states without having to obtain additional licenses (NCSBN, 2019b). A map of which states recognize the NLC and related rules can be found at www.ncsbn.org/compacts.htm.

- **Certified Medication Aide (CMA) or Technician (CMT):** Similar to the fashion in which PAs and APRNs emerged in the wake of physician shortages or maldistribution, this category of healthcare paraprofessional first developed to complement the role of licensed nurses with administering routine medications. In addition to meeting the requirements for becoming a certified nursing assistant/aide (CNA) or state-registered nursing assistant/aide (SRNA), a CMA/CMT receives training in fundamental pharmacology and relevant observation protocols so they can recognize and report to a nurse any symptoms of negative drug interactions. Not all states provide for this category, but it has become increasingly popular among those with vast rural areas or communities with an undersupply of licensed nurses.

- **CNA or SRNA:** The training required for this credential provides basic information about human physiology and common chronic conditions, with emphasis on tasks that assist patients with performing their activities of daily living (ADLs). CNAs provide direct care and emotional support in a variety of senior living settings. All states regulate nurse aides who work in nursing homes due to a federal mandate. Preparation in some jurisdictions exceeds the federal minimum of 75 hours, reaching the 120-hour minimum recommended by the Institute of Medicine or even higher. Regardless, it culminates with both passing a written exam and demonstrating satisfactory proficiency in performing essential practical skills (NursingLicensure.org, 2019b), such as:

- measuring a patient's vital signs (temperature, blood pressure, pulse, and respiration rate);

- providing personal care (oral care, bathing, and personal hygiene); and

- completion of related tasks (changing the linens on an occupied bed, lifting or transferring a patient using proper body mechanics and/or assistive devices, hand washing, or following universal precautions).

Another member of the clinical IDT is typically the medical records technician or coordinator. Especially with the advent of electronic medical records (EMRs), having someone on the team who is proficient in medical coding and relevant computer applications contributes significantly to successfully managing the flow, retention, and retrieval of patient information. A medical records technician compiles, processes, organizes, and maintains medical records in a manner consistent with applicable medical, administrative, regulatory, and ethical standards. After completing a 2-year associate degree in health information management, the two most widely recognized credentials for this position are registered health information technician from the American Health Information Management Association (AHIMA, 2019) or certified professional coder (CPC) from the American Academy of Professional Coders (AAPC, 2019). If the staff person charged with managing the organization's medical records has neither of these qualifications, retaining a medical records consultant who does can prove a wise investment.

An assessment coordinator—someone who serves as the clinical IDT's quarterback—might serve in some other capacity already, such as a nurse, depending on the size of the organization. If there is enough volume, as determined by size or length of stay, a provider might assign the role exclusively. The tools for assessment and care planning vary by setting (see Care Planning and Documentation).

Finally, the director of nursing (DON), also referred to as the director of nursing services (DNS), is the operational coordinator and clinical team leader in most senior living settings. If providing skilled nursing care, the DON must be an RN; some states also require the DON in other postacute environments to be an RN. They typically have administrative responsibility for developing and implementing policies and procedures related to healthcare services, including departmental staffing and performance evaluation, training, quality assurance, and regulatory compliance. The American Association of Directors of Nursing Services (AADNS) and the National Association of Directors of Nursing Administration/Long-Term Care (NADONA/LTC) also offer a variety of relevant professional certifications for a nurse serving in a key leadership position of a postacute care organization (AADNS, 2019; NADONA/LTC, 2019). In assisted living, this position may be referred to as the health and wellness director.

Rehabilitative/Restorative Therapies

The foundational therapy disciplines in senior living that apply across the postacute care continuum include physical therapy (PT), occupational therapy (OT), speech therapy or speech-language pathology (ST or SLP), and audiology. Each one requires a licensed health professional, with specific formal education in the applicable discipline, providing services in either an inpatient or outpatient setting. In larger practices, therapist **extenders**—specialized assistants or aides—work under the direct supervision of the licensed therapist, more commonly in PT or OT. Other related disciplines continue to develop but are not yet as widely recognized by regulators or third-party payers.

PT has five subspecialties, one of which is **geriatric** PT. It focuses on the unique movement needs and capabilities of older adults. Geriatric PT aims to restore or enhance a person's mobility and ability to perform activities of daily living (ADLs), reduce their pain, and increase physical fitness—primarily by improving strength, endurance, balance, and range of motion. It may also include fitting and training a patient on the proper use of a prosthesis (artificial limb), cane, or walker.

A **physical therapist** (the credential for which is also **PT**) specializes in treating someone's functional decline related to (a) bones, joints, spine, and soft tissue (musculoskeletal issues, such as a fracture or osteoporosis); (b) the brain or nervous system (neuromuscular issues, such as a stroke); (c) cardiopulmonary problems; or (d) a severe wound (Singh, 2016). States issue a PT license to someone who completes a graduate academic program—typically accredited by the Commission on Accreditation in Physical Therapy Education (CAPTE)—and passes a comprehensive, standardized exam administered by the Federation of State Boards of Physical Therapy (FSBPT). Although becoming a PT previously required a master's level education, a DPT degree has become required for new students to receive a license (American Physical Therapy Association [APTA], 2019a, 2019b).

Helping to implement selected components of the treatment plan might be a **physical therapist assistant (PTA)**, who works under the PT's direct supervision. The PTA's duties typically also include collecting information related to the interventions provided and recommending modifications for enhancing outcomes or ensuring a patient's safety or comfort. All states require a PTA to become either licensed or certified by receiving an associate degree from an appropriately accredited academic program and passing a state-approved approved exam (APTA, 2019c; U.S. Bureau of Labor Statistics, 2019).

The **physical therapist aide** works under the direct supervision of either a PT or PTA and is commonly responsible for keeping the treatment area clean and organized in preparation for each patient's therapy, transporting or escorting a patient, and assigned documentation within the scope of practice. A physical therapist aide usually has a high school diploma or general education diploma (GED) and receives on-the-job training. However, the National Career Certification Board (NCCB) offers a competency-based credential called certified physical therapy aide specialist (CPTAS) that provides an employer with assurance of a person's relevant knowledge and skills (U.S. Bureau of Labor Statistics, 2019).

For an **occupational therapist, OTR/L** is the standard credential. This signifies that the professional is both *registered* by the National Board for Certification in Occupational Therapy (NBCOT) and *licensed* by at least one state. According to the NBCOT:

> ... *occupational therapy focuses on helping people participate in the meaningful activities they need and want to do after an injury, disability, or other health condition. It uses a holistic approach to look not only at why a client's participation in activities has been impacted but also at the client's roles and environment. Treatment strategies include wellness promotion, rehabilitation, and habilitation. The occupational therapy professional assists the*

client in regaining function or adapting to changes by assessing and addressing all aspects of recovery, not just the physical. (NBCOT, 2019)

At a minimum, an OTR/L earns a master's degree from an academic program accredited by the Accreditation Council for Occupational Therapy Education (ACOTE), an affiliate of the American Occupational Therapy Association (AOTA); passes a national competency-based exam; and receives professional license from the state in which they practice.

A **certified occupational therapist assistant (COTA)** works collaboratively with and under the direct supervision of an occupational therapist by performing specified treatments, documenting therapeutic interventions, and providing feedback on the patient's progress. Becoming a COTA requires an associate degree from an appropriately accredited academic program and passing an approved, standardized exam. Most states license COTAs (NBCOT, 2019).

Therapies aimed at improving speech, language, and hearing can wind up bundled because they are so closely related. They even share the same national professional society: the American Speech-Language-Hearing Association (ASHA). However, they are distinct disciplines: SLP addresses conditions related to the first two functions, and audiology pertains to hearing. An **SLP**, also referred to as a speech therapist, assesses, diagnoses, and treats communication, swallowing, and cognitive disorders. An SLP holds a master's degree in the discipline, a professional license issued by the state in which they practice, and a national credential through ASHA called a Certificate of Clinical Competence in Speech-Language Pathology (CCC-SLP). All licensing boards require an SLP to complete prelicensure professional experience requirements, and some now require having the CCC-SLP, as well (ASHA, 2019).

An **audiologist** works to prevent, identify, and treat hearing, balance, and other auditory disorders. Since 2012, a doctoral degree in audiology (AuD, PhD, EdD, or ScD) is required to become licensed. The two most widely recognized advanced practice credentials come from either ASHA, called the Certificate of Clinical Competence in Audiology (CCC-A; ASHA, 2019), or the American Board of Audiology (ABA), referred to simply as board-certified in audiology (ABA, 2019).

Other therapy disciplines have also begun to emerge in various senior living settings by demonstrating measurable, positive outcomes affecting ADL or cognitive performance, comfort, or life satisfaction. However, payment by public programs or commercial insurance carriers for the therapies listed in Table 2.1 has not kept pace with the mounting evidence of their efficacy.

Dining Services and Nutrition

In congregate senior living settings, the dining services department is likely to either be second in size to only the nursing department (e.g., IRF, SNF, or continuing care retirement facility [CCRC]) or may even be even the largest department (e.g., RC, AL, independent living, or CCRC). There is a professional on the IDT focused on assessing each resident's nutritional needs, including in the plan of care approaches for meeting those needs, and coordinating implementation of the plan through the IDT. According to the Association of Nutrition and Food Service Professionals (ANFP, 2019), a **dietary manager** can prepare for the position to manage the department either by earning an associate degree in general dietetics and becoming a **registered dietetic technician** or by completing the requirements for becoming a **certified dietary manager (CDM)**. In assisted living and other settings, chefs are being hired that will consult with an RD.

TABLE 2.1 Emerging Therapy Disciplines in Senior Living

Therapy Discipline	Preparation	State License	Professional Certification	Resource
Aquatic	Graduate degree	No	Yes	Aquatic Therapy and Rehab Institute www.atri.org (and multiple proprietary continuing education sponsors)
Aroma	Continuing education	No	Yes	Aroma Therapy Council www.aromatherapycouncil.org (and multiple proprietary continuing education sponsors)
Art	Graduate degree	Yes *(Minority)*	Yes	Art Therapy Credentials Board www.atcb.org
Drama	Graduate degree	Yes *(Minority)*	Yes	North American Drama Therapy Association www.nadta.org
Family	Graduate degree	Yes	Yes	American Association for Marriage and Family Therapy www.aamft.org
Massage	Varies by state	No *(Majority)*	Yes	American Massage Therapy Association www.aamtamassage.org
Meditation	Continuing education	No	Yes	International Meditation Teachers Association www.meditationteachers.org (through several association members and multiple proprietary continuing education sponsors)
Music	Bachelor's degree (+)	Yes *(Minority)*	Yes	American Music Therapy Association www.musictherapy.org
Pet or animal-assisted	Continuing education	No	Training and Resources	*~Health standards for pets in most jurisdictions* ~Animals and Society Institute www.animalsandsociety.org or ~Animal-Assisted Therapy of the Triangle www.animalassistedtherapyofthetriangle.com (and multiple proprietary continuing education sponsors)

(continued)

TABLE 2.1 (*continued*)

Therapy Discipline	Preparation	State License	Professional Certification	Resource
Reminiscence	Continuing education	No	Training and Resources	~National Association of Activities Professionals www.naap.org or ~Therapeutic Recreation Directory www.recreationtherapy.com (and multiple proprietary continuing education sponsors)
Tai Chi or Qigong	Continuing education	No	Training and Resources	Amirian Tai Chi and Qigong Association www.americantaichi.org (and multiple proprietary continuing education sponsors)
Yoga	Continuing education	No	Training and Resources	Yoga Alliance www.yogaalliance.org (and multiple proprietary continuing education sponsors)

Although HCBS staff may not have an active role in preparing food, there is a typically comparable professional involved with similar responsibilities. The logistics may be different from a more institutional setting—ranging from menu planning, safe food storage, and handling to contracting for catered meal service—but the charge is the same. Whether in a person's private residence or in a nonresidential, congregate meal site, such as an adult day center or multpurpose senior center, overseeing the delivery of an appropriate and effective nutrition program is a vital contribution.

Additionally, professional input by a **registered dietitian (RD)** is required by Medicare, Medicaid, and many commercial insurers. An RD completes at least an undergraduate degree at a program accredited by the Commission on Accreditation for Dietetics Education, completes a 6- to 12-month practicum, and passes a national exam. Nearly all states license or regulate RDs. The relevance of the greater preparation rises with the acuity or complexity of the elders served. An RD adds depth to the IDT when an increasing potential for multiple chronic conditions, polypharmacy, drug–food interactions, special diets, and cognitive impairment combine in complicating ways. Except in organizations large enough to hire an RD internally, this gets accomplished through a professional consulting contract (Academy of Nutrition and Dietetics, 2019).

Social Services and Chaplaincy

The organization's **social services director** wears many hats, from concierge and advocate to counselor, with the primary charge of addressing each client's psychosocial needs in ways that enhance the person's quality of life. A social worker is fundamentally a professional matchmaker, linking people with social support needs to service providers that can meaningfully and effectively address those needs. According to the National Association of Social Workers (NASW, 2019), that means working collaboratively—and proactively—with varying combinations of the care recipient, family members, others on the clinical IDT and staff from other departments, as well as with relevant outside agencies and resources.

Federal law (42 CFR 483.15) requires SNFs to provide "medically related social services to attain or maintain the highest practicable resident physical, mental and psychosocial well-being." The same regulation stipulates that a bachelor's degree in social work is required to serve in this role in an SNF with more than 120 beds, but not for serving in a smaller one. The NASW published "Standards for Long-Term Care" in 2003, which recommended that a nursing home social worker have no less than a bachelor's degree in social work from an accredited school of social work that is licensed, certified, or registered by their state (National Social Work Policy Institute, 2019). Regulation of this discipline varies by state.

Social services professionals working in other senior living settings aim to provide similar assistive and counseling services to help clients cope with circumstances or changes that might cause stress, grief, conflict, or emotional discomfort (Singh, 2016). The primary goal remains facilitating a person's adjustments to life changes and enhancing their self-defined quality of life.

A full-time **chaplain** is more common in a senior living organization with a not-for-profit, faith-based sponsor, but many senior living providers arrange for part-time pastoral care support from clergy living in the surrounding community—either with a stipend or voluntary. A chaplain is ordained or endorsed by a faith group to provide chaplaincy care in a range of settings, including *all* senior living lines of service. According to the Association of Professional Chaplains (APC, 2019), this means "emotional, spiritual, religious, pastoral, ethical, and/or existential care" through relationships with patients/clients, family, and staff. The Board of Chaplaincy Certification, an affiliate the APC, offers a credential as a board-certified chaplain (BCC) to someone who holds a master's degree in theology, completes four units of clinical pastoral education (CPE), receives endorsement from a sponsoring faith group, and demonstrates knowledge and skill proficiency in at least 31 professional competencies.

Activities and Life Enrichment

The **activities director** in most senior living organizations plans, initiates, and coordinates events and interactions designed to engage each client—based on their unique interests and capabilities—in activities ranging from entertainment, crafts, and celebrating special holidays to discovery, connecting with the surrounding community, and volunteering. The National Association of Activities Professionals (NAAP) provides resources for entry-level training programs that prepare someone to get started in this field. NAAP's affiliated National Certification Council for Activities Professionals (NCCAP) is the only independent standards and certification body recognized by the CMS regarding quality of life, activities, and engagement certification across all care settings. Although the most widely used title remains "activities" director or coordinator, progressive providers have experimented with a variety of substitutes to replace the unintended image of "busy-ness broker" with a greater emphasis on the benefits enjoyed by care recipients, such as "life enrichment director" (NAAP, 2019).

Consumer: Patient / Resident / Client / Participant / Family or Responsible Party

The most significant stakeholder is the care recipient, of course, and this often includes a family member or responsible party—particularly if the care recipient has some form of cognitive impairment. Including the consumer's perspective in the IDT's discussions not only improves the quality and depth of the information on which to rely in framing interventions, it promotes an atmosphere of dignity and respect for the individual served. It also opens the door for effectively negotiating an agreement—a "social contract"—to embrace the approved plan of care as a *member* of the clinical IDT.

Key Consultants

The **medical director** for a senior living provider is a licensed physician who typically serves as an independent administrative contractor to:

- oversee and coordinate all medical care;
- develop and monitor the effectiveness of medical care policies and procedures;
- participate in regulatory inspections, including the development and implementation of corrective action plans, if warranted;
- educate staff members about high impact practices and new developments in caregiving approaches; and
- serve as the provider's liaison with attending physicians and clinical consultants.

Depending on the size and licensure level of the provider, the medical director might also serve as the attending physician for many (sometimes *all*) of the clients. At a minimum, they should be available to become the attending physician for anyone added to the client roll without having one.

The Society for Post-Acute and Long-Term Care Medicine (PALTC; formerly known as the American Medical Directors Association) has developed a model medical director agreement and job description that is available on its website: https://paltc.org. These documents include recommended language for clearly addressing key responsibilities of the medical director, such as duties and time commitment, qualifications, professional liability insurance, confidentiality, employment status (employee or contractor), compensation, renewal, and termination.

The Society for Post-Acute and Long-Term Care Medicine also offers a competency-based certification program—awarding the credential "Certified Medical Director" (CMD)—that requires a physician to demonstrate knowledge and skills regarding geriatric medicine, relevant regulatory compliance, and the administrative functions of a contemporary medical director (PALTC, 2019). Laura Morton, MD, CMD, associate professor in the University of Louisville's Department of Family and Geriatric Medicine, recommends that a senior living organization consider the following qualifications as "ideal" for a medical director:

1. Board-certified geriatrician or other related specialties (American Board of Family Medicine, American Board of Internal Medicine, or American Board of Hospice and Palliative Care)
2. Certified medical director (CMD)

3. Member: Society for Post-Acute and Long-Term Care Medicine (and state affiliate)

4. Clinical experience in postacute and long-term care medicine (Morton, 2019)

The **consultant pharmacist (RPh for registered pharmacist)** is licensed by the state and provides the IDT with invaluable information about medications ordered by attending physicians and referred specialists, both regarding safety of use and effectiveness for treatment. They evaluate each patient's medication profile, taking into account the complex interrelationships among disease states, nutrition, medications, and other variables. The consultant pharmacist also contributes to many policies and procedures, such as the contents of the "emergency kit" (medications, supplies, instruments, and equipment that do not have a physician's order for use with a particular patient, but for which there is a reasonable probability of need in the event of a common medical emergency, such as cardiac arrest, seizure, or stroke) and its restocking after use.

According to the American Society of Consultant Pharmacists (ASCP, 2019), the consultant pharmacist in senior care:

> … counsels patients, provides information and recommendations to prescribers and caregivers, review patients' medication regimens, presents in-service educational programs, and oversees medication distribution services…[with] focus on the special pharmacotherapeutic challenges of the senior citizen.

Two hot health policy topics in recent years have been the need to curb inappropriate use of psychotropic drugs in long-term care and the chain of custody, administration, and disposal of controlled substances (narcotics). The consultant pharmacist adds expertise and insight to shaping the senior living organization's policies and procedures related to both.

Since 2000, a doctoral degree (PharmD) has been required to become an RPh. In order to avoid the potential for a conflict of interest, some states prohibit a consultant pharmacist from also working for the provider pharmacy that supplies medications, durable medical equipment, and/or other related goods to the senior living organization (Council on Credentialing in Pharmacy, 2014).

Other disciplines that commonly provide direct services—via contract or referral—and thereby might intermittently appear on the clinical IDT include the following:

- **Dentistry:** Oral health is closely tied to one's overall wellness, and this is particularly true for seniors (American Dental Association, 2019). More people than ever are reaching advanced years with the majority of their natural dentition in place. Unfortunately, public and private payment models for dental care remain provider-centric, limiting the types of procedures that can be performed outside of a dental office. Some states have expanded the scope of practice for dental hygienists to allow them to address preventive care. Transporting patients to and from a dental practice is still the main challenge of facilitating treatment or restorative dental care. A dentist completes a graduate program awarding either a DMD or DDS, passes a national exam, and is licensed by the state in which they practice. Some may also complete post-graduate studies in geriatric dentistry.

- **Podiatry:** The risks associated with providing foot care rise with the age of the patient. Circulatory inefficiency and sensory decline in the lower extremities (peripheral neuropathy) are common by-products of type II diabetes, the incidence of which increases exponentially with advancing age (National Institutes for Health, National Institute of neurological Disorders and Stroke [NIH/NINDS], 2019). The most reported foot disorders of older adults are corns and calluses, nail conditions, and toe deformities. A doctor of podiatric medicine (DPM) is qualified to diagnose and treat conditions affecting the foot, ankle, and related structures of the leg. A podiatrist completes 4 years of training in a podiatric medical school and three years of hospital-based residency training, similarly to that of physicians, passes a national exam, and is licensed by the state. Some may go on to complete fellowship training following their residency. A podiatrist's instruments are more transportable than a dentist's, making on-site and in-home treatment even more achievable (American Podiatric Medicine Association, 2019).

- **Vision Care:** In congregate senior living settings, vision exams and some related procedures can be performed on-site by either a physician trained as an ophthalmologist or an optometrist (OD). The former completes medical school plus a 4-year ophthalmology residency and then passes a national exam. They diagnose and treat diseases of the eye, perform eye surgery, and prescribe corrective eyeglasses or contact lenses, as indicated. An optometrist graduates from an accredited graduate academic program in optometry, passes a national exam, examines eyes for vision and health problems, corrects refractive errors by prescribing eyeglasses or contact lenses, and refers patients who may require services outside of this scope of practice. Both are licensed by the state, sometimes by the same board and sometimes by separate boards (American Association of Ophthalmology [AAO], 2019a, 2019b). The most common conditions identified and treated by these vision care professionals are cataracts (clouding of the lens), macular degeneration (sight erosion due to deterioration of the macula, a small area of the retina), and diabetes-related conditions, such as glaucoma (optic nerve damage) and diabetic retinopathy (decline of the retina's functionality). Setting up a private area for performing routine vision exams is relatively easy, and the instruments needed are typically transportable (Howley, 2019).

- **Hair Care:** The requirements for training and licensing, as well as the services performed by, a barber and a cosmetologist overlap considerably (NextInsurance.com, 2019). Requirements vary by state: training programs for becoming a barber average between 1,500 and 2,000 hours of instruction and practicum; training for becoming a cosmetologist is similar but more varied among states depending on which subjects are required (Beauty Schools Directory [BSD], 2019; National Barbers Association [NBA], 2019). Women outlive men by an average of 5 years. According to the American Association for Long-Term Care Insurance (AALTCI), over 70% of nursing home residents and more than 75% of AL residents are female (AALTCI, 2019). In our culture, looking good is a highly valued component of feeling good and self-worth—regardless of gender. A barber predominantly serves men by washing, cutting, or shaping their hair and grooming their facial hair. Although women could certainly use a barber's services, older women generally prefer to go to a licensed cosmetologist or hairstylist instead, who performs a broader range of services (e.g., hair care *plus* skin treatments, manicures, pedicures, facials, makeup application, or scalp treatments). There is also a social consideration—for both genders—favoring interaction with the other customers in a familiar setting reminiscent of earlier routines. The senior living organization generally retains either (or both) as an independent contractor. An invitation to participate in the *clinical* IDT typically calls for reporting observed changes in the client's behavior, capacity, or condition.

Coordination

Members of the clinical IDT share information in a variety of ways to create the most complete profile possible of each patient and to coordinate their collective effort toward planning, implementing, and evaluating treatment. Selecting which disciplines to include on the clinical IDT typically begins with a core group and is completed by adding others specific to the needs of each patient. The clinical IDT's core group is often broader in a more medically intense environment, such as IRF or SNF, than in service lines with less acuity, such as AL or congregate housing.

Members of the clinical IDT confidentially share information about each resident with one another from each member's disciplinary perspective, building a more complete picture of the whole person, their needs, and what actions the IDT agrees to perform. Higher resident acuity generally calls for more frequent interaction and greater involvement by the physician. Although the physician appears as a clinical IDT member in most of the service lines shown in Table 2.2, their role is most often approval—sometimes with modifications—of the plan of care developed by the rest of the team's members. Involving a physician assistant (PA) or advanced nurse practitioner (ANP) who works in tandem with an attending physician has become an increasingly popular approach, particularly in the IRF, SNF, home health, and hospice service lines.

The IDT might meet in various member constellations over time, depending on a resident's changing condition or the applicable regulatory expectations for the service line. It could meet in person, virtually or via a hybrid of both formats. The keys to success are establishing an optimal mix of IDT members, scheduling that fosters participation, and accessing appropriate resources to develop a comprehensive plan of care with clearly stated goals, approaches, timelines, and assignments—for each care recipient. The tools utilized for accomplishing this, which vary by service line, are outlined later in this chapter.

Computer software to facilitate capturing and using patient information has been developed for each senior living lines of service, most commonly in personal computer (PC) platforms. Computer-assisted health records management aids the clinical IDT by fostering information sharing, analysis, and collaboration in:

1. Assessing each resident's medical condition and needs
2. Planning a coordinated approach for addressing each identified condition or need
3. Documenting progress toward fulfilling the goals of each resident's care plan

TABLE 2.2 Contemporary Clinical Interdisciplinary Team—Core Disciplines

Setting	Disciplines
Inpatient rehabilitation facility Or Skilled nursing facility	Physician (order required for admission), nursing (licensed and paraprofessional), social services, dining services, activities Consultant pharmacist or medical records (as needed) (As ordered by the physician): Therapies and consulting direct care providers (dental, podiatric, vision care, etc.) Consumer/representative
Assisted living	Nursing/wellness, social services, dining services, activities, consultant pharmacist (as needed) (As ordered by the physician): Therapies, consulting providers (i.e., dental, podiatric, vision care, etc.) Consumer/representative (Primary care physician *apprised*)
Home health and hospice	Physician (order may be required for services), nursing, social services Consultant pharmacist (as needed) (As ordered by the physician): Therapies, consulting providers (i.e., dental, podiatric, vision care, etc.) Consumer/representative
Adult day	Physician (order may be required for services), nursing, social services, activities (As ordered by the physician): Therapies, consulting providers (i.e., dental, podiatric, vision care, etc.) Consumer/representative
Congregate housing/independent living	Social services, dining services, and activities Consumer/representative (Primary care physician *apprised*)

4. Evaluating the outcomes of executing the care plan (often leading to refining the care plan further)

The clinical IDT engages in QAPI activities concerning both individual residents and groups of them (by location, diagnosis, or some other classifying characteristic). In concert with addressing regulatory compliance matters, QAPI efforts typically target issues concerning:

- safety—preventing falls, other injuries, or elopement;
- quality—reducing the risk of pressure ulcers, weight loss, incontinence, infections, or preventable hospital readmissions;
- comfort—minimizing or eliminating restraints, catheters, or distractions that might negatively affect cognitively impaired residents, such as overhead paging; or
- life satisfaction—residents' self-esteem, engagement, and contentment.

Sanitation and Infection Control and Prevention

A common thread woven into the very fabric of a provider's QAPI program is the importance of cleanliness, whether it concerns the physical environment, people, or anything with which they come in contact. Older or disabled adults commonly have compromised immune systems or other underlying health conditions that can place them at a higher risk for contracting communicable diseases while having less capacity for battling them. That is why direct and indirect caregivers are expected to have current immunizations against easily transmitted diseases, such as tuberculosis (TB), and often against the flu or pneumonia.

In addition to the sanitation procedures followed by personnel performing their duties in dining services, housekeeping, and laundry to provide food safety and maintain a clean environment, it is essential to train clinical and nonclinical staff how to respond when they might come into contact with either airborne germs or any bodily fluids. "Universal Precautions" were developed to prevent the transmission of blood-borne pathogens, such as HIV or hepatitis B virus, when providing healthcare services or first aid. They typically applied when there was the potential for coming into contact with blood and other body fluids containing visible blood, and they presumed that those fluids were potentially infectious. They included frequent, thorough handwashing, wearing personal protective equipment (PPE), and discarding needles in puncture-resistant containers (Broskey, 2019). Although home health agencies are required to follow, at a minimum, Universal Precautions, most go beyond those by adopting applicable elements of "Standard Precautions," discussed further in the following (Gonzalez, 2014).

Building on the platform of Universal Precautions, the CDC introduced in the 1990s **Body Substance Isolation (BSI) protocols**. This expanded the list of recommended PPEs to include plastic aprons, medical gloves, hair and shoe covers, safety goggles, surgical masks, and N-95 respirators, and called for handwashing before patient care as well (Garner, 1996).

We have witnessed in just the past two decades devastating illness caused by the Ebola, West Nile, severe acute respiratory syndrome (SARS) and Zika viruses, avian flu, COVID-19, and even isolated incidents of biological warfare. The current set of safety procedures, called "Standard Precautions," are designed to reduce the risk of transmitting microorganisms from both recognized and unrecognized infection sources. They apply when there is a reasonable probability of coming into contact with blood or other bodily fluids (regardless of whether they contain visible blood), nonintact skin, and mucous membranes. Enhancements added on top of the BSI standards include (Segal, 2018; Siegel et al., 2019):

1. Handwashing before and after patient contact, whether or not gloves are worn
2. Wearing clean
   a. Gloves
   b. (Nonsterile) protective gown
   c. Mask, eye protection, or face shield
3. Respiratory hygiene and cough etiquette
4. Careful handling of soiled equipment and linens
5. Cleaning and disinfecting environmental surfaces (i.e., doors, hardware and door frames, countertops, and other "high-touch" areas)

No infection control event in the memory of most people alive compares, of course, with the worldwide pandemic caused in 2020 by the COVID-19 (also "Novel Corona-19") virus. Efforts by the CMS and public health officials to prepare providers to prevent contact with and transmission of a wholly new strain of human pathogen were initially dwarfed by the robust nature of the virus' ability to spread human-to-human, quickly and exponentially. Officials from the CDC observed that people who showed no visible symptoms could also serve as sources of infection transmission and that the virus could survive for several hours on hard surfaces, from counter tops to delivered boxes. Separation by "social distancing" surfaced as an initial defense, but that turned into recommended—or even government-mandated—protective quarantines in many communities. Barriers alone did not appear to be sufficient for completely preventing the community spread of the disease.

Lessons learned from the rapid rise of—and society's recovery from—the COVID-19 pandemic will likely inform the next set of precautions, from the micro- to macro-level. However, two constants seem likely to remain with respect to infection control: (a) an ounce of prevention is worth a pound of cure and (b) expect the unexpected.

Policies and Procedures—Corporate Compliance

In addition to complying with regulatory expectations and professional standards of practice, it is imperative to monitor how closely the clinical IDT adheres to approved organizational policies and procedures in fulfilling its responsibilities. This is a form of "corporate compliance," consistently following internally developed values, priorities, and protocols. Striving for corporate compliance applies to all areas of the operation, but *clinical* corporate compliance is arguably the most complex subset.

INTERDISCIPLINARY TEAMS: SUPPORT SERVICES

Due to their routine interaction with patients fulfilling indirect care roles, employees from other departments often have information valuable to the clinical IDT. Inviting them to participate by sharing their observations or assisting with implementing appropriate parts of the care plan can enhance the provider organization's effectiveness. Developing a culture that values and welcomes input from the non-clinical staff is not always easy. The disciplines mentioned thus far typically require more formal education than most of the support services areas, sometimes causing low expectations in both groups. However, expanding the variety of people who develop "skin in the game" has the dual benefit of (a) adding information regarding the care recipient to the IDT's process and (b) broadening interdisciplinary ownership of the care plan.

Housekeeping and Laundry

In most congregate senior living settings, employees in these departments may have the most direct contact with a resident without an assignment of performing any direct care. They arrive with the charge of doing something for the resident, not to the resident. In many instances, that difference can make the relationship between employee and resident a little less threatening and seem a little less hurried or frantic. Nonclinical observations about a resident's change in disposition, attitude, balance, strength, or even cognition can help affirm (or question) clinical assessments of the same metrics.

Maintenance and Security

Many of the same dynamics mentioned earlier regarding housekeeping and laundry staff apply to maintenance and security personnel. One chief difference is that members of these departments tend to be male, and that is less true in housekeeping and laundry departments. The prominence of female residents throughout senior living service lines can play a role in both the nature of this staff/resident relationship and the nature of observations offered by the employee to the clinical IDT.

Transportation

Drivers—whether internally or externally employed—have a hybrid set of interactions with the clients they transport. Their tasks may involve physically assisting the client in boarding and exiting a vehicle, escorting them to and from the vehicle, or observing and monitoring their behavior before, during, and following travel. They can often provide helpful information about a client's capabilities, from strength and stamina to balance and cognition.

Administration

Some of the following departments may appear in a different column than administration on a particular provider's organizational chart, but people working in each can also serve as a valuable resource to the clinical IDT, as needed.

- **Marketing and Admissions:** Usually the first staffmember to meet the client and/or client's family, input from this department can often prove useful to inform discussions about the initial assessment, as well as to compare that baseline information with observations later. There also might already exist a level of trust and familiarity that adds to the consumer's confidence that the clinical IDT has an accurate picture of the person at arrival.

- **Accounting or Business Office:** Paying for senior living services and qualifying for public programs or commercial insurance benefits are important concerns for consumers. Although not "clinical" in the strictest sense, the accuracy of billing and payments received closely ties to how well the provider captures complete and accurate information about each client. Involving someone from this operational area in the clinical IDT's conference improves the odds of closing any gaps in information needed about financial matters related to the resident, from billing and benefits eligibility to administration of resident trust accounts.

■ **Human Resources:** Matching personnel who possess the most applicable knowledge and skills to the unique set of needs associated with each resident is mainly the purview of each department's director. However, the HR professional may have the widest view of staff capabilities, backgrounds, and interests across departmental lines. Special circumstances can arise when a nontraditional assignment may very well make the most sense (e.g., relying on a laundry employee who speaks Spanish fluently to serve also as an interpreter for a memory care resident whose native tongue is Spanish and who has very limited command of English).

PERSON-CENTERED CARE AND CULTURE CHANGE

The term *person-centered care* has emerged to describe a consumer-oriented philosophy of care growing in popularity over the past three decades throughout senior living's lines of service. It started in the sphere of nursing homes, replacing a traditional institutional model of care with one that elevated the importance of consumer needs, expectations, and autonomy. Instead of viewing a long-term care facility as a healthcare institution, proponents of person-centered care have advocated reshaping them as person-centered homes offering chronic care and postacute rehabilitation services. Instead of making operational decisions that directly affect the patient experience—schedules, menus, activities, or even décor—based on the *provider*'s goals for achieving optimal aggregate efficiency, they have championed the notion that such decisions should become the sum of each *individual* patient's needs and preferences (Tellis-Nayak & Tellis-Nayak, 2016).

An important derivative term of person-centered care is "person-*directed* care," which adds emphasis on the importance of soliciting, respecting, and honoring the perspectives of elders and those who serve them most directly. Values that an organization pursuing a more person-directed care model must embrace include choice and self-determination, dignity and respect, purposeful living, and relationship (Pioneer Network, 2019a).

The resulting movement in senior living toward adopting a more person-centered model of care has expanded to other service lines, and it has broadly become known as "culture change" (Koren, 2009). A national coalition of like-minded senior living providers and aging services professionals, consumers and advocates, regulators and policy makers, and educators and researchers, called the "Pioneer Network," has grown dramatically in its scope since its inception in 1997 (Pioneer Network, 2019b). It supports the creation of senior living environments—in both congregate community-based settings—where both older adults and their caregivers can express choice and practice self-determination in meaningful ways at every level of daily life. The Pioneer Network now serves as a tremendous resource portal for any organization or person interested in learning more about culture change, person-centered and person-directed care, including training materials, current research, and high-impact practices. (Learn more about the Pioneer Network at www.pioneernetwork.net.)

The applicable core principles and practices have steadily evolved, shaped by shared concerns among consumers, policy makers, and providers. They have shown promise in improving both quality of life and quality of care in each senior living setting. Policy makers have embraced their value through regulation, reimbursement, public reporting, and other mechanisms. Providers have applied and refined them. Consumers and advocates have been diligent in keeping the movement's momentum. Box 2.1 displays what the Pioneer Network (2019c) considers the fundamental, core principles and practices for framing sustainable, positive culture change in senior living.

BOX 2.1 Core Values and Principles of Culture Change

1. Know each person.
2. Each person can and does make a difference.
3. Relationship is the fundamental building block of a transformed culture.
4. Respond to spirit, as well as mind and body.
5. Risk-taking is a normal part of life.
6. Put person before task.
7. All elders are entitled to self-determination wherever they live.
8. Community is the antidote to institutionalization.
9. Do unto others as you would have them do unto you.
10. Promote the growth and development of all.
11. Shape and use the potential of the environment in all its aspects: physical, organizational, psycho/social/spiritual.
12. Practice self-examination, searching for new creativity and opportunities for doing better.
13. Recognize that culture change and transformation are not destinations but a journey, always a work in progress.

Source: Pioneer Network. (2019c). *What is culture change?* Retrieved from https://www.pioneernetwork.net/about-us/mission-vision-values/

The Stages of Culture Change

The Commonwealth Fund supported a study to examine the key elements of culture change that identified at least four stages of its development in congregate living settings (Haran, 2006):

1. **Institutional Model:** Traditional medical/institutional model without permanent assignments for direct care staff members.
2. **Transformational Model:** Initial phase when awareness and knowledge of (and interest in) culture change spreads among direct care workers and the leadership team.
3. **Neighborhood Model:** Reorganizes traditional care units into smaller living areas and introduces resident-centered dining.

4. **Household Model:** Consists of self-contained living areas with 25 or fewer residents who have their own fully functional kitchen, living room, and dining room. Staff work in multidisciplinary self-directed work teams.

Key Outcomes of Successful Culture Change

Much of the justification offered by proponents of culture change for embracing it may seem intuitively attractive. While empirical evidence has not yet solidly established a clear direction forward, the most promising areas appear to be the following:

1. **Customer Satisfaction:** Consumers (and their advocates) who feel respected, valued, and have retained some self-determination experience a greater

   a. quality of life—physical, mental, emotional, and psychosocial wellness; and

   b. sense of purpose—contributing to the well-being of another; not just *receiving* care.

2. **Staff Retention:** Empowered employees tend to become engaged team members, stakeholders involved in the success of the organization. This has at least two benefits:

   a. **Continuity of Care:** Consistent assignments foster relationship development, which in turn bolsters resident confidence *and* reduces the risk of error due to unfamiliarity with the resident.

   b. **Productivity Increase (Cost Decrease):** Familiarity contributes positively to both speed and accuracy, and the burden of working short-staffed or the added cost of covering the schedule with overtime or temporary agency staff vanishes with a stable, engaged staff.

There certainly remain questions to answer, of course, such as, "What is the most appropriate and useful role of

- government (federal, state, and local) in promoting culture change through regulation, reimbursement, or both?"

- researchers in examining which components of culture change lead to clinically significant quality of life outcomes, whether their cost represents a good investment, and what are the chief barriers to (and facilitators of) their implementation?"

- payers in developing performance metrics that recognize valid, reliable evidence that supports costs associated with culture change?"

- consumers in determining in the marketplace whether this is worth demanding or simply nice to have"? (Zimmerman, Shier, & Saliba, 2014, S3)

The historic transition of our healthcare system from volume-based outcomes to value-based outcomes should be welcomed by all. Finally, we have the incentives well-aligned between quality and economy of care. This transition does come at a price though: This transition is placing a lot of burden on the frontline team members. The required overhaul in processes and expectations is quite disruptive. This is where healthcare leaders need to shine. They need to focus on team well-being by investing in strategies to motivate and inspire. They need to ensure that team members truly believe that the organization is well aligned with their own noble vision and mission and that there are resources for self-improvement. Simple, carrot-and-stick accountability systems will not suffice. The complexity of the care and tasks require that teams feel supported at every aspect of change.

Arif Nazir, MD, CMD, President,
SHC Medical Partners

CARE PLANNING AND DOCUMENTATION

The clinical IDT's chief charge is to collaboratively develop, implement, and evaluate a plan of care for each client. Sharing the client's medical and social histories and an initial assessment of their current condition through the respective lens of each discipline forms the foundation for identifying problems. Cross discussion—in live meetings, virtual interaction through an EMR/EHR, or a hybrid of both—lead to selecting interventions for most effectively addressing each identified problem. This avoids conflicting approaches or duplication of effort and fosters coordination, efficiency, and effectiveness.

Documentation that is complete and accurate is vital for providing clinical guidance, regulatory compliance, and reimbursement validation. (Rule of thumb to follow: If not documented, it might as well not have happened.) Each record is typically organized by discipline, with some mechanism for capturing information throughout the process—assessment, plan of care, progress notes concerning achievement of the goals in the plan of care, and refinement of the care plan. Generally, the higher the medical nature of the care setting, the more likely the information will be managed electronically. However, the availability of EMR systems designed to meet the unique needs of each senior living service line has improved dramatically. The most useful ones share relevant patient information with a compatible financial module that enables accurate and timely billing.

Two operational issues that have emerged due to the exponential rise in senior living's reliance on EMR technology are the importance of health informatics and cybersecurity. The U.S. Library of Medicine defines "health informatics" as "the interdisciplinary study of the design, development, adoption, and application of IT-based innovations in healthcare services delivery, management, and planning" (Health Information Management and Systems Society, 2019). We have mastered collecting a tremendous amount of information about each resident, so how can we now best *use* it to benefit them?

Cybersecurity is a rising risk management concern in all aspects of contemporary business operations, not just in senior living. In addition to facing mounting challenges in protecting the confidentiality of PHI, the threat continues to rise of becoming the victim of a "ransomware" attack. Just like a kidnapper demands a ransom in exchange for the safe return of the victim, a cybercriminal hacks a provider's computer and installs a malicious software that blocks access to the computer's data until the provider pays a fee to the attacker (Proofpoint. com, 2019).

> **Note:** The FBI and many cybersecurity experts advise against paying such a ransom to keep from encouraging the ransomware cycle; one-half of those who pay the ransom experience repeat ransomware attacks. For more information, visit the No More Ransom Project at www.nomoreransom.org/en/about-the-project.html.

Assessment: Skilled Nursing

In an SNF certified by Medicare and Medicaid, the federally mandated process for performing a comprehensive clinical assessment of each resident relies on utilizing a standardized screening tool of health status known as the Minimum Data Set (MDS). The process builds a picture of the whole person and helps identify problems or needs so that approaches and treatments can most effectively address each one. An MDS assessment form is completed for each resident, regardless of payment source, upon admission and then periodically, within specific guidelines and time frames. Care planning typically requires developing action plans with measurable goals, associated timelines, and specific assignments based on the information entered in the MDS concerning each of the areas set forth in Table 2.3.

TABLE 2.3 Sections of Minimum Data Set (MDS)

1. Identification Information	9. Bladder and Bowel	17. Restraints
2. Hearing, Speech, and Vision	10. Active Diagnoses	18. Participation in Assessment and Goal Setting
3. Cognitive Patterns	11. Health Conditions	19. Care Area Assessment (CAA) Summary
4. Mood	12. Swallowing/ Nutritional Status	20. Correction Request
5. Behavior	13. Oral/Dental Status	21. Assessment Administration
6. Preferences for Customary Routine and Activities	14. Skin Conditions	
7. Functional Status	15. Medications	
8. Functional Abilities and Goals	16. Special Treatments, Procedures, and Programs	

Source: U.S. Center for Medicare & Medicaid Services. (2019c). *Minimum data set 3.0 resident assessment instrument manual.* Retrieved from https://www.cms.gov/Medicare/Quality-Initiatives-Patient-Assessment-Instruments/NursingHomeQualityInits/MDS30RAI Manual

Once completed, the MDS information:

1. forms the foundation for developing the clinical plan of care;

2. assigns each resident to one of 44 acuity classifications, known as resource utilization groups (RUGs), according to their activity level, primary diagnosis, complexity of care needs, cognitive status, and other relevant care variables (primarily for determining reimbursement, as discussed in Chapter 4, Financial Management in Senior Care); and

3. is transmitted electronically by the provider to the MDS database in each state, and sequentially to the national MDS database at the CMS, where it feeds into the Certification and Survey Provider Enhanced Reports (CASPER) system, the agency's operational data resource for monitoring the status of a provider's short- and long-term quality measure rates and the effectiveness of applied improvement strategies (CMS, 2019a). Similar systems are also in place for the patient assessments described in the following for Medicare/Medicaid-certified IRFs and HHAs.

The importance of the HSE™ understanding how the MDS and RUGs relate to both clinical outcomes and reimbursement cannot be emphasized enough. The archaic attitude of separating the clinical enterprise from the organization's financial performance is unjustifiably risky—even irresponsible—in the current reimbursement environment. A basic familiarity with this process is required to become a licensed administrator, but effective leadership in this setting calls for a commanding knowledge of the mechanics and consequences of accurate, thorough, and timely utilization of the MDS tool. Advanced training on this is frequently offered by trade and professional associations, and it does not require having a clinical background to grasp the logistics. Those who leave this responsibility solely to the clinical IDT can expect to regret that decision.

The MDS tool is updated periodically by the CMS, so we are not including here a sample form. However, the most current coding requirements for completing the MDS can be found in the Resident Assessment Instrument User's Guide (see Care Recipient Assessment in the Additional Resources section at the end of this chapter).

Assessment: Inpatient Rehabilitation Facility

The tool comparable to the MDS that is used in an IRF is known as Patient Assessment Instrument (PAI), generated by the CMS as part of its Quality Reporting Program for IRFs participating in Medicare and Medicaid. It has a very similar purpose, design, application, and workflow but geared toward patients with higher acuity and/or medical complexity than typically found in an SNF (see Care Recipient Assessment in the Additional Resources section at the end of this chapter).

Assessment: Home Health

The CMS developed as the centerpiece of its Home Health Quality Reporting Program a patient assessment tool for evaluating people receiving skilled nursing care at home: the Outcome and Assessment Information Set (OASIS). According to its website, the CMS uses the data for multiple purposes, "including calculating several types of quality reports which are provided to home health agencies to help guide quality and performance improvement efforts." Revisions and new items were added in 2019 to align more closely with the MDS and PAI assessment sets; it is known as the OASIS-D. (See Care Recipient Assessment in the Additional Resources section at the end of this chapter.)

Assessment: Assisted Living

Although there are no federally mandated resident assessment instruments for use by AL communities, there are several variations of a similar process that are collectively most widely referred to as Individual Service Plans (ISP). They typically focus on supporting emotional, psychosocial, and spiritual wellness; on addressing cognitive impairment; and on accessing appropriate community resources. (See the link to a sample format from LeadingAge listed in the Additional Resources section at the end of this chapter.)

Assessment: Adult Day Center

Participants in an adult day center's program may have a wide variety of needs that generally fall into one of three service models and/or licensure levels: social, health/medical care, or memory care. In some states, these levels blend or overlap. Regardless, there is not yet a standardized, federally mandated assessment tool for this service line, so providers rely on excerpting features of the ones already described and applying them to their environment. One notable exception is when a day care program is a partner in a Medicare/Medicaid-certified PACE (Program of All-inclusive Care for the Elderly). The PACE model utilizes an adult day program as the hub of the wheel for an HCBS-oriented IDT that coordinates housing, medical, and social supports for people who meet the Medicaid eligibility requirements for nursing home care. The National PACE Association acts as a clearinghouse for its members to share successful innovations, including participant assessment tools (NPA, 2019).

Like technology, healthcare continues to rapidly evolve to reflect every changing consumer preference, market competition, and breakthroughs in practice and policy. Accordingly, healthcare providers and practitioners must constantly consider new, and more effective and efficient, methods for organizing, delivering, and marketing our services. Staying the same will assuredly guarantee our irrelevance or failure. We must increasingly understand, plan for and develop services for the seniors of tomorrow.

Shawn Bloom, President,
National PACE Association

QUALITY ASSURANCE AND PERFORMANCE IMPROVEMENT

Two mutually reinforcing facets of a quality management system—whether in industry or services—are quality assurance (QA) and performance improvement (PI). A section of the Affordable Care Act enabled the CMS to launch in 2011 its effort to serve as a catalyst for taking what it described as a "systematic, comprehensive, and data-driven approach to maintaining and improving safety and quality in nursing homes." A central feature of blending the two components was the expectation of involving all levels of caregivers in practical and creative problem-solving.

QA calls for specifying quality standards and codifying organizational processes for ensuring that care meets or exceeds them. PI (also called quality improvement) is the ongoing study and improvement of those processes in order to enhance healthcare outcomes and resident quality of life, as well as to reduce the risk of developing problems. Weaving them together as QAPI represents more than a federal requirement for Medicare/Medicaid-certified senior living providers; it sets the stage for senior living providers to engage in an ongoing, organized method of conducting business to achieve optimum results (CMS, 2019d).

QAPI is at the center of all we do. It is a critical thinking process that requires us to intervene and act proactively on our areas of greatest risk. With a team focus on quality assurance, continually auditing and monitoring, we expect to have improved outcomes – and generally achieve them. QAPI replaces the quick fix approach that does not last. Teams highly engaged in QAPI are dedicated to being more strategic, innovative and forward thinking by always focusing on improving their performance in key areas.

Donna Kelsey, CEO,
American Senior Communities

CMS: Five Elements of QAPI

Although the CMS has strived to avoid becoming overly prescriptive in order to encourage the development of QAPI innovations among providers, it does expect at least the five elements described in Box 2.2 to be effectively addressed in a provider's QAPI program. Although it may not be required outside of participating in Medicare or Medicaid, the benefits of maintaining a solid QAPI program are innumerable.

Measuring Quality

"Quality"—everyone wants it, of course! However, effectively measuring it has been an elusive goal in healthcare in general, and in senior living in particular. The medical/scientific metrics we have relied on to determine quality are the most definitive and quantifiable ones, such as successful medical or care *outcomes*. Consumer expectations have begun to creep into the picture, though, influencing discussions about quality to place a greater emphasis on the patient *experience*. We

BOX 2.2 - Five Elements of Quality Assurance and Performance Improvement (QAPI)

1. **Design and Scope:** A QAPI program must be ongoing and comprehensive, dealing with the full range of services offered by the facility, including the full range of departments. When fully implemented, the QAPI program should address all systems of care and management practices; include clinical care, quality of life, and resident choice; aim for safety and high quality with all clinical interventions; emphasize autonomy and choice in daily life for residents (or residents' agents); and utilize the best available evidence to define and measure goals. A Medicare/Medicaid-certified provider must have a written QAPI plan adhering to these principles.

2. **Governance and Leadership:** The governing body and/or administration develops a culture that involves leadership seeking input from facility staff, residents, and their families and/or representatives. The governing body ensures adequate resources exist to conduct and sustain QAPI efforts, including designating one or more persons to be accountable for QAPI; developing leadership and facility-wide training on QAPI; and ensuring staff time, equipment, and technical training as needed. Responsibilities include setting expectations around safety, quality, rights, choice, and respect by balancing safety with resident-centered rights and choice. The governing body ensures staff accountability, while creating an atmosphere where staff is comfortable identifying and reporting quality problems or opportunities for improvement.

3. **Feedback, Data Systems, and Monitoring:** Implement systems to monitor care and services, drawing data from multiple sources. Feedback systems actively incorporate input from staff, residents, families, and others as appropriate. Use performance indicators to compare a wide range of care processes and outcomes to benchmarks and/or targets the facility has established for performance. Track, investigate, and monitor adverse events, and implement action plans designed to prevent recurrences.

4. **Performance Improvement Projects (PIPs):** A concentrated effort on a specific problem in either one area or organization-wide. Systematically gather information to clarify issues or problems and intervene for improvements. Conduct PIPs to examine and improve care or services in areas the provider identifies as needing attention (depending on the unique scope of services offered).

5. **Systematic Analysis and Systemic Action:** Use a systematic approach to determine when in-depth analysis is needed to fully understand the problem, its causes, and implications of a change. Use a thorough and highly organized/structured approach to determine whether and how identified problems may be caused or exacerbated by the way care and services are organized or delivered. Develop policies and procedures and demonstrate proficiency in the use of root cause analysis. Systemic actions look comprehensively across all involved systems to prevent future events and promote sustained improvement. Focus on continual learning and continuous improvement.

Source: U.S. Centers for Medicare & Medicaid Services. (2019d). *Quality assurance and performance improvement.* Retrieved from https://www.cms.gov/Medicare/Provider-Enrollment-and-Certification/QAPI/qapidefinition

are currently somewhat "stuck in the mud" between the respective value placed on objective versus subjective feedback. We tend to focus on measuring the decline or absence of bad things (reduction in falls, infections, bed sores, medication errors, or preventable rehospitalizations), which eerily resembles how total or continuous quality improvement looked in manufacturing decades ago, reducing variance, error, or rework. However, applying sound psychometric techniques in determining patient/family satisfaction—in real time—has provided meaningful data for improving quality in other industries. The best approach is probably not to exclusively rely on either, but rather to find a way to blend them.

In 2014, Congress passed the Improving Medicare Post-Acute Care Transformation (IMPACT) Act, requiring the submission of standardized patient assessment data by providers of several senior living service lines, including SNFs, IRFs, and HHAs (CMS, 2019f). The resulting quality reporting program requires the submission of data pertaining to quality measures (i.e., MDS, PAI and OASIS-D), resource use and other domains. The primary objective is facilitating the exchange of the data among postacute providers and other healthcare providers to improve Medicare beneficiary outcomes through shared decision-making, effective care coordination, and enhanced discharge planning. All three service lines submit their data to the CMS and view reports concerning quality indicators and CASPER via the agency's Internet Quality Improvement and Evaluation System (IQIES).

Additionally, the CMS developed a program intended to assist *consumers* in comparing senior living providers participating in the Medicare and/or Medicaid programs—the "Five-Star Quality Rating System." It is very similar to third-party rating models aimed at prospective students considering applying for college, such as the program offered annually by *U.S. News and World Report* (USNWR), evaluating organizational performance on a series of metrics determined by the reporting entity as important and relevant (USNWR, 2019). Each provider within a designated service line receives a rating between one and five stars concerning each of a few significant criteria, as well as an overall score. Those with five stars are considered by the CMS to have outperformed those receiving fewer stars. Table 2.4 provides an overview of how nursing homes and HHAs are addressed by the CMS for this purpose.

TABLE 2.4 Center for Medicare & Medicaid Services' Five-Star Quality Rating System (Medicare.gov)

Service Line	Components
Skilled nursing facility: Nursing home compare	**Compliance:** The three most recent Medicare/Medicaid certification inspections (and complaint investigations, if any), with greatest weight given to the more recent survey findings.
	Staffing: The number of hours of care provided on average to each resident per day by nursing staff, considering variances in the acuity and complexity of residents' care needs.
	Quality Measures: Information on 15 physical clinical measures for nursing home residents (CMS, 2019e).

(continued)

TABLE 2.4 (*continued*)	
Service Line	**Components**
Home health agency: Home health compare	**Process Metric:** Timely initiation of care.
	Outcome Metrics: Improvement in ambulation, bed transferring, bathing, management of oral medications; reduction in pain interfering with activity, shortness of breath, and acute care hospitalization.
	Plus (separate)
	Patient Survey: Based on the patient experience of specified care measures (CMS, 2019b).

Source: U.S. Centers for Medicare & Medicaid Services. (2019b). *Home health five-star quality rating system.* Retrieved from https://www.cms.gov/Medicare/Quality-Initiatives -Patient-Assessment-Instruments/HomeHealthQualityInits/HHQIHomeHealthStarRatings; U.S. Centers for Medicare and Medicaid Services. (2019e). *SNF five-star quality rating system.* Retrieved from https://www.cms.gov/Medicare/Provider-Enrollment-and-Certification/ CertificationandComplianc/FSQRS

POLICIES AND PROCEDURES

Establishing written policies and procedures that address the purposes, roles, and expectations of the clinical IDT, including how complementary internal and external resources can be incorporated, is vital. They should also include training standards concerning applicable assessment tools, EMR systems in place, and developing clinical IDT member familiarity with the quality metrics monitored for regulatory compliance and the relationship between clinical documentation and reimbursement.

SUMMARY

Leaders need to have a solid understanding of all of the care and service elements of an organization. They also need to make sure their team is both qualified and competent to perform their jobs. One of the critical elements of leadership is to model a good teamwork approach because it is an essential need for all of these talented professionals to work together. At the end of the day, the best quality care and service is delivered when everybody respects each other and the disciplines appreciate the contributions of all. An effective leader also ensures that all of the support and systems are in place to enable a collaborative and efficient care and service delivery approach.

KEY POINTS

1. People serving older adults should learn something about them—changes in physical, mental, emotional, and spiritual wellness, loss and grief, and trends in family dynamics.

2. Technology promises to provide a host of new solutions for enhancing an elder's safety, comfort, social engagement, care coordination, and options for where to live.

3. The clinical IDT blends the expertise of people with complementary professional backgrounds, knowledge, and skills to:
   a. Thoroughly assess a person's condition
   b. Identify problems or needs
   c. Develop approaches and interventions to meaningfully address those problems or needs in a plan of care
   d. Implement that plan
   e. Continuously evaluate how well the approaches worked
   f. Periodically adjust the plan of care accordingly

4. The IDT's membership should reflect the licensure level of the service line and complexity of the care recipient. For SNF, IRF, and HHA services, the constant core members are typically a physician (or licensed designee), nurse, social worker, therapist (PT/OT/ST), and dietitian. Nonclinical disciplines often provide complementary and relevant information, as well.

5. Key licensed professional consultants typically include medical director, pharmacist, dietitian, dentist, podiatrist, ophthalmologist or optometrist, and barber/cosmetologist.

6. Coordination of the IDT is paramount—scheduling, information sharing, assigning, and monitoring workflow and documenting progress—for establishing and achieving clinical care goals and for regulatory compliance.

7. Person-centered care and culture change have entered the contemporary lexicon of senior living and now influence the expectations of both consumers and regulators.

8. Care planning and documentation can be organized with various formats by service line, but the foundational premise to embrace is that without a written account, *any* event—whether positive or negative—might as well not have happened.

9. Accurate and timely documentation is required to ensure quality care, evaluate opportunities for performance improvement, and validate reimbursement rates.

10. Quality should be reimagined as more than the absence of bad things. We keep trying new approaches to measure it and to share that data in ways that are useful to consumers, providers, and regulators. The quest continues.

11. Understanding and following the CDC's "Standard Precautions" is essential to sound infection control and prevention.

LEADERSHIP ROLES

The HSE™ sets the tone for setting and upholding high standards. Consistently promoting and fostering a corporate culture that embraces person-centered care and striving for exceeding minimal requirements is a common thread among successful leaders in our field. It is most important for the HSE™ to facilitate the work effort of the IDT by equipping them with the tools they need to succeed, clearly articulating expectations and providing support and time for meaningful collaboration. The progressive HSE™ capitalizes on the data generated by the various assessment and quality metric reports available to frame and implement performance improvement strategies.

HIGH-IMPACT PRACTICES

1. **Reimagine:** Scope of service.

   a. **Medical Director:** Many senior living employees either do not have a primary care physician or face barriers to access, such as transportation or work schedules. Occupational medicine has become popular in manufacturing settings—offering healthcare at the work site increases access, and healthy staff members tend to have higher rates of attendance, productivity, engagement, and retention. This also strengthens the business relationship with the medical director.

   b. **Multidisciplinary Treatment Room:** Furnish space that can accommodate the care delivery needs for providing onsite dentistry, podiatry, or vision exams. With some modest modification, a reclining dental chair or barber chair can serve this purpose.

2. **Engaging Family in IDT:** Provide livestreaming videoconferencing opportunities for a resident's family member(s) to participate in care planning and related care conferences as contributing stakeholders. With the advent of commercial smart phone apps for this purpose, such as FaceTime® or DUO®, special equipment is no longer needed to offer this option in most settings.

3. **Break Down the Traditional Silo Between IDT and Business Office:** Most contemporary EMR systems are intimately linked to a provider's financial reporting system, so why not mirror that with training for the people regularly working in each sphere about how their information affects the other? Be prepared to hear, "I had no idea!"

4. **Gerontology for All:** Knowing more about aging is not just good for caregivers; the people we serve may also be curious about what happens and why. The learning experience can transcend the course content when caregivers and care recipients step out of their respective roles and become students together.

QUESTIONS FOR DISCUSSION

1. Meadow View Health and Rehabilitation Center is licensed for 100 SNF beds, all of which are dually certified for participation in Medicare and Medicaid. Although it remains full most of the time, its Medicare Part A volume has risen steadily in recent years from less than 10% to just over 25% of all resident days. What impact is this trend likely to have on each of the following aspects of the operation, and why?

   a. Average length of stay

   b. Discharge planning

   c. Revenue

   d. Expense

   e. Gross margin

   f. Staff recruitment and retention

2. How can a HHA's IDT most effectively share information about a client and collaborate on developing an effective plan of care?

3. What disciplines are typically included in the IDT in each of the following settings?

   a. Adult day center

   b. SNF—postacute rehabilitation

   c. Home health

   d. SNF—long-term care

   e. Hospice

   f. Assisted living

4. Describe "person-centered care" and what you find most attractive about it?

5. Which core value or principle of "culture change" do you think would be the hardest to uphold? Why?

6. Name two ways through which technology seems likely to provide new solutions for allowing elders to remain in their homes; explain how this would be achieved.

CASE PROBLEMS

1. The clinical IDT of Greentree Rehabilitation Center was having difficulty fitting its care planning into the allotted time, no matter what day of the week or time of day. The MDS coordinator's frustration was driven mainly by the inconsistent compliance of the members with agreed-upon deadlines for completing their respective portions of the MDS prior to the conferences, so that their time together could be focused on refining the plan of care instead of creating it. By moving to a shared leadership model—each member of the core team taking responsibility for leading the IDT for 2 weeks at a time—the team reached a new level of stakeholder ownership and mutual accountability.

   Questions:

   a. What are two key barriers to coordinating time and workflow for a clinical IDT?

   b. How would you propose to address them?

2. A common—and avoidable—misstep for clinicians who change practice settings within senior care is "over-medicalizing" the assessment and care planning process in a setting that has less stringent documentation requirements. Atlas Assisted Living Community nipped this in the bud by attaching to each professional consultant's affiliation agreement a position description for members of the IDT.

   Questions:

   a. Describe an example of a health professional "overmedicalizing" their service approach in a senior living setting that does not require that level of intensity.

   b. What basic elements should be included in the position description for contracted health professionals who serve on the IDT?

3. Establishing, updating, disseminating, and monitoring compliance with IDT policies and procedures can easily become a never-ending task, largely

because of the dynamic nature of related regulations. T-Rex Apothecary, an institutional pharmacy, partnered with a senior living software developer to include in its maintenance agreement a provision assuring the contracting provider organization of ongoing regulatory compliance with all relevant reporting requirements of the CMS (across all applicable service lines).

Questions:

   a. What, if any, potential conflicts of interest might T-Rex Apothecary's strategy pose?

   b. Under such an arrangement, would the provider that contracted with T-Rex Apothecary be responsible for a cited survey deficiency? Why or why not?

4. Navigator Home Health was recently acquired by Anchor Care Centers, a senior living organization that previously operated solely SNFs. In the interest of standardization and following the same patient across multiple lines of service, Anchor Care Centers' IT department set out to build a proprietary EMR system that would appropriately populate both the OASIS-D and MDS assessment tools.

Questions:

   a. What obstacles to success would you anticipate?

   b. Describe an alternate strategy for pursuing this operational goal.

NAB DOMAINS OF PRACTICE

10 CUSTOMER CARE, SUPPORTS, AND SERVICES

10.01 Establish care recipient service policies and procedures that comply with federal and state laws, rules, and regulations.

10.02 Ensure plans of care are evidence-based, established, implemented, updated, and monitored based on care recipient preferences and assessed needs.

10.03 Ensure the planning, development, implementation/execution, monitoring, and evaluation of admissions/move-in process, including pre-admission/pre-move information, to promote a quality experience for care recipients.

10.04 Ensure the planning, development, implementation/execution, monitoring, and evaluation of discharge/move-out process to promote a quality experience for care recipients.

10.05 Ensure the planning, development/execution, implementation, monitoring, and evaluation of programs to meet care recipients' psychosocial needs and preferences.

10.06 Ensure the planning, development, implementation/execution, monitoring, and evaluation of care recipients' activities/recreation to meet social needs and preferences.

10.07 Ensure the planning, development, implementation/execution, monitoring, and evaluation of a health information management program to meet documentation requirements in compliance with federal and state regulations.

10.08 Ensure the planning, development, implementation/execution, monitoring, and evaluation of medication management that supports the needs of the care recipient.

10.09 Ensure the planning, development, implementation/execution, monitoring, and evaluation of a rehabilitation program to maximize optimum level of functioning and independence for care recipients.

10.10 Ensure the planning, development, implementation/execution, monitoring, and evaluation of systems for coordination and oversight of contracted services.

10.11 Ensure the planning, development, implementation/execution, monitoring, and evaluation of policies and procedures for responses to care recipient-specific incidents, accidents and/or emergencies.

10.12 Ensure the planning, development, implementation/execution, monitoring, and evaluation of housekeeping and laundry services for care recipients.

10.13 Ensure the planning, development, implementation/execution, monitoring, and evaluation of education intended for care recipients and their support networks.

10.14 Ensure the planning, development, implementation/execution, monitoring, and evaluation of nutritional needs and preferences of care recipients.

10.15 Ensure the planning, development, implementation/execution, monitoring, and evaluation of dining experience that meets the needs and preferences of care recipients.

10.16 Ensure care recipients' rights and individuality within all aspects of care.

10.17 Integrate support network's perspectives to maximize care recipients' quality of life and care.

10.18 Ensure transportation options are available for care recipients.

10.19 Ensure the provision of a customer service culture that leads to a quality experience for care recipients.

A summary of the related knowledge, skills, and core expectations across service lines—and unique features of each service line—is available at www.nabweb.org/filebin/pdf/Annotation_of_Tasks_Performed_Across_LOS_in_LTC.pdf.

Source: Reproduced with permission from National Association of Long-Term Care Administrator Boards. (2016). *Annotation of tasks performed and knowledge and skills used across lines of service in long term care.* Retrieved from https://www.nabweb.org/filebin/pdf/Annotation_of_Tasks_Performed_Across_LOS_in_LTC.pdf

REFERENCES

Academy of Nutrition and Dietetics. (2019). *Commission on dietetic registration.* Retrieved from https://www.cdrnet.org/

Allan, C., Valkanova, V., & Ebmeier, K. (2014). Depression in older people is underdiagnosed. *Practitioner, 258*(1771), 19–22.

American Academy of Professional Coders. (2019). *Medical billing and coding certification.* Retrieved from https://www.aapc.com/certification/

American Association for Long-Term Care Insurance. (2019). *Long-term care: Important information for women*. Retrieved from https://www.aaltci.org/long-term-care-insurance/learning-center/for-women.php

American Association of Directors of Nursing Services. (2019). *Director of nursing services—Certified (DNS-CT)*. Retrieved from https://www.aadns-ltc.org/Education/DNS-CT-Certification

American Association of Ophthalmology. (2019a). *What is a doctor of optometry?* Retrieved from https://www.aoa.org/about-the-aoa/what-is-a-doctor-of-optometry

American Association of Ophthalmology. (2019b). *What is an ophthalmologist?* Retrieved from https://www.aao.org/eye-health/tips-prevention/what-is-ophthalmologist

American Board of Audiology. (2019). *American Board of Audiology® certified*. Retrieved from https://www.boardofaudiology.org/board-certified-in-audiology/

American Dental Association, Health Policy Institute. (2019). *Oral health and well-being among seniors in the United States*. Retrieved from https://www.ada.org/~/media/ADA/Science%20and%20Research/HPI/Files/HPIgraphic_0916_2.pdf?la=en

American Health Information Management Association. (2019). *AHIMA certified coding specialist*. Retrieved from http://www.ahima.org/

American Physical Therapy Association. (2019a). *Licensure of physical therapists*. Retrieved from http://www.apta.org/Licensure/

American Physical Therapy Association. (2019b). *Physical therapy academic programs*. Retrieved from http://aptaapps.apta.org/ptcas/programlist.aspx

American Physical Therapy Association. (2019c). *Role of a physical therapy assistant*. Retrieved from https://www.apta.org/PTACareers/RoleofaPTA/

American Podiatric Medicine Association. (2019). *Is podiatry for me?* Retrieved from https://www.apma.org

American Society of Consultant Pharmacists. (2019). *What is a senior care pharmacist?* Retrieved from https://www.ascp.com

American Speech-Language-Hearing Association. (2019). *Certificates of clinical competence*. Retrieved from https://www.asha.org/certification/

Association for Nutrition and Food Service Professionals. (2019). *Certifying board for dietary managers*. Retrieved from https://www.cbdmonline.org/

Association of Professional Chaplains. (2019). *Board of certification for professional Chaplains*. Retrieved from http://www.professionalchaplains.org

Beauty Schools Directory. (2019). *Cosmetology school*. Retrieved from https://www.beautyschoolsdirectory.com/programs/cosmetology-school

Broskey, E. (2019). *The purpose of universal precautions*. Retrieved from https://www.verywellhealth.com/universal-precautions-3132819

Center for Aging Services Technology, Leading Age. (2011). *The state of technology: Executive summary*. Retrieved from http://hweb.leadingage.org/State_of_Technology_Executive_Summary.aspx

Council on Credentialing in Pharmacy. (2014). Credentialing and privileging of pharmacists: A resource paper from the council on credentialing in pharmacy. *American Journal of Health-System Pharmacy, 71*(21), 1891–1900. doi:10.2146/ajhp140420

Dahlke, D., Lindeman, D., & Ory, M. (2019, November 7). *Technology could be the solution to caregiver shortage for seniors*. Retrieved from https://www.considerable.com/home/technology/technology-caregiver-shortage-seniors/

Darling, L. (2019, December 11). Is there a medical cure for loneliness? *AARP*. Retrieved from https://www.aarp.org/home-family/friends-family/info-2019/medical-cure-for-loneliness.html

Etkin, K. (2019, December 4). *Which technology giants have their eye on the longevity economy prize?* Retrieved from https://www.thegerontechnologist.com/which-tech-giants-have-their-eye-on-the-longevity-economy-prize/

Fagin, C., & Pargament, K. (2011). Strengthened by the spirit: Religion, spirituality and resilience through adulthood and aging. In B. Resnick, L. Gwyther, & K. Roberto (Eds.), *Resilience in aging: Concepts, research and outcomes* (pp. 163–180). New York, NY: Springer Publishing Company.

Garner, J. S. (1996). Guideline for isolation precautions in hospitals. The Hospital Infection Control Practices Advisory Committee. *Infection Control and Hospital Epidemiology, 17*(1), 53–80. doi:10.1086/647190

Gonzalez, E. (2014). *Home health infection control: A manual for compliance and quality.* Danvers, MA: Beacon Health.

GraduateNursingEdu.org. (2019) *Gerontological nurse practitioner.* Retrieved from https://www .graduatenursingedu.org/gerontological-nurse-practitioner/

Haran, C. (2006). *Transforming long-term care: Giving residents a place to call home.* New York, NY: The Commonwealth Fund. Retrieved from https://www.commonwealthfund.org/ publications/publication/2006/apr/transforming-long-term-care-giving-residents-place -call-home

Harris-Kojetin, L., Sengupta, M., Lendon, J. P., Rome, V., Valverde, R., & Caffrey, C. (2019). Long-term care providers and services users in the United States, 2015–2016. National Center for Health Statistics. *Vital Health Statistics, 3*(43), 1–88. Retrieved from https://www.cdc.gov/ nchs/data/series/sr_03/sr03_43-508.pdf

Health Information Management and Systems Society. (2019). *Health informatics.* Retrieved from https://www.himss.org/who-we-are

Health Level 7 International. (2019). *About HL7.* Retrieved from http://www.hl7.org/about/ index.cfm?ref=nav

HIPAA-Journal.com. (2017, February 13). *Majority of healthcare organizations struggling with EHR interoperability.* Retrieved from https://www.hipaajournal.com/majority -healthcare-organizations-struggling-with-ehr-interoperability-8686/

Hooyman, N., Kawamoto, K., & Liyak, H. A. (2015). *Aging matters: An introduction to social gerontology.* Upper Saddle River, NJ: Pearson Education.

Howley, E. (2019, September 13). *Eye exams in nursing homes: Our eyes change with age; keeping up with routine eye care is important.* US News and World Report. Retrieved from https:// health.usnews.com/best-nursing-homes/articles/eye-exams-in-nursing-homes

Joint Commission on Accreditation of Healthcare Organizations. (2019a). *Long term care accreditation requirements.* Retrieved from https://www.jointcommission.org/ accreditation/long_term_care_accreditation_requirements.aspx

Joint Commission on Accreditation of Healthcare Organizations. (2019b). *Medical staff essentials: Clarifying medical staff standards.* Retrieved from https://www.jointcommission.org/the _view_from_the_joint_commission/medical_staff_essentials_clarifying_medical_staff _standards/

Koren, M. J. (2009). Person-centered care for nursing home residents: The culture-change movement. *Health Affairs, 29*, 2. Retrieved from https://www.healthaffairs.org/doi/ full/10.1377/hlthaff.2009.0966

Morton, L. (2019, October 8). Author Interview with Laura Morton, MD, CMD, Associate Professor in the University of Louisville's Department of Family and Geriatric Medicine.

National Association of Activities Professionals. (2019). *Professional certification.* Retrieved from https://naap.info/

National Association of Directors of Nursing Administration/Long-Term Care. (2019). *Certification exams.* Retrieved from https://www.nadona.org/exams/

National Association of Social Workers. (2019). *About NASW.* Retrieved from https://www .socialworkers.org/

National Barbers Association. (2019). *About NBA.* Retrieved from https:// nationalbarbersassociation.com

National Board for Certification in Occupational Therapy. (2019). *What does it meant to be an OTR or COTA?* Retrieved from https://www.nbcot.org/en/Public/Occupational -Therapy

National Council of Certification of Physician Assistants. (2019). *About NCCPA.* Retrieved from https://www.nccpa.net/

National Council of State Boards of Nursing. (2019a). *NCLEX and other exams.* Retrieved from https://www.ncsbn.org/nclex.htm

National Council of State Boards of Nursing. (2019b). *Nurse licensure compact.* Retrieved from https://www.ncsbn.org/nurse-licensure-compact.htm

National Institutes for Health, National Institute of Neurological Disorders and Stroke. (2019). *Peripheral neuropathy fact sheet.* Retrieved from https://www.ninds.nih.gov/Disorders/Patient-Caregiver-Education/Fact-Sheets/Peripheral-Neuropathy-Fact-Sheet

National PACE Association. (2019). *Understanding the PACE model of care.* Retrieved from https://www.npaonline.org/start-pace-program/understanding-pace-model-care

National Social Work Policy Institute. (2019). *Social work services in nursing homes: Toward quality psychosocial care.* Retrieved from http://www.socialworkpolicy.org/research/social-work-services-in-nursing-homes-toward-quality-psychosocial-care.html

NextInsurance.com. (2019). *Barber license vs cosmetology license: New opportunities and legal limitations.* Retrieved from https://www.next-insurance.com/blog/barber-license-vs-cosmetology-license/

NursingLicensure.org. (2019a). *Certified nursing assistant.* Retrieved from https://www.nursinglicensure.org/cna/nursing-assistant.html

NursingLicensure.org. (2019b). *Why do California and Texas use the title licensed vocational nurse?* Retrieved from https://www.nursinglicensure.org/articles/lvn-lpn.html

Pioneer Network. (2019a). *Core values and principles of culture change.* Retrieved from https://www.pioneernetwork.net/about-us/mission-vision-values/

Pioneer Network. (2019b). *Overview of the pioneer network.* Retrieved from https://www.pioneernetwork.net/about-us/overview/

Pioneer Network. (2019c). *What is culture change?* Retrieved from https://www.pioneernetwork.net/culture-change/what-is-culture-change/

Proofpoint.com. (2019). *Ransomware is big business.* Retrieved from https://www.proofpoint.com/us/threat-reference/ransomware

RegisteredNursing.org. (2019). *Nursing school accreditation commission guide.* Retrieved from https://www.registerednursing.org/guide/nursing-school-accreditation/

Segal, P. (2018). *The evolution of standard precautions.* Retrieved from https://www.infectioncontroltoday.com/standard-precautions/evolution-isolation-precautions

Siegel, J., Rhinehart, E., Jackson, M., Chiarello, L., and the Centers for Disease Control and Prevention Healthcare Infection Control Practices Advisory Committee. (2019). *2007 guideline for isolation precautions: Preventing transmission of infectious agents in healthcare settings.* Retrieved from https://www.cdc.gov/infectioncontrol/guidelines/isolation/index.html

Singh, D. (2016). *Effective management of long-term care facilities* (3rd ed.). Burlington, MA: Jones and Bartlett.

Society for Post-Acute and Long-Term Care Medicine. (2019). *Certified medical director.* Retrieved from https://paltc.org

Tellis-Nayak, V., & Tellis-Nayak, M. (2016). *Return of compassion to healthcare.* Conneaut Lake, PA: Page Publishing.

U.S. Bureau of Labor Statistics. (2019). *Occupational outlook: Physical therapy assistants and aides.* Retrieved from https://www.bls.gov/ooh/healthcare/physical-therapist-assistants-and-aides.htm

U.S. Centers for Medicare & Medicaid Services. (2019a). *Certification and survey provider enhanced reports (CASPER).* Retrieved from https://www.cms.gov/cms-search?search=casper&field_date%5Bmin%5D=&field_date%5Bmax%5D=&sort_by=search_api_relevance&items_per_page=10

U.S. Centers for Medicare & Medicaid Services. (2019b). *Home health five-star quality rating system.* Retrieved from https://www.cms.gov/Medicare/Quality-Initiatives-Patient-Assessment-Instruments/HomeHealthQualityInits/HHQIHomeHealthStarRatings

U.S. Centers for Medicare & Medicaid Services. (2019c). *Minimum data set 3.0 resident assessment instrument manual.* Retrieved from https://www.cms.gov/Medicare/Quality-Initiatives-Patient-Assessment-Instruments/NursingHomeQualityInits/MDS30RAIManual

U.S. Centers for Medicare & Medicaid Services. (2019d). *Quality assurance and performance improvement.* Retrieved from https://www.cms.gov/Medicare/Provider-Enrollment-and-Certification/QAPI/qapidefinition

U.S. Centers for Medicare & Medicaid Services. (2019e). *SNF five-star quality rating system.* Retrieved from https://www.cms.gov/Medicare/Provider-Enrollment-and-Certification/CertificationandComplianc/FSQRS

U.S. Centers for Medicare & Medicaid Services. (2019f). *SNF quality reporting program overview*. Retrieved from https://www.cms.gov/Medicare/Quality-Initiatives-Patient-Assessment-Instruments/NursingHomeQualityInits/Skilled-Nursing-Facility-Quality-Reporting-Program/SNF-Quality-Reporting-Program-Overview

U.S. News and World Report. (2019). *U.S. news best colleges*. Retrieved from https://www.usnews.com/best-colleges

Zimmerman, S., Shier, V., & Saliba, D. (2014). Transforming nursing home culture: Evidence for practice and policy. *The Gerontologist, 54*(Suppl. 1), S1–S5. doi:10.1093/geront/gnt161

ADDITIONAL RESOURCES

1. **GERONTOLOGY OVERVIEW**

An easy-to-read introduction to the field of aging services, addressing all aspects of social gerontology from theories to practice.

Hooyman, N., Kawamoto, K., & Liyak, H. A. (2015). *Aging matters: An introduction to social gerontology*. Upper Saddle River, NJ: Pearson Education.

2. **AGING SERVICES TECHNOLOGY**

- **LeadingAge's CAST (Center for Aging Services Technology)** produces and publishes a comprehensive portfolio of hands-on resources that help providers—and consumers—understand, plan for, select, implement, and adopt the appropriate technology for a variety of needs. They range from electronic health records (EHRs), telehealth and health information exchanges (HIE), to safety, medication management, and remote patient monitoring (RPM). Retrieved from https://leadingage.org/technology-selection-tools

- **The Thrive Center** is a not-for-profit technology innovation center designed to enhance the quality of life for seniors, featuring innovative technology, specialized programming to enhance elder wellness, and a series of educational programs for the community. Learn more at https://www.thrivecenterky.org

3. **CULTURE CHANGE AND PERSON-CENTERED CARE**

Resource sites of organizations that have led with innovative programming in this movement:

- Action Pact: http://actionpact.com
- Center for Positive Aging: http://www.centerforpositiveaging.org
- Eden Alternative: https://www.edenalt.org
- Green House Project: https://www.thegreenhouseproject.org
- Pioneer Network: https://www.pioneernetwork.net

4. **CARE RECIPIENT (RESIDENT/PATIENT/CLIENT/PARTICIPANT) ASSESSMENT**

- Skilled Nursing Facility (MDS Manual): https://www.cms.gov/Medicare/Quality-Initiatives-Patient-Assessment-Instruments/NursingHomeQualityInits/MDS30RAIManual
- Inpatient Rehabilitation Facility (PAI Manual): https://www.cms.gov/Medicare/Quality-Initiatives-Patient-Assessment-Instruments/

IRF-Quality-Reporting/IRF-PAI-and-IRF-PAI-Manual

- Home Health (OASIS-D Requirements): https://www.cms.gov/Medi care/Quality-Initiatives-Patient-Assessment-Instruments/HomeHealth QualityInits/Home-Health-Quality-Reporting-Requirements

- Assisted Living/Other (ISP Sample From LeadingAge): https://www .leadingageny.org/home/assets/File/ISP%20DAL%20Addressing%20 EH%20annual%20functional%20assessment(1).pdf

5. **QUALITY ASSURANCE AND PERFORMANCE IMPROVEMENT (QAPI):** https://www.cms.gov/Medicare/Provider-Enrollment-and-Certification/ QAPI/Downloads/qapifiveelements.pdf

6. **CMS STAR RATINGS (Details on Performance Metrics Utilized)**

- Skilled Nursing Facility: https://www.cms.gov/Medicare/Provider -Enrollment-and-Certification/CertificationandComplianc/FSQRS

- Inpatient Rehabilitation Facility: https://www.cms.gov/Medicare/ Provider-Enrollment-and-Certification/CertificationandComplianc/ InpatientRehab

- Home Health Agency: https://www.cms.gov/Medicare/Quality -Initiatives-Patient-Assessment-Instruments/HomeHealthQuality Inits/HHQIHomeHealthStarRatings

7. **RANSOMEWARE**

- No More Ransom Project: https://www.nomoreransom.org/en/about -the-project.html

Operations

Section II offers a foundational framework for three domains of professional practice that the National Association of Long Term Care Administrator Boards (NAB) identifies for the health services executive: human resources, finance, and environment. Although treated individually, they weave together like fabric. Each chapter closes with a summary of key points, a brief discussion of the leader's role with respect to the domain, examples of high-impact practices, recommended discussion questions and case studies, and additional resources for further reference.

The healthcare and human services field, in general, and its senior living component, in particular, are labor-intensive and high-touch by their very nature. Human resources (Chapter 3, Human Resources) is the practice domain that encompasses the full range of effectively pursuing the organization's mission through the actions of its people. In addition to needing to identify, attract, and employ qualified and motivated personnel, it is essential to train and develop, reward and compensate, and engage and support them in order to *retain* them. Retention not only reduces cost but also strengthens continuity of care and quality of services. The same concepts and techniques can apply to volunteers (*unpaid* personnel).

Whether operating a not-for-profit or proprietary enterprise, financial performance (Chapter 4, Financial Management in Senior Care) drives the long-term viability of the organization. "No money, no mission" is a popular phrase that captures this reality. Accurate and timely financial reporting matters for both internal management purposes (i.e., monitoring actual performance against budget or managing cash flow) and meeting external requirements (i.e., billing and reimbursement, tax returns, or cost reports). Establishing and adhering to policies and procedures that reflect generally accepted accounting principles (GAAP) serve to enhance a provider's regulatory compliance, accountability, and public confidence. Financial management entails more than accounting and reporting—it can also include financing, fundraising and grantseeking, merger and acquisition, investments, and managing financial risk.

Although the word "environment" (Chapter 5, Environment) can trigger thoughts of the great outdoors, sustainability, or energy conservation, it refers here to the physical surrounding of the care/service recipient—across service lines. Here it can mean house, condominium, or apartment; congregate housing, assisted living, or skilled nursing community; or continuing care retirement community or life plan community. The issues that permeate this domain include standards for a structure's construction and stability, occupant safety and comfort, as well as policies and procedures addressing disaster preparedness, preventive and corrective maintenance, cleanliness, and groundskeeping. The environment domain also includes legal and regulatory matters, from the organization's governance and compliance with applicable laws, regulations, and standards to its liability for negative outcomes that harm people. A myriad of government regulatory agencies, private accrediting bodies, and even payers both set and enforce rules for their respective purposes. Finally, we live in an increasingly litigious society, as evidenced by the rise in the frequency with which families engage personal injury attorneys to settle grievances about postacute care through the court system.

Human Resources

INTRODUCTION

Serving elders and/or disabled adults—and their families—is a "people business," people helping others in need. It is an enterprise that relies on consistently having enough committed, motivated, qualified, and competent team members to perform the services needed by our customers. An effective leader focuses on harnessing and leveraging the collective knowledge, skills, creativity, and sense of purpose of the work team to produce high-quality services in a cost-effective manner. In short, people are the most valuable assets of a postacute care provider organization.

The key challenges in this core element of the operation include finding the right people (recruiting), attracting them (screening and hiring), onboarding them (orienting), fostering their growth (training and talent development), organizing their effort (staffing and scheduling), and *keeping* them (retention). Establishing and maintaining a culture of transparency, respect, fairness, and equal treatment is paramount and relevant to each phase.

Human resource management is referred to by some organizations as personnel management or employee relations (Singh, 2016). In a larger setting, there typically is a designated position for addressing human resources management duties. If affiliated with a larger corporate entity, such as a hospital or management company, an operation might receive human resources management support externally. In a smaller organization, those responsibilities may in part belong to the local site administrator.

RECRUITING

Finding and hiring persons with an optimal balance of skills, knowledge, motivation, personality, and professionalism (and keeping them) is paramount to sustaining the success of any postacute care organization. It also is becoming more challenging in an increasingly competitive market, with the pool of available workers failing to keep pace with the exponential growth in potential clients. The combination of the graying of America and little growth in the pool of available workers has resulted in the ratio of potential caregivers to recipients trending downward (Pratt, 2016).

The expanding economy during the second decade of this century has exacerbated the situation. While there is good reason for most to celebrate a decline in the unemployment rate that typically accompanies a period of economic expansion, it makes recruiting new employees even tougher because fewer people are available or looking for work.

Senior living does not compete only with other postacute provider organizations for staff members. For licensed professionals—primarily nurses and therapists—we also compete with hospitals, outpatient clinics, manufacturers (occupational health), and even school systems and insurance companies, and they often offer higher compensation packages (pay and benefits), more attractive shifts, or both. For paraprofessionals, the competition matrix is even broader, including employers offering a wide array of services and those operating fast-food restaurants or manufacturing plants. Few of the competing employers have as many constraints on their revenue streams as the continuum of long-term care providers that rely heavily on Medicare and Medicaid reimbursement.

Presenting a whole new set of hurdles for organizations providing direct services is the anticipated emergence of a "gig" economy—a free market system in which temporary positions are common and organizations contract with independent workers for short-term engagements. The success and explosive growth of companies such as Uber, Airbnb, and TaskRabbit is expected to further reduce the availability of potential workers by attracting them instead to fruitful vocations with greater flexibility than jobs that have more traditional, fixed schedules and more rigid workplace expectations (Sundararajan, 2015).

Fishing in the Right Pond With the Right Lure

The days of simply placing a HELP WANTED ad in the local paper when there is an opening to fill in the organization, and then waiting for the phone to ring or for the applications to pile up awaiting review and completing reference checks are behind us. There is a multitude of other ways in which people seeking new opportunities go about finding them. Many employers and prospective team members rely on Internet-based, third-party employment facilitators, such as Indeed or ZipRecruiter. Employers also increasingly rely on a full range of recruiting software or services, such as Fountain or BreezyHR, that feature not only applicant resourcing but resume parsing (ranking each resume by the extent to which it aligns with the position specifications submitted by the employer) or providing interview guidance for hiring managers (Capterra, 2019). Finally, word-of-mouth referral is a time-tested and often effective recruitment method (see High-Impact Practice 1 at the end of this chapter).

SCREENING

Once a candidate is identified—through recruiting efforts or because of a submitted inquiry or application—it is important to establish that they meet the organization's minimum requirements for employment and have the appropriate qualifications to perform the duties of the position.

An employment application can be completed on a paper form or online. Each has its advantages. If it is filled out in person, a paper form enables a team member to meet the applicant as well as to possibly observe the applicant's reading and writing proficiency (because it is not getting completed by someone else and then turned in). However, applying online can prove much more convenient for the prospective employee, which can positively impact the speed of attracting and hiring new talent.

Most postacute care providers maintain similar minimum standards for hiring. Some of them are governed by law, such as U.S. citizenship (or lawful alternative). Others may be either conditions of participation in Medicare or Medicaid, such as a prohibition against hiring a convicted felon, or another federal, state, or local law or regulation relating to an applicant's criminal record. Depending on the position, there may also be good reason to complete a credit check. The results can be relevant for anyone handling money, of course, but they can also provide information about an applicant's financial stresses or even trustworthiness.

Increasingly, provider organizations also expect an applicant to pass a pre-employment drug test. They also disclose that passing randomly selected employee drug testing is a condition of continuing employment. The nature and expense of providing accurate and timely drug testing in-house is generally cost prohibitive, so most postacute care providers rely on an outside clinical lab to perform the actual tests and report the results confidentially to the employer. Some perform this step as part of the screening process, whereas others make it a final condition of employment in the job offer.

TABLE 3.1 Summary of Popular Pre-employment Drug Test Panel Options

Panel	Drugs Detected	Advantages/Disadvantages
5	Opiates, PCP, cocaine, amphetamines, and marijuana	+ Most cost-effective + U.S. Department of Transportation utilizes for safety-sensitive positions (-) Scientific limitations are "impaired" threshold for marijuana
6	(Panel 5) without (PCP) + (methamphetamines and benzodiazepines)	+ Adds two popularly misused drugs (-) Omits PCP
7	(Panel 5) + (benzodiazepines and barbiturates)	+ Adds two popularly misused drugs (-) Omits methamphetamines
8	(Panel 6) + (Panel 7)	+ Addresses wider range of misused drugs (-) Cost:benefit
12	Opiates, PCP, cocaine, amphetamines, benzodiazepines, barbiturates, methadone, methaqualone, propoxyphene, ecstasy, oxycodone, and marijuana	+ Most comprehensive + Misuse of prescription painkillers (-) Cost:benefit

PCP, phencyclidine.

Caution: Testing positive for THC, the active ingredient in marijuana, has some limitations as far as a disqualifying criterion. First, the scientific evidence is weak so far for determining a standard level of concentration in a person's system that causes impairment, unlike thresholds established for alcohol (Gurston, 2019). Furthermore, some states are permitting the medical and/or recreational use of marijuana, which could make maintaining a "zero tolerance" policy for hiring or retaining staff more difficult than it has been before.

Source: Adapted from TOMO Drug Testing. (2015, November 4). *What are the different panel drug tests?* Retrieved from https://www.yourdrugtesting.com/what-are-the-different-panel-drug-tests/

The most cost-effective method is a urine sample test—known as the "5-panel drug test" because it detects five drugs that can impair a worker on the job—which includes the following set of disqualifying substances: opiates, phencyclidine (PCP), cocaine, amphetamines, and marijuana. This is the test used by the U.S. Department of Transportation for safety-sensitive positions regulated by its affiliated agencies. There is a multitude of recognized panel options, up to a 12-panel test (see Table 3.1).

An applicant's work history is typically disclosed in the applicant screening stage, revealing how long they have stayed in previous positions, why there was a change in employer, what kinds of responsibilities were fulfilled, and compensation. The practice of verifying this information and checking with the people listed as references is more than established form—it has pragmatic implications. First, it is important to determine if the information is accurate and complete. If the applicant misrepresents anything on the signed application, that is often considered grounds for disqualification; further investigation might be necessary. Second, an enthusiastic recommendation from a former employer or other reference can enhance the probability of success for this hiring decision.

Increasingly, employers are opting to provide *only* a former employee's dates of hire and departure, rather than any qualitative assessment of their performance. This approach is a risk management technique intended to reduce the probability that a former employee who is rejected for employment sues the former employer for contributing to that outcome by providing feedback that is either inconsistent with the application or negative.

HIRING

Having satisfactorily completed a diligent and thorough screening process, it is time to meet the applicant—now considered a "candidate"—for an in-person interview. This gives the hiring team member an opportunity to assess the candidate's presentation and demeanor as well as clarify any responses entered on the employment application. It also provides the candidate an opportunity to ask further questions about the organization, position responsibilities, potential for growth and advancement, schedule, or other concerns.

When there are multiple openings for similar positions, some organizations engage in an initial group interview, interacting with two or more screened candidates at the same time. This is certainly efficient, and more people hear answers at the same time to questions they may also have, but it erodes the personal connection that can come from a one-on-one interview.

If there is more than one qualified candidate for a single opening, the challenge becomes selecting the person with the best probability of success. Although there are many instruments and metrics available to narrow the choices and flesh out the candidate with the closest alignment to the organization's mission, most relevant and highly developed technical skills, and greatest likelihood to stay, there is still a significant element of executive judgment in determining the best fit. It is a science-*enhanced* art, but not foolproof.

Senior living organizations vary widely on their approach to framing a job offer. Generally, the larger the organization, the more prescriptive the policy governing what to include in a written offer. Regardless, consistency within the organization is essential, just as it is for administering *any* of its operating policies and procedures. Key elements of a job offer include position title (and sometimes a brief description), work shift and location, starting date, compensation (wages and benefits), and an acceptance line for the candidate to sign and return. There may also be additional conditions to sealing the deal, such as passing a pre-employment drug test or physical capacity test (for physically demanding positions).

It is common to find established pay ranges for positions, often differentiated by shift, with a floor, median, and ceiling. Some organizations recognize prior experience when setting the hiring salary, whereas others start everyone at the same rate for the same position. How frequently a provider adjusts its pay ranges can impact its competitive position in the market served, not only for attracting new employees but retaining those it already has. When it is adjusted, consideration must also be given to the current staff's compensation, or there is a risk of bringing in newly hired team members who earn than more for performing the same job.

Pre-Employment Reinforcement

The period between a candidate's acceptance of a job offer and starting date can be a risky one for an employer. Although the offer was accepted, they may not remain convinced about the decision—much like buyer's remorse. Keeping a candidate engaged in the interim is wise, such as (Handrick, 2018):

- Staying in touch with the candidate and continuing to sell the value of joining your company
- Calling, texting, or emailing to reassure them that you are looking forward to their first day
- Sending a map of where employees park as well as a public transportation route map and schedule that connects the home address on the application with the work site
- Sending a special gift bearing the company logo, such as a pen, small flashlight, or mock name badge

ORIENTING

The candidate who accepts the job offer and meets any remaining conditions of employment reports for the first day of work. Where are the welcome banners, the parade, the band, and confetti dropping from the ceiling? Well, the very best way to provide their equivalent is to equip the new employee with the tools needed to succeed in their new role. Orientation is the organization's opportunity not only to reinforce for the new employee all the reasons an application was submitted but to launch this new career with feelings of confidence and support (Handrick, 2018).

Sometimes the urgency associated with filling a vacant position causes a manager to rush, shorten, delay, or bypass altogether a new employee's thorough orientation. This is most certainly a recipe for disaster, either in the short term or later. "Sink or swim" is simply not a rallying cry of true leaders! The evidence supports that investing in optimizing every team member's probability of success pays handsome dividends for continuity of care, quality of life and clinical care, staff retention and productivity, and cost-effectiveness (Bishop et al., 2008; Kemper, Brannon, Barry, Stott, & Heier, 2008).

The field of senior living has a notoriously poor history when it comes to employee retention. Turnover in America's skilled nursing facilities (SNFs) has been estimated at as high as 75% annually (Scales, 2018), over 70% among assisted living facilities (McKnight's Long-Term Care News, 2012; Yee-Melichar, Boyle, & Flores, 2011), and over 60% in home healthcare (Mozga, 2015). For a frame of reference, consider that in 2016 the overall turnover rate in the healthcare and social assistance sector was about 32%, according to data from the Bureau of Labor Statistics' Job Openings and Labor Turnover Survey (JOLTS) program, while the average turnover rate for all U.S. industries stood at 42% (Argentum, 2018). Contributing factors to this include the significant physical and emotional demands of the work, relatively low wages and benefits, ease of finding alternative employment, either within or outside the field (Browning, 2017; Quilter, 2019).

A solid orientation can serve as one of the very best techniques for preventing employee turnover (aka *enhancing* employee retention), especially since a disproportionate share of departure occurs during the first 90 days of employment. Provide every new hire with adequate information about the company's:

- mission and history: its purpose and track record of advancing the mission;
- values and culture: what the organization stands for and considers its norms;
- vision: the aspirational future to be gained by fulfilling the mission;
- policies and procedures: approaches and techniques for performing assigned duties;
- performance expectations for the position: metrics for defining success; and
- hands-on training: concerning equipment and supplies that will be used in discharging the duties of the position.

To ensure each new staff member receives the same information (except for job-specific training), it is a common practice to follow an orientation checklist. It should include all the tasks required to make sure the employee has a memorable experience joining the organization. Following a checklist also prevents missing basic hiring process steps—such as payroll and compliance paperwork or a security badge—or the most important task: welcoming the newest member of the team. The main goal of the first day is to convince the newly hired employee that they made a great decision by joining your organization.

New Hire Paperwork

Here is a list of the documents and forms an employee typically completes, reviews, and/or signs to help make onboarding easier to manage.

- **I-9 Form (Employment Eligibility Verification):** Used to verify citizenship and employment eligibility; ask the employee to bring on day one a government-issued photo ID, such as a driver's license or passport (U.S. Department of Homeland Security, Citizenship and Immigration Service, 2019)
- **W-4 (Wage and Tax Statement):** Used to gather employee tax withholdings (U.S. Treasury/IRS, 2019a); there may be a state tax version of the W-4 that also needs to be completed
- **Employee Handbook:** Have the employee review and sign an acknowledgment of receiving and agreeing to abide by the employee handbook
- **Other Policies:** If there are policies unique to the site, service line, department, or job that are not addressed in the employee handbook, explain them

and have the employee sign a document acknowledging they read and understood it

- **Direct Deposit Form:** Used to gather banking information for payroll disbursement (if offered)
- **Employee Data Sheet:** Emergency contact information
- **Signed Offer Letter**

> **Practical Tip:** Consider pacing the paperwork review throughout the first few days instead of handing the new hire a stack of documents and disappearing. Review each item together to prevent them from becoming overwhelmed. For instance, complete payroll and I-9 and IRS documentation on the first day, benefits and payroll documentation on day two, and policies and the employee handbook on day three.

ONBOARDING

The most effective onboarding experiences are those that make a big deal about the new hire's first day. Day 1 on the job is when the new, and often nervous, hire needs to know that everyone celebrates their arrival. Whether in person, via teleconference call or prerecorded video, or by personal letter, it is helpful for someone as highly situated on the organizational chart as possible to connect with every new hire.

The first week on the job is nerve-wracking for most people. It is vital to make each newcomer feel welcome and encouraged so that they will be able to learn the organization's processes, system, and culture and to contribute meaningfully to advancing its mission.

Many providers also link an experienced staff member to each newly hired person to serve as a mentor, either for some prescribed period or until the mentor approves them as proficient enough in the position to no longer need a mentor. This is generally someone holding a similar job or who at least works in the same area. Even if there is not a formal mentoring program, it is beneficial to choose a peer to check in with the new hire each day for the first few weeks. That person can be a reliable resource for the new hire to ask questions and an ambassador for the organization's culture.

> **Practical Tip:** To help a new employee feel welcome, consider asking a peer to invite them to lunch each day during the first week. If meals are served on site, provide a voucher for the new hire and host. Use that first week to help the newcomer build relationships with coworkers.

By the end of the first month, performance expectations should have become clear. This is the perfect time to check on their perception of the following:

- How training is coming along; would more training be helpful? (If so, about what?)

- How well coworker relationships are forming; are there any early issues to address?

- Whether policies, procedures, or work practices are easy to follow; is anything confusing?

- If there are any tools or resources needed to be more productive

- If a struggle still exists with anything (identify who can help resolve it)

- The performance management process

Enrollment for many fringe benefits, such as health insurance coverage, also typically occurs within the first 30 days. The first 90 days on the job is a period when the new employee, coworkers, residents, and their families are all assessing whether the newcomer will be a good fit. The new staff member may continue to receive follow-ups from job applications made prior to accepting this position, so keep reinforcing their decision to join *this* team.

Practical Tips: Some of the most effective activities utilized by leading organizations for engaging and inspiring new employees to help them want to stay include the following (Handrick, 2018):

Training: On-the-job training is highly valued for learning the new job's tasks. Investing in training for the employee demonstrates commitment to their growth and success, and it is a great way for them to develop valuable skills that ensure continuity of care and consistency.

Performance Review: Why wait for the annual review? A 90-day feedback session, and even another at 6 months, is a great way to share what stands out about the new employee's performance. Some organizations even check weekly for the first 3 months. Ask what they still need to progress. (This is **not** a time to give the employee a B grade; it is an opportunity to clarify performance expectations and goals and to find out what the employee needs to meet or exceed those goals.)

Team Building: Provide opportunities for team members to build strong coworker relationships. Consider ways to help build trust and appreciation among team members. (Remind existing staff that they were new once, too.)

Projects: Once your employee has begun to understand the specific job, explore ways in which they can contribute to projects and encourage that involvement. Projects expose them to others in the organization and help build relationships. This can be as simple as decorating for a holiday event or as complex as implementing a new software system.

Feedback: The new hire has probably observed much in the first 90 days; ask them to share what opportunities for improvement—big or little—they have discovered. Giving and asking for feedback is an effective way to make the new hire feel important, valued, and encouraged to keep contributing.

Onboarding should not end once a newly hired employee passes the 90-day mark. Many companies make that mistake, which is probably why an estimated one third of new hires do not make it to the 6-month mark (Handrick, 2018). Continuing with onboarding activities throughout the employee's first year improves the odds of retention and of fostering their motivation, engagement, and productivity.

At the end of the first year, celebrate each new hire's onboarding success with an announcement and perhaps a 1-year anniversary gift. The first hire date anniversary marks a transition from a new hire to an experienced employee.

TRAINING AND TALENT DEVELOPMENT

Talent acquisition is an event, and talent development is a journey. Creating and fostering a culture that places a premium on the value of lifelong learning—aimed at growing both professionally and personally—is an effective strategy for attracting and retaining today's most promising candidates.

Like any planning process, this starts with an assessment of each employee's current knowledge, skills, and interests. Identifying growth opportunities and goals can provide the basis for crafting a personal development plan (PDP), which is similar to a resident's plan of care; a road map for career advancement and/or personal fulfillment. It is beneficial to align the employee's interests and aspirations with the opportunities available within the organization (or at least within the field) for the PDP to offer meaning and motivation. The extent to which this is achieved generally predicts the probability of success.

Learning Organization

A learning organization is one that applies the concepts of continuous quality improvement by embracing the inherent value of ongoing training for its employees (Senge, 2000). This can mean promoting and resourcing both informal and formal continuing education efforts across a variety of content categories:

- **Knowledge:** Relevant information about one's own discipline, others with which they may commonly interact, or the broader field and forces that might impact it
- **Skills:** Job-specific tasks or skill sets that are either new or unfamiliar and, once mastered, can enhance one's probability of advancement
- **Internal Dynamics:** Establishing relationships with people across departments or locations and increasing one's awareness of internal issues or concerns that are on people's minds
- **External Dynamics:** Forming external connections and becoming knowledgeable about issues and trends that have the potential for affecting the organization

STAFFING AND SCHEDULING

Having found, recruited, screened, hired, oriented, and trained a promising new staff member, the ongoing challenge becomes organizing the work effort and assignments that the people with the most skin in the game—the residents—are optimally served. It is a 24-7/365 (24 hours per day, 7 days per week, and 365 days per year) operation. This may seem somewhat lessened for home- and community-based services (HCBS), but there is an "on-call" expectation among clients and their families that a provider must be constantly ready to adapt to their changing needs, sometimes abruptly.

What is the right number of people to have on duty? Of course, the main driver of the answer is the "case mix" of the care recipients—the collective scope and intensity of their needs. Models have been developed for most postacute care settings to predict minimal and/or optimal staffing levels for clinicians (RN, LPN, certified nursing assistant [CNA], registered dietitian [RD], therapists, etc.) based on the blend of their respective interventions and time required to satisfactorily complete them. Other disciplines may vary less with changes in resident acuity, such as maintenance, housekeeping, and administrative staff.

The assertion by advocates of implementing minimum staffing ratios for postacute care providers to follow that ratios would improve client outcomes has met with mixed reviews. The attraction is the potential simplicity of enforcement. However, requiring a ratio of staff-to-residents based on anything other than the residents' actual care needs has limitations. For instance, any given resident's needs change over time, perhaps suddenly with an unexpected adverse event, such as a stroke. Furthermore, many residents leave—returning to home after a successful rehabilitative stay, going to a hospital for treatment of an acute care episode, or due to death—and they are often replaced by new residents with different health profiles.

Over three decades ago, the Institute of Medicine (IOM) conducted a study of staffing needs among SNFs participating in the Medicare and Medicaid programs. In its final report, "Improving the Quality of Care in Nursing Homes," it suggested stronger governmental oversight and some basic standards that would apply to all facilities receiving these funds (Institute of Medicine Committee on Nursing Home Regulation, 1986). However, there was not an ideal standard identified that would appropriately meet the care needs of residents across all venues, regardless of their acuity case mix (the composite level of care needed, based on each resident's condition).

Fifteen years later, the Centers for Medicare & Medicaid Services (CMS) performed a follow-up study that concluded that for each of the quality measures studied, "there was a pattern of incremental benefits of increased staffing until a threshold was reached, at which point there were no further significant benefits with respect to quality when additional staff were utilized." The following thresholds provide staffing levels below which facilities were more likely to have quality problems and above which quality rates were not improved by increasing staffing ratios (Feuerberg, 2001). See Table 3.2 for resident ratio thresholds.

Proponents of moving toward a more prescriptive standard have relied heavily on the findings of the CMS study as the place to start (Bowblis, 2011). Many states

TABLE 3.2 Skilled Nursing Facility Nursing Personnel: Resident Ratio Thresholds

Nursing Staff Category	Threshold	
	Short-Stay (Hours per Resident per Day)	Long-Stay (Hours per Resident per Day)
Nurse aide	2.40	2.80
Licensed (all)	1.15	1.30
RN	0.55	0.75

have at least experimented with that approach, but with disappointing results: More money was spent by some providers on bringing staffing levels up to the minimum, but the quality measures included in the study did not show statistically significant improvement (Feuerberg, 2001). An unexpected consequence was that some providers appear to have responded to the new requirements by reducing staffing levels, since there was new evidence that staffing above the thresholds was both inefficient and ineffective (Dellefield, Castle, McGilton, & Spilsbury, 2015).

A review of the efficacy of minimum staffing ratios in long-term care facilities was performed by the Urban Institute for the U.S. Department of Health and Human Services (Tilley, Black, & Ormond, 2003). The authors found that the consensus among state officials responsible for overseeing compliance with the minimum staffing ratios agreed that while "adjustment of the ratios to take into account resident case mix would be ideal," it would likely add more complexity calculating the ratios, and few had suggestions about how to form a case mix–adjusted ratio. However, just because it may be difficult, linking staffing levels to the aggregate acuity of the residents—adjusting the blend of direct caregiver levels to mirror changes in residents' collective care needs—is a current practice of some organizations and holds promise for the future.

While the debate continues, the standard that is operative in the SNF arena, at least for now, is found in the federal regulations governing Medicare and Medicaid: The facility must have sufficient nursing staff to provide nursing and related services to attain or maintain the highest practicable physical, mental and psychosocial well-being of each resident, as determined by resident assessments and plans of care (42 C.F.R. Section 483.30, 2020). First, this provision is mandatory, as it says *must* have sufficient staff. Second, it refers to the highest state of well-being. Third, there is what appears to be a balancing provision of practicable. While one-on-one care would most likely provide the highest level of well-being, it simply is not feasible.

Responsibility for scheduling staff coverage and distributing assignments often varies by size of the department, site, or company. In most nonclinical departments, it is common for the department supervisor to have this duty. Having a designated staff scheduler in nursing and other clinical services (therapies and HCBS) is often found. There is an abundance of specialized software to aid in this process, which can minimize the risk of burning out those who are the most willing to work extra hours (and the associated costs of overtime pay), as well as optimally filling shifts with people in accordance with their prestated preferences.

A trend with increasing support in practice is the emergence of self-directed work teams—staff members collaborating to set the work schedule among themselves, without a master scheduler. The empowerment and accountability that accompany this strategy combine to make it attractive to employers and employees alike.

Any organization that embraces true staff empowerment opens doors for individuals to grow in experience and knowledge. It enhances "stakeholdership"—the ability to develop and build a culture of shared devotion to reaching the organization's goals and advancing its mission.

Daniel J. Suer, LNHA, FACHCA
Administrator, Hillebrand Nursing and
Rehabilitation Center

RETENTION

Now that the newcomer has been hired and oriented, the challenge becomes keeping them engaged. Staff retention—the inverse of employee turnover—is highly correlated with high-performance and high-quality outcomes (Cirillo, 2018a). Experienced employees tend to be more efficient because of their familiarity with policies and procedures as well as with the people served.

A key term in health services and senior living is **person-centered care**, providing safe and high-quality services in such a fashion that honors and respects people's choices and preferences. Consistent care (also known as **continuity of care**) can only come when a caregiver has enough time to get to really know the people for whom they care every day...their personalities, likes and dislikes, routines, and especially their life stories. Retaining workers is not only good for the bottom line, but also it is a quality imperative.

Why People Stay: Six Keys to Retention (Cirillo, 2018a)

1. *Competitive Compensation:* According to the National Nursing Assistant Survey, satisfaction with wages had the second strongest association with intrinsic job satisfaction and overall job satisfaction. The higher the intrinsic job satisfaction, the lower the probability of departure.

2. *Affordable and Accessible Health Insurance:* Nursing home and home health workers enrolled in their employer-sponsored health plan have a significantly higher retention rate than workers who are eligible but not enrolled.

3. *Empowering Culture:* When there is a culture that emphasizes addressing the employee experience first, that positively affects the customer experience. Certain job satisfiers generally accompany such an environment: training, mentoring, relationship building, career ladders (more on this later), and empowerment.

4. *Job Design and Competent Supervision:* Some of this may flow from embracing culture change: recognition and feedback, appropriate staffing and effective scheduling, career advancement, and paths to follow, respect for each position, job flexibility, leadership development, greater autonomy, and teamwork.

5. *Training:* The federal government requires nurse aides and home health aides working in Medicare/Medicaid-certified agencies to have 75 hours of initial training. Many states have established additional training requirements. The IOM has recommended that the minimum federal requirements for CNAs and home health aides be raised to 120 hours and include a demonstration of competence in caring for older adults as part of certification. Studies have shown that staff who were more satisfied with the quality of their training also had higher job satisfaction and were more likely to stay on the job (Feuerberg, 2001).

6. *Career Advancement Opportunity:* Over 3,000 employees from 50 nursing homes, 39 home care agencies, 40 assisted living facilities, and 10 adult day services in five states participated in a survey that showed "the perceived lack of opportunity for advancement and the perception of work overload were most significantly related to intent to leave, particularly among home care agency and skilled nursing home staff" (Stott, Brannon, Vasey, Dansky, & Kemper, 2007).

Proactively developing strategies for addressing any of the six keys listed requires an investment of money and time, and a deep commitment to sustaining the effort. The health services executive who invests in recruiting and retaining the best workforce—and who understands that it will lead to better care—will not only survive, but *thrive*, in the arriving era of accountable care organizations and managed care. As third-party payers look to tighten referral networks based on performance, long-term care providers with the highest outcome measures are predicted to prevail.

Career Ladder

Related to a PDP is the notion of a career ladder. It is simply a structured sequence of positions through which a person can progress in an organization, to advance in scope of responsibility, professional competence, and/or pay by "climbing" up the ladder. While common in many industries, services for the aging have been slower to embrace this concept.

Traditionally, a career ladder encourages, recognizes, and rewards employees who demonstrate their acumen for their job role and desire for professional growth and advancement. A career ladder can be a vertical progression, but not necessarily. Progressive organizations also map lateral and advanced positions that a person could naturally fit in based on their background. Consistently successful performance and acquisition of additional skills through education or training can prepare an individual for the next job level or a new career path (Cirillo, 2018b).

This tends to work best in an organization that is large enough to have a matrix of related occupations *and* enough opportunity (through growth and/or turnover) to allow for advancement. However, a smaller organization can depend on its employees to identify potential opportunities and foster mentoring by experienced employees.

Moving through the steps of a career ladder typically requires more than simply accumulating time and seniority in an organization. It is common to expect an employee to demonstrate competence at a new skill, apply newly acquired knowledge to a relevant situation, and exhibit readiness to accept new responsibilities. Indeed, a career ladder may very well evolve into a career "lattice," with several opportunities to grow in a variety of directions rather than up a single vertical trajectory.

HUMAN RESOURCES AND OPERATIONS

In addition to assisting department directors with finding, screening, hiring, orienting, onboarding, and retaining qualified and motivated staff members, human resources professionals support and coordinate other key functions that touch all employees.

Performance Expectations and Appraisal

Performance expectations are most effectively conveyed in a clearly written job description, one that stipulates essential duties of the position, reporting relationships, work site location, physical demands, and an acknowledgment that the employee understands its content and agrees to perform the duties described and to abide by all applicable policies, procedures, laws, and regulations.

The most effective performance appraisal formats provide meaningful feedback to an employee that reward them for meeting or exceeding expectations and identify opportunities for growth and improvement. Some organizations include both job-specific performance measurements (i.e., timely and complete task completion and accurate documentation) and adherence to company policies and procedures (i.e., attendance and punctuality, protecting confidentiality, or avoiding conflicts of interest). Progressive providers also incorporate—or at least synchronize with the appraisal cycle—a review of the employee's goals that were set during the prior period and a discussion about goals for the ensuing period. This can range from a specific project assignment to professional development.

Traditionally, performance appraisals would occur toward the end of a new employee's orientation and onboarding experience—60 to 90 days—as a "pulse check" regarding how well they are integrating into the new role. Some organizations would also connect again during the first year, at 6 or 9 months, recognizing that it takes some time for a new hire to perform at the same level as an experienced employee. It was considered better to focus during the first year—whatever the evaluation intervals—on learning and mastery, rather than on meeting numbers-based performance goals. An annual performance appraisal on the employee's hire date anniversary, and then annually thereafter, was the most widely followed practice.

An increasingly popular approach to evaluating performance involves providing more immediate and ongoing feedback than annually. Contemporary leaders are finding that replacing traditional supervisory techniques with "coaching" interventions gets better results concerning productivity, employee engagement, and retention. Today's workers desire more frequent—even ongoing—feedback about their performance and contributions. (Shaw, 2013).

Compensation and Benefits

Most people equate the term compensation with wages or salary. Offering competitive wages is certainly an important consideration in attracting (and keeping) staff. Human resources often assists with gathering benchmark information about competitors, analyzing the data, and recommending pay ranges for each position that reflect the organization's compensation strategy.

A pay range sets a wage floor, ceiling, and midpoint for any given position, sometimes with subranges within the overall span. An organization's compensation strategy, starting with pay, can be characterized as:

- **aspirational:** striving to consistently land at a targeted goal in comparison with the wages paid for similar jobs among its peers locally, regionally, or even nationally, such as at least the 75th percentile among benchmark competitors; or

- **market driven:** determining pay ranges based on the availability of qualified workers in a particular location and the intensity of competition for those people among area employers.

The two models are not necessarily mutually exclusive. The extent to which one influences the other is often determined by changes that occur over time in an area's economy, housing availability and price, unemployment rate, and public transportation. Furthermore, an organization's ability to adjust the time it takes to adjust its compensation strategy to meaningfully respond to any of those changes can be as important as the adjustment itself. The window of opportunity for gaining a competitive edge in attracting and retaining employees is sometimes narrow. It is not unusual for an organization to get caught up in the "paralysis of analysis," finding that, by the time action is taken, the opportunity disappeared.

Compensation is not limited to salary or pay. Fringe benefits constitute a form of compensation for the services provided by employees. A fringe benefit is sometimes referred to as a "PERK," which is simply short for the term *perquisite*. This as "an incidental payment, benefit, privilege, or advantage over and above regular income, salary, or wages" (Dictionary.com, 2020). Benefits can cover a wide array of rewards and incentives. Some are considered by the Internal Revenue Service (IRS) as tax-free to the employer that provides them (indicated by an * in the list that follows) and an employee who shares in the purchase of the benefit may qualify to do so applying pretax dollars. PERKs that are commonly valued—and often *expected*—by prospective employees include the following:

Insurance

Medical (aka Health) Insurance: This has become nearly as important to many people as monetary pay, given the rising costs of medical care, the rising financial risks associated with a single catastrophic health event, and the growing limits imposed on access to care without it.

- *Employer Plan*:* Since employer-provided health insurance became tax-advantaged nearly eight decades ago, it has evolved into a wide range of options. In recent years, rising costs have motivated employers to explore ways in which employees participate in paying a greater share for medical insurance protection as well as in making informed decisions about both their own wellness behaviors and selection of health providers. The emergence of "high-deductible" medical insurance plans has been widespread during the past decade, and many carriers have tightened their provider networks (participating doctors, hospitals and clinics, pharmacies, etc.), negotiating lower prices in exchange for higher volumes of patient referrals. By sharing more of the costs with employees, organizations reduce their risk of absorbing spiraling healthcare costs and the potentially negative impact on financial performance.

- *Individual Coverage:* Under provisions included in the Affordable Care Act, different rules apply to organizations with under 50 employees with respect to what is required of an employer's medical insurance plan. To remain competitive with larger employers, some smaller providers adjust their pay ranges to provide sufficient resources for employees to purchase this protection in the individual insurance market. Even larger providers have at least begun evaluating the feasibility of following suit—dropping health insurance as a benefit. (Although there is a substantial federal penalty for doing so, it may cost the company less to pay the fine while bolstering wages by enough to enable staff to buy health insurance individually.)

Disability Insurance*: This insurance provides income replacement for an employee who is unable to work due to illness or a nonoccupational injury. It is offered as a bridge to financially sustain an employee until they fully recover or partially recover or until they are declared permanently disabled by the Social Security Administration. Some plans also include insurance premium continuation so there are

---

*The asterisk indicates that these are tax-free to the employer that provides them to employees.

no lapses in an employee's other insurance coverages in place. Disability insurance is categorized by the time period of the employee's disability: short term (30–180 days) or long term (beyond a short-term disability [STD]).

- **Short-term disability (STD)** benefits typically provide 60% to 75% of a full-time employee's normal gross wage. It is standard practice to require that an employee be unable to perform their job duties for a minimal time frame—called an "elimination period"—to qualify for receiving this benefit, such as 30 consecutive calendar days of disability. Example: If the maximum length of the STD period is 6 months, it generally comprises a 1-month elimination period plus 5 months of STD benefits.

- **Long-term disability (LTD)** benefits are usually designed to trigger when an employee is continuously disabled for 6 months after the disability began. It is common for the benefit level to be lower than STD payments and for it to gradually diminish until permanent disability has been determined.

- **Partial disability job (PDJ) program** returns to work an STD or LTD recipient who can perform gainful employment but not capable of performing their prior duties. An employee who is able to perform PDJ assignments is expected to accept and perform them when they are available.

- **Part-time disability program** is a hybrid approach that enables an employee whose recovery allows returning to their original job on a part-time basis at some point, and at least temporarily receiving compensation that blends regular salary for hours worked with the appropriate disability benefit for hours missed due to the disability.

Life Insurance*: Up to $50,000 in group term life insurance benefits can be provided without affecting an employee's taxable income. Many organizations also make additional term life insurance available for purchase at rates much lower than an employee could find individually, but with after-tax dollars (Miller, 2019). There is a variety of factors that contribute to why this may be the only life insurance coverage many long-term care workers have. Employees who witness the impact it has on the family of a coworker who dies understand and appreciate its potential importance for their own families. Note: There are special IRS guidelines regarding face value limits that apply to top wage earners in an organization (U.S. Treasury/IRS, 2019c).

Mandatory Insurance Coverages

- **Workers compensation insurance** in most states provides at least five basic benefits for a staff member who is injured on the job, and the premiums are paid by the employer (Priz & Priz, 2010).
  1. Medical care to help them recover.
  2. Temporary disability benefits to replace lost wages if the work-related injury prevents them from returning to work while recovering.
  3. Permanent disability benefits if they do not recover completely.
  4. Supplemental job displacement benefits to help pay for retraining or skill enhancement if they do not recover completely and cannot return to the same employer.

---

*The asterisk indicates that these are tax-free to the employer that provides them to employees.

5. Death benefits to their family if a work-related injury or illness results in death.

   The volume and value of an organization's claims drives its premium rate in subsequent years—sometimes referred to as its "experience rating"— with the most recent years weighted more heavily. Proactive programs that promote and foster safety in the workplace help reduce the risk of escalating worker's compensation premiums and lost productivity resulting from job-related injuries or illness.

- **Unemployment insurance** provides limited income benefits to an eligible worker who becomes unemployed through no fault of their own and meets other eligibility requirements. The U.S. Department of Labor (DOL) sets minimum standards for determining who qualifies, and some states expand them. Extended unemployment insurance benefits may also be made available to workers who have exhausted regular unemployment insurance benefits during periods of high unemployment. Consistent and timely enforcement of an organization's policies and procedures that are tied to progressive disciplinary steps, as well as thorough documentation that supports a decision leading to an involuntary termination of employment, must demonstrate that the separation was justified due to the employee's noncompliance with those policies and procedures, refuting that they lost the job "through no fault of their own."

   Example: Attendance is one of the most common expectations in postacute care settings, but exceeding an organization's prescribed limit for absences is among the most common causes of involuntary separation in the field. It is imperative that the system for tracking absences triggers timely counseling for each employee who misses an assigned shift, including documented sanctions, which are consistent with the organization's employee handbook. Doing otherwise invites a successful—avoidable— unemployment insurance claim.

- The **Family Medical Leave Act (FMLA)** allows an eligible employee to take *unpaid* leave for a serious health condition of either the employee's or an immediate family member for up to 12 weeks during a 12-month period. For an employee who qualifies to receive FMLA benefits, time off from work under either a disability program or worker's compensation is typically counted concurrently with FMLA (Bossart, 2016).

Optional Insurance Coverages

Another way to bolster the fringe benefit package is to offer additional insurance protections that mitigate an employee's risk of financial exposure. That risk could be getting named individually in a lawsuit brought against the employer. It might be more personal, such as needing long-term care services that are not addressed in the health insurance plan. Optional insurance coverages may be paid for by the employer or offered at a price lower than available in the individual market.

- **Supplemental professional liability insurance** protects an employee whose job role makes them a potentially attractive target for inclusion in a legal action filed against the employer. An employer's professional liability insurance policy often has a "shared limit," which means that multiple employees are covered under the same aggregate (total annual) limit. If one employee is involved in a claim and uses the insurance, it could exhaust the limit of the policy or leave too little leftover to cover any other claims that may arise for another employee. Furthermore, an employer's policy typically covers events occurring during working hours (Miller, 2019). Staff members who regularly engage in direct caregiving roles, and higher wage-earning nonclinical staff, might find greater value in such a benefit than others. Purchasing a personal, supplemental policy provides

- flexibility in choosing coverage limits, greatly reducing the risk of being underinsured;
- coverage that applies *around* the clock, not just while *on* the clock; and
- protection if they change employment—most policies are either portable (when the employee pays the premiums) or transferable (if partially or fully paid for by the employer).

- **Long-term care insurance** is one of the most overlooked elements of any family's estate plan. We consider it important enough to insure ourselves against the risks of losing our home due to a fire or natural disaster, personal, and financial devastation caused by a catastrophic health event or unable to provide for our families due to becoming disabled or even dying. Although we observe every day the financial drain endured by the people we serve—and their families—long-term care insurance has not yet graduated to the list of core fringe benefits described earlier. Recent changes in federal and many state income tax laws aimed at encouraging more people to purchase this protection are expected to make this increasingly valued by employees. Much like health insurance, long-term care insurance coverages vary, and pricing is often difficult to compare. However, key elements that are typically offered, either a la carte or bundled in different combinations, include the following:

  - Underwriting Risk Rating: Age, gender, family health history, and current health exam all contribute to premium determination.
  - Care Setting: SNF, assisted living facility or personal care home, home health (medical or nonmedical), hospice/palliative care, or adult day center.
  - Benefit Determination (per episode and/or lifetime limits): Determined by the number of days (or units of care, such as shifts or hours per day) multiplied by the charged (or insured) rate, with an aggregate ceiling (maximum amount allowed).
  - Payment Model: Direct payment to the provider (assignment) or reimbursement to the insured of approved expenses, subject to policy limits.
  - Renewal: Not all policies offer the owner *guaranteed* renewal (although competition has moved this to the norm).
  - Premium Waiver: Forgiveness of the premium during an insured benefit period.

Some carriers have experimented with blending long-term care insurance with products that address more familiar risks, such as life insurance or disability insurance (Marquand, 2019; Sullivan, 2016). Combining premiums and benefits for multiple, related risks is not uncommon in the realm of insuring vehicles or homes, so this trend may continue.

Business Purpose Benefits

Reimbursement of Expenses

Reimbursing an employee for approved business-related expenses is a widely accepted practice. It is important to clearly define in the employee handbook how expenses qualify for reimbursement, the process to follow for approval, and how to submit a request for reimbursement.

- *Meals and entertainment* is a commonly used line item description for expenses incurred when an employee incurs expenses for dining or meeting with people as assigned by the employer. At a minimum, it is important that receipts submitted to support the request for reimbursement have written on them (a) with whom the meeting was held and (b) the main business purpose and topic discussed. Many organizations limit the amount available for reimbursement of meals according to the time of day (breakfast, lunch, or dinner); others provide a predetermined flat rate per diem and expect the employee to manage the assignment within that budget.

- *Travel and mileage* covers any mode of transportation used to meet an approved business purpose, but not for getting to and from work (exception: commuter benefits, which are discussed later in this chapter). It is typically treated in similar fashion to meals and entertainment, including expectations about supporting receipts and accompanying documentation. Providing a vehicle, either owned or leased by the employer, is more common in the home health care arena than in the other postacute care service lines. However, it is sometimes included as part of a benefits package for key leadership personnel. The IRS publishes guidelines concerning upper limits on reimbursing mileage for an employee's use of their personal vehicle for business purposes that factor in fuel consumption, vehicle wear and tear (tires, engine, etc.), and depreciation, as well as rules to follow in tracking and reporting business use versus personal use of a company-owned vehicle (U.S. Treasury/IRS, 2019f).

- *Professional development and continuing education* represent investments in the most important resource of the organization—its people. Supporting an employee's professional growth enhances not only their relevant knowledge and skills, as well as opportunities for advancement, but the probability of overall success. Creating and sustaining an organizational culture of continuous quality improvement helps draw talented people. Paying for their ongoing development typically pays direct and indirect dividends, from job performance to loyalty and retention. (Some organizations prefer to track all expenses related to training separately, so meals, lodging, travel, and tuition fees are posted under this heading.)

- *Formal education* refers to a course of study that results in the awarding of an academic degree beyond high school or general equivalency diploma (GED). Examples include an associate's degree in medical records management, a bachelor's degree in accounting, a master's degree in social work, or a doctorate in physical therapy. Many clinical disciplines also are licensed by each state, and the level of licensure is sometimes tied to the highest degree attained. Nursing is the most complex health profession when it comes to matching formal education and licensure level. An associate's degree in nursing is required for a person to become an LPN, sometimes referred to as a licensed vocational nurse; an RN can hold either a state licensure board–approved associate's degree or a bachelor's, master's, or doctoral degree. For either credential, the eligible person must pass a discipline-specific examination to become licensed. Whether providing direct scholarships and grants or reimbursement for formal education, there are other considerations to evaluate in designing a program. Will any of the following criteria apply to qualify?

1. Is the subject or discipline relevant to the operation?

2. How will we prioritize applications if the demand is greater than the budget?

3. How will we recognize the employee's new level of credential if there is not a position open for them to fill after graduation?

4. Will the employee (be expected to) commit to working here after graduating?

5. For how long?

6. What are the consequences of not doing so?

7. Are scheduling accommodations needed to attend classes?

8. Will that require replacement and associated costs?

9. What is the most tax-advantaged way we can support this effort?

10. How does our program compare with what competitors offer?

- *Informal continuing education* includes seminars, workshops, webinars, courses, and other professional development activities that do not result in a formal degree, but a certificate of completion or professional certification. Nearly all licensed professions have minimum expectations for continuing education for the licensing entity to approve renewal. Professional associations that offer advanced practice certifications typically require proof of continuing education units (CEUs) as well. This investment can generally touch more different employees because the duration and cost per training are less than an entire degree-granting course of study. Because the length of commitment is so much shorter, there is more flexibility over a year to adjust resources allocated to this endeavor. Sending five people to a 3-day workshop on wound treatments may cost less than underwriting one LPN to complete a course of study to become an RN. Most of the same questions listed earlier under formal education apply here as well. Regardless, informal continuing education builds more than skills and knowledge in someone selected to participate. It can also develop self-confidence and strengthen loyalty by showing the organization values their contributions and potential.

Qualified Employee Benefit Plans

The most familiar qualified employee benefit plans are profit-sharing or stock option programs, both of which are governed by the Employee Retirement Income Security Act (ERISA). They have the same rules for eligibility, allocation of benefits and vesting, and contributions to either type of plan are tax deductible. Providing an opportunity for each employee to have additional "skin in the game" for the overall operational success of the organization has been successful in other business sectors for decades, but it has been slow to emerge in postacute care—even though a supermajority of the provider organizations have proprietary ownership. (This is not available to not-for-profit, tax-exempt provider organizations.)

Some fundamental rules apply to both profit-sharing and stock option or stock bonus plans (Rosen, 2014):

- Governance: A plan trustee must operate the plan for the exclusive benefit of the plan participants.

- Eligibility and Vesting: Rules are generally the same as for other defined contribution plans.

- Investment: No minimum requirement.

- Fiduciary Oversight: Subject to close scrutiny by the U.S. Department of Labor (USDL) regarding compliance with valuation and transaction rules.

A proprietary provider organization can realize some handsome tax advantages and enhance its fringe benefits package by offering either a profit-sharing or stock option bonus plan, such as:

- tax deduction for up to 25% of eligible compensation, and

- employees are taxed in the same way as other defined contribution plans, based on distributions from the plan that are not otherwise rolled over to another qualified plan or IRA.

Incentive Programs

Employee incentive programs are a way of compensating and motivating employee performance with pay and benefits. There is an impressive body of evidence that suggests employees are not inspired by money alone to do their best. At the end of this chapter, some examples of high-impact practices that have produced positive results in a variety of settings are described, most of which rely on the collective performance success of the team. Here are a few of the ones with little or no downside financial risk, but potential for positive dividends (Handrick, 2018):

1. Advancement Access: Give top-rated employees first choice on job openings.

2. Preferred Parking: Reserve a parking space near the entrance that recognizes an employee for high achievement.

3. Payroll Period: Shorten the frequency of payroll for a calendar quarter (from biweekly or semimonthly to weekly) for employees who meet or exceed an operational goal or objective, such as perfect attendance and punctuality or project specific.

4. Safety First: Distribute a portion of the premium savings when a reduction in the organization's experience rating for worker's compensation insurance lowers the cost.

5. Express Gratitude: Whether via a handwritten note ("old-school," but highly effective), letter, email, phone call, or text message, showing sincere appreciation for any job well-done builds relationships and honors achievement in ways few other techniques surpass.

Nonsalary Economic Benefits

Tax-Advantaged Employee Savings Methods: There are several options available to an employer for offering ways an employee can use pretax earnings to set money aside to meet certain kinds of expenses. In some instances, the employer may contribute to the savings instrument, too, as an additional and effective retention tool.

Saving for retirement is an important activity for everyone and ideally should complement an employee's Social Security contributions and any other form of savings accumulated throughout their career, such as savings accounts, investments, or equity in a home. Retiring from work is a relatively new phenomenon in the history of humankind, but it is an integral part of contemporary American culture and a widely held expectation.

During much of the 20th century, the most prevalent retirement savings programs were pension plans, funded primarily by employer contributions. In exchange for long-time service, a company would promise an employee who provided long-time service some form of continuing income after retiring—for the rest of their *life* (and often some benefit for a surviving spouse, too). This is known as a "defined benefit" retirement pension, because it pledged a retirement income level and the employer accepts responsibility for resourcing the payments through pension fund investments.

During the first two decades of the 21st century, to shift more of the responsibility for retirement saving to employees, "defined *benefit*" pensions have been steadily replaced by "defined *contribution*" savings plans. Rather than guaranteeing a future payment level, this approach incentivizes saving for retirement by *deferring* income taxes on the earnings deposited by an individual in a special account for this purpose. Taxes are instead paid when the funds are withdrawn during retirement (at a presumably lower rate because the person's income is likely to be lower when no longer working full-time).

Defined contribution programs have different advantages and governing rules and generally bear the name of either their enabling legislation or relevant section of the IRS Code. Different rules apply to each. For tax-favored status, a plan must be operated in accordance with the applicable rules. Therefore, it is important that the employer be familiar with the special rules that apply to its plan, so it is administered in accordance with those rules. The complexity of options available makes consulting a retirement planning professional extremely worthwhile. An overview of the most widely used plans appears in Table 3.3 (not intended to be all-inclusive).

Savings for meeting healthcare expenses, such as health savings accounts (HSAs), enable an employee covered by a high-deductible health plan (HDHP) to receive tax-preferred treatment of money they save for medical expenses. An HSA reduces an employee's out-of-pocket costs, lowers their income tax liability, rolls over from year-to-year, and lowers an employer's payroll taxes (Handrick, 2018).

Although designated for health expenses, funds from an HSA may be withdrawn and used for nonmedical expenses—but they will be taxed. In fact, if the employee is under 65 years old, there is also an early withdrawal penalty for using HSA money for non–medical-related expenses (U.S. Treasury/IRS, 2019d). An HSA is also portable—it can go with the person, regardless of the nature of their departure. It can continue to be used to pay for valid medical expenses and can accumulate interest. However, if the former employee no longer has an HDHP, no more contributions can be added.

A flex spending account (FSA) is a short-term savings account that enables an employee to set aside pretax money each month for approved dependent care expenses in that year, such as medical copays, in-home healthcare for a family

TABLE 3.3 Overview: Defined Contribution Retirement Plan Options

Plan Type	Description
401(k)	An employee can make contributions from their paycheck either before or after tax, depending on the options offered in the plan (there are over 450 variations). The contributions go into a special 401(k) account, with the employee often choosing the investments based on options provided under the plan. In some plans, the employer also makes contributions, such as matching the employee's contributions up to a certain percentage.
401(k) Traditional	A traditional 401(k) plan allows an eligible employee to make pretax elective deferrals through payroll deductions. The employer also has the option of making contributions, making matching contributions based on the employee's elective deferrals, or both. These employer contributions can be subject to a vesting schedule, which provides that an employee's right to employer contributions becomes nonforfeitable after some period or must be vested. To ensure that the plan satisfies all requirements, the employer must perform annual tests, known as the actual deferral percentage (ADP) and actual contribution percentage (ACP) tests, to verify that deferred wages and employer matching contributions do not discriminate in favor of highly compensated employees.
401(k) SIMPLE (Savings Incentive Match Plan for Employees)	Created so that small businesses (100 or fewer employees) could have an effective, cost-efficient way to offer retirement benefits to their employees. This option is not subject to the annual nondiscrimination tests that apply to traditional 401(k) plans. The employer is required to make contributions that are fully vested. An employee who is eligible to participate may not receive any contributions or benefit accruals under any other plans of the employer.
401(k) Safe Harbor	Similar to a traditional plan, any employer contributions are fully vested when made. These contributions may be employer matching contributions, limited to an employee who defers, or employer contributions made on behalf of all eligible employees, regardless of whether they make elective deferrals. This type of plan is not subject to the complex annual nondiscrimination tests that apply to traditional 401(k) plans but must each year give written notice of the employee's rights and obligations under the plan.
403(b) or Tax-Sheltered Annuity (TSA)	Offered by public schools and certain tax-exempt organizations only. Generally, these annuities are funded by elective deferrals made under salary reduction agreements and nonelective employer contributions.
IRA (Individual retirement arrangement or account)	An IRA is an investing tool for retirement savings. It can consist of a range of financial products such as stocks, bonds, or mutual funds.
IRA Traditional	An employee can open and make contributions to a traditional IRA if they (a) received taxable compensation during the year and (b) are less than age 70½ by the end of the year. Contributions may be partially or fully deductible, depending on whether the employee (or spouse) is covered by another employer retirement plan.

(continued)

TABLE 3.3 (*continued*)

Plan Type	Description
IRA—Roth	Contributions are not tax deductible, but qualified *distributions* are tax free; as the account grows, there are no taxes on investment gains, nor are there any on withdrawals during retirement. The IRS sets additional income limits for married couples filing separately, single filers, and heads of household.
IRA—SIMPLE (Savings Incentive Match Plan for Employees)	Follows the same taxation rules for withdrawals as a traditional IRA. An employee can make contributions, and the employer is *required* to make contributions, too. All the contributions are tax deductible, potentially pushing the business or employee into a lower tax bracket.

Source: U.S. Department of the Treasury, Internal Revenue Service. (2019e). *Retirement plan options*. Retrieved from https://www.irs.gov/retirement-plans

member, or childcare expenses. An FSA can be offered instead of health insurance or in addition to the existing healthcare plan to help save on out-of-pocket costs. Like an HSA, using an FSA lowers the employee's taxable income and the organization's payroll taxes. An employer can contribute to an employee's FSA account, subject to limits published by the IRS that are typically adjusted annually.

An FSA is different from an HSA in that (a) the employer owns an FSA, while the employee owns an HSA (i.e., if the employee leaves or is terminated, they forfeit any unused FSA funds, but an HSA balance follows the employee), and there is no alternate option in the marketplace for an employee to set up an FSA; (b) the employee needs to use the FSA funds during the plan year or risks losing them (although an employer may opt to offer a grace period of up to 2-1/2 months to allow an employee to apply any balance remaining); and (c) in addition to an FSA for healthcare expenditures, FSA funds can also be applied to qualified dependent care costs through the dependent care assistance account program (DCA or DCAP). Examples include expenses for childcare and after-school care for children under 13 years old, in-home or institutional care for disabled or seriously ill dependents of any age, or even adoption services.

Section 125 Cafeteria Plans (named for section 125 of the IRS Code) offer a way for an employer to allow a staff member to select the combination of benefits that best suits their family's needs from a *menu* that typically includes the organization's available insurance coverages and other employee benefits, or sometimes to even opt out and receive that value as compensation (Hopkins, 2017). Each employee receives the same amount of money through a deposit to a personalized savings account setup for this express purpose. They can customize their plan, regardless of whether the funds are applied to purchasing benefits that are eligible for pretax payments (i.e., health-related insurance premiums or retirement account contributions), to taxable benefits (i.e., supplemental disability of life insurance above basic coverage), or in taxable wages.

The plan must include at least one qualified benefit, eligible for payment with pretax dollars. It must also include at least one taxable benefit option, which means the government views it as part of the employee's salary. Although having a Section 125 Plan is not the same as *providing* health insurance, it offers a blend of vehicles for an employee to prudently meet life expenses based on their unique family circumstances and priorities.

Commuter benefits, sometimes called transit or transportation benefits, can help reduce an employee's commuting expenses. Such a program spans public transit, vanpooling, bicycling, and/or work-related parking expenses. As a pretax payroll deduction, this can reduce employee income taxes and employer payroll taxes. Some municipalities have enacted commuter benefit laws that make offering them mandatory, but those are still the exception. In an era of increasing awareness about energy conservation and sustainable ecology, commuter benefits have an additional appeal among younger workers as well (Handrick, 2018).

Employee assistance programs (EAPs) are designed to assist an employee in resolving personal problems that may be adversely affecting their performance. EAPs were first introduced to assist workers with issues such as alcohol or substance abuse, but many now address a broader range of issues, such as child or elder care, relationship challenges, financial or legal problems, wellness matters, and traumatic events (i.e., workplace violence, a natural disaster, or family tragedy). EAP services are typically delivered at no cost to the employee by contracted EAP vendors or providers. Services are often delivered via phone, video-based counseling, online chatting, email interactions, or face-to-face (Society for Human Resource Management, 2019).

EAP services are usually free to the employee and their household members (spouse, children, and nonmarital partner living in the same household). *Note:* An EAP that offers medical benefits such as direct counseling and treatment rather than just referrals for counseling and treatment is regulated under ERISA and subject to the Comprehensive Omnibus Budget Reconciliation Act of 1985 (COBRA; Clark, 2015).

Paid time off (PTO): According to the U.S. Department of Labor's Bureau of Labor Statistics (2018), over 70% of American employees receive paid days off from work for sick or vacation time. However, there at least eight other circumstances for which an increasing number of employers also offer PTO. Taking time off is often critical for managing life away from work. Providing financial support that enables an employee to address those needs typically fosters morale, engagement, and productivity and loyalty.

Some organizations specify a certain number of hours or days they will pay an employee's wages for time away from scheduled work, based on the reason for the absence. Others offer a lump sum of days—much like a cafeteria plan, but for PTO—that an employee can elect to use annually, based on their greatest need. This is often referred to as a PTO plan, and it has grown in popularity in recent years because of the ability to personalize the benefit.

Operationally, the true cost of any benefit that pays wages for time away from work is influenced by whether the employee's position is one that must be filled by someone else, such as a direct caregiving role, effectively doubling the expense. Such replacement costs can be difficult to manage, especially if the number of available substitutes is limited and the options become paying an inflated rate for either overtime or temporary labor.

It is vital to clearly explain in the organization's employee handbook its policy regarding PTO, including who is eligible for which benefit, how much time off can be supported with wages and at what rate of pay (regular or reduced), when it is available to use, and what happens to unused time at year-end. Ten of the most widely utilized PTO benefits are outlined in Table 3.4.

TABLE 3.4 Overview of Paid Time Off Benefits

Reason	Benefit Pays During
Holidays	New Year's Day, Memorial Day*, Independence Day*, Labor Day*, Thanksgiving, and Christmas. (*Some federally declared holidays are most often recognized on the nearest Monday; the others listed are typically recognized on the actual holiday date.) Also popular: Martin Luther King, Jr. Day*, Easter, Christmas Eve and New Year's Eve, or a religious holiday to substitute for Christmas. ***Related:*** *Paying double time for working on an included holiday or allowing a scheduled day off with pay within a specified time frame before or after the holiday worked.*
Vacation	Break from work to refresh, either in one period or split among several short periods. Policy should explain rules governing approval for payment, such as notification requirements and how competing requests are considered. ***Related:*** *Seventy-seven percent of full-time employees receive paid vacation (U.S. Department of Labor Bureau of Labor Statistics, 2018); unused vacation pay is typically paid at termination unless otherwise restricted (i.e., involuntary termination for cause).*
Sick leave	Illness or non-work-related injury; may require a qualifying period (1–3 days off) before starting; can serve as an infection control function by encouraging sick employees to stay home rather than exposing others; typically earned and accrued per pay period; some jurisdictions have *mandatory* sick leave laws (Blakely-Gray, 2017). ***Related:*** *Capping stored sick pay time helps mitigate the risk of an extended liability of paying sick time pay to an employee who does not have long-term disability coverage (i.e., 3 weeks or 240 hours), as well as annually paying out unused sick time above that limit; unused sick pay is generally* not *paid at termination.*
Personal day	Time off to handle personal commitments or needs, such as a medical appointment or attend a parent-teacher conference—without tapping into vacation time. ***Related:*** *Recognition day(s)—birthday, hire date anniversary, or milestone anniversary (1-, 2-, 5-, 10-, 15-, 25-year work anniversary).*
Parental leave	Time away from work for maternity/paternity leave or adoption. Related: *Paid parental leave is generally coordinated with vacation and sick leave, and then unpaid time off through FMLA benefits.*
Public service	• **Military Duty:** For either active duty or training; employers must follow the USERRA, which requires also offering at least an *unpaid* leave of absence to military personnel for up to 5 cumulative years (U.S. Department of Labor, Veterans Employment and Training Service, 2019). • **Jury Duty:** For responding to a summons to serve, regardless of whether selected for a trial or not; most jurisdictions pay a nominal stipend to jurors, regardless; some states require employers to offer jury duty pay. ***Related:*** *Paying the difference between the employee's normal pay and the jury duty stipend awarded.* • **Voting:** For voting in presidential, state, or local election; generally limited to a few hours; some states require either paid or unpaid time off to vote. ***Related:*** *almost one-half of employers offer employees paid time off to vote* (Wessels, 2018).

(continued)

TABLE 3.4 (*continued*)

Reason	Benefit Pays During
Bereavement leave	Time for grieving the loss of a family member or friend—to cope with the employee's loss, make funeral arrangements, or attend memorial activities; generally tied to the employee's relationship (sanguinity) to the deceased, and sometimes to distance. ***Related:*** Explicitly describe what relationship qualifies, maximum days per year, and acceptable documentation (obituary, funeral program, etc.).
Compensatory time	Scheduled time off in lieu of paying overtime, (available *only* to an *exempt* employee; compensatory time off rules apply to avoid violating the FLSA (Kappel, 2017).

FLSA, Fair Labor Standards Act; FMLA, Family Medical Leave Act; USERRA, Uniformed Services Employment and Reemployment Rights Act.

Discounts on Services Provided

Similar to an automobile manufacturer offering a discount on the purchase price of a new vehicle that is built by the company, providing employee access to the services a postacute care organization delivers every day—at a favorable rate—can have multiple positive outcomes. First, the employee saves money while receiving needed goods or services from trusted coworkers. Second, this practice introduces new revenue streams that can enhance the organization's financial performance.

Services that lend themselves to this idea include inpatient, outpatient, or home health therapies (physical, occupational, or speech), nursing or related health services, and social services. Postacute care providers typically access a broad range of licensed health professionals to care for their customers, either as employees or consultants, but overlook and underutilize them as potential providers of valued services for staff members. Examples include physicians, dentists, podiatrists, and dietitians.

Goods that can be offered for resale to staff (sometimes subject to state or local sales tax), include items the organization buys in bulk, and can pass along at lower prices than available to the general public, such as food (raw or prepared), baby formula or disposable diapers, paper and office supplies, or linens.

De Minimis Fringe Benefits

The term *de minimus* is a Latin expression meaning "about minimal things." For the purpose of determining the taxability of a fringe benefit, the IRS exempts from taxation an employee benefit "for which, considering its value and the frequency with which it is provided, is so small as to make accounting for it unreasonable or impractical" (U.S. Treasury/IRS, 2019b).

Section 132(a)(4) of the IRS Code sets forth the rules governing such exemptions, and it includes items that are not specifically excluded under other sections of the Code. Examples of de minimis benefits include gift debit cards, traditional awards (such as a retirement gift), birthday or holiday presents, and event tickets.

Two key determinants of whether a benefit can be considered de minimis are its frequency and its value. It must be provided infrequently, and it must not be a form of disguised compensation. As recently as 2018, the IRS has ruled that items with a value exceeding $100 could not be considered de minimis. Also, if a benefit is determined to be too large to be considered de minimis, the entire value of the benefit is taxable to the employee, not just the excess over a designated de minimis amount.

Affinity Programs

Whether leveraging an organization's business relationships or negotiating favorable pricing in exchange for purchase volume, affinity programs that enhance an employee's access to goods or services that they value are a great way to demonstrate an employer's commitment. This can range from no direct cost to the employer, except time devoted to distribution, to low cost to the employer (with a potentially big return on investment):

A. No Cost: Discounted group pricing for:

1. Goods: Groceries, medications, uniforms, or gasoline

2. Services: Auto repair or home maintenance (plumbing, electrical or HVAC [heating, ventilation, and air conditioning] work, roofing, landscaping, or tree care)

3. Membership/admission: Community activities (a concert, performance or sports event) or entertainment destination (amusement park, zoo, or museum)

B. Low Cost: providing a membership for a discount department store, such as COSTCO or Sam's Club.

PAYROLL

The importance of an accurate and timely payment system for employee compensation cannot be overemphasized. Receiving the correct wages on time is generally one of an employee's core expectations. Establishing and maintaining systems that consistently produce those results, along with compliance with applicable federal, state, and local laws and regulations, is a key responsibility of the Health Services Executive.

Exempt or Nonexempt? That Is the Question

The federal Fair Labor Standards Act (FLSA) was originally enacted in 1938 to protect worker rights, establish a minimum wage, and govern overtime pay. The FLSA pertains to full- and part-time hourly employees and establishes criteria for salaried workers. It is amended periodically to reflect changes in related business laws and inflation (McKay, 2017). Under FLSA, there are two classifications of employee that determined which set of rules with which the organization must comply, based mainly on whether the employee is entitled to overtime pay: An employee may be exempt (from eligibility for overtime pay) and nonexempt (eligible). An employer is required to pay at least minimum wage for up to 40 hours in a work week (or for up to 80 hours in a 2-week period, if qualified, further described later), and overtime pay at least 1.5 times the employee's regular rate for any additional time unless the employee falls into an exempt category.

The FLSA allows certain health services providers another option, known as the "8 and 80" system because it replaces the standard 40 hours/week test with triggers

TABLE 3.5 Fair Labor Standards Act (FLSA) Employee Classifications Summary

Exempt Employee	Nonexempt Employee
Ineligible for overtime pay	Entitled to 1.5 times regular pay rate for work in excess of either: (a) 40 hours/week or (b) 8/days or 80 hours/14 days
Salaried for any pay period worked	Hourly
Performs executive, administrative, or professional duties. *(Categories are purposefully broad to encompass many types of jobs.)* Based on tasks performed, not job title.	Does not meet any of the qualifying tests for exemption listed in column 1.
• *Executive:* Primary duty is managing the enterprise or one of its departments; customarily and regularly directs the work of at least two employees; authority to hire, fire, or change the status of other employees (or recommendation materially affect the same).	Some states and companies may have FLSA-allowable variations (but must at least adhere to the federal minimums), such as: • Higher minimum wage • Decreased full-time work week hour designations • More generous overtime policies
• *Administrative:* Primary duty of performing office or nonmanual work directly related to management or operations, including the exercise of discretion and independent judgment concerning matters of significance.	
• *Professional:* Primary duty requires knowledge of an advanced type in a field of science or learning, customarily acquired by prolonged, specialized, intellectual instruction and study, or must specialize in a few other similarly, highly specialized fields, such as teaching, computer analytics, or engineering.	
Other: (2019) Earns over $455/week; $23,660/year	Other: (2019) Earns less than $455/week; $23,660/year
Examples: Administrative, executive, and professional staff; salespeople; STEM (science, technology, engineering, and math) staff	Examples: Direct caregivers, nonsupervisory or nonlicensed staff in dining services, environmental services or activities

at 8 hours/day or 80 hours/14 days (biweekly). This alternative has three qualifying criteria (DOL, 2009):

1. The employer and employee must have an agreement to use the 8 and 80 system before any work is performed. (The employee handbook should clearly

indicate that the 8 and 80 system will be used, and this should be emphasized in orientation.)

2. Overtime rate applies to every hour worked in excess of 8 hours per day, regardless of how many total hours are worked during the 14-day work period.

3. Overtime must be paid for every hour worked more than 80 hours during the 14-day work period. (Credit can be taken for any overtime paid in excess of 8 hours per day.)

Most states have their own wage and hourly rate laws that have even more requirements to follow. There are also other federal and state laws related to other kinds of workers, such as interns and workers-in-training, independent contractors, temporary employees, foreign workers and volunteers. It is wise to check with the state's department of labor for the overtime and minimum wage provisions currently in effect. Table 3.5 provides an overview of the main qualifying criteria applied to determining whether an employee is properly classified for payroll purposes (Doyle, 2019).

To properly calculate wages owed to nonexempt employees, having a reliable and user-friendly time recording system is vital. It also serves as backup documentation in the event of an audit by a government agency, such as the federal or state labor department. Furthermore, for any SNF participating in Medicare or Medicaid, a new system was implemented by the CMS in 2016 for facilities to electronically submit direct care staffing information (including agency and contract staff) along with its census. It is called a "Payroll-Based Journal" (PBJ) because it relies on regularly extracting data from the organization's payroll as well as other auditable data. When combined with census information, PBJ reports can be used to monitor an SNF's staffing level, but also to analyze employee turnover and retention, which has been shown to impact the quality of care delivered (U.S. Department of Health and Human Services, Centers for Medicare & Medicaid Services, 2019).

There is a multitude of commercially available time record systems available, and new ones get introduced every year. Whether it is a conventional time clock that imprints an employee's check-in and checkout times, one with biometric reader capability (i.e., fingerprint, hand shape, or retinal scan) for employee identification, or one that enlists the smart phone of an employee, having a system that records time worked accurately, seamlessly reports it for approval and payroll processing, and provides an effective audit trail is both good business and good for employee relations.

CONFLICT RESOLUTION STRATEGIES

When conflict happens in the workplace, it is important to address it head on and not allow it to distract people from pursing the organization's mission—*together*. Resolving conflict eases stress and focuses collective energy on achieving shared goals. Preparing supervisors to effectively manage conflict among employees—or with care recipients and their families, visitors, vendors, or volunteers—is an effective strategy for ensuring an environment conducive to cohesiveness, productivity, and continuity of care. Human resources consultant Deb Peterson (2018) offers 10 recommendations for resolving conflicts peacefully and successfully:

1. **Prepare:** Start by checking your own behavior. Take responsibility for your part in the conflict. Then plan what you want to say—it often helps to visualize the conversation.

2. **Timing:** Do not wait! Ignoring the conflict does not make it go away; it may even make it fester and tougher to resolve later. If a specific behavior or event has caused the conflict, promptness gives you an example to cite, and it gives the other person the best chance of understanding the subject for discussion.

3. **Place:** Find a location to meet that is both private and neutral. The goal is to eliminate the tension created by conflict, and privacy helps. Try to minimize physical barriers, such as a desk or table between people, to make the office as neutral as possible.

4. **Nonverbal Language:** Know what unspoken message you are sending with your posture and expression … show sincerity and interest. Maintain eye contact; relax your neck and shoulders; use a neutral and conversational tone and moderate speed and volume; and avoid absolutes, such as *always* or *never*.

5. **Feelings:** The vast majority of conflicts originate with *feelings*, not facts, owning one's feelings and caring about someone else's matter when resolving conflict. It is generally beneficial to concentrate on a behavior, not someone's personality. It also helps to use "I" statements, such as "I feel really frustrated when you…" rather than "You make me so angry."

6. **Problem Identification:** Confirm how the other party views the situation; do not assume that perceptions match. Discuss what contributed to the conflict and establish whether there is missing information or incorrect facts, and then reach agreement about a desired outcome and expectations.

7. **Actively Listen:** Remember that appearances can deceive—things are not always what they seem. Remain open to hearing and objectively considering the other person's explanation as well as the possibility of learning new information that might influence the discussion. Be ready to respond with compassion.

8. **Solution Mining:** Resolving conflict is not about changing another person; it should focus on reaching agreement about how to best prevent recurrence. Acknowledging the other person's ideas first often increases their personal commitment. If you have ideas the other person does not mention, suggest them afterward. Then discuss and reasonably consider each proposed solution.

9. **Action Plan:** Verify what is expected to happen differently going forward and how success will be measured, pledge your commitment to supporting the plan, and ask the other party to do likewise. Set a follow-up date to discuss progress.

10. **Confidence:** Thank the other person for earnestly participating, and express optimism and confidence that your work relationship will grow stronger as a result.

Remember: Very few people start their day actively seeking a conflict with someone else. Even fewer are interested in the stress associated with a workplace conflict continuing, or worse yet, escalating. Following the advice of the TV character Deputy Sheriff Barney Fife on the "Andy Griffith Show" nearly a half-century ago is a good practice: "Nip it! Nip it in the bud!"

STAFF SATISFACTION AND ENGAGEMENT

A key part of any continuous quality improvement process is to periodically test how well things are working, whether it is a policy or procedure, a strategy or tactic, or an initiative or corrective action. A solution to a given challenge may make sense to those who developed it but has the situation improved after implementation? Meaningfully measuring success in the human resources arena often relies on simply *asking* employees—as internal customers—about their assessments, perceptions, attitudes, and ideas.

Fostering movement toward a more contemporary workplace culture—one that embraces person-centered care and employee empowerment—is a key responsibility of the Health Services Executive. Staff members offer the very best source of information concerning cultural climate, including topics ranging from employee morale and trust to mission alignment and engagement.

> *As the competition for compassionate and qualified staff only continues to grow fiercer, a thriving culture is no longer just a nicety; it is a necessity. Culture is defined as "the way things work around here." It impacts staff engagement, turnover, and customer loyalty. Understanding the culture of an organization goes beyond just reading the sign posted in the lobby about mission—it involves understanding the current values that staff are acting on each day.*
>
> Denise Boudreau-Scott, MHA, LNHA
> President, Drive, Inc.

Although the two terms are sometimes used interchangeably, we refer to engagement here as meaning more than satisfaction when it comes to evaluating corporate culture. Rather than merely *satisfying* each employee's needs, the goal becomes creating an environment in which everyone gives their very best effort every day—embracing the organization's mission and values and *engaging* in the successful pursuit of its goals and vision for the future. The organization flourishes in such an environment because this enhances its employees' sense of well-being and purpose.

Employee engagement is typically more robust when a leader consistently and convincingly demonstrates their commitment to fundamental core values that build trust, such as integrity, transparency, honesty, inclusiveness, fairness, and equal treatment. An engaged employee does more than reliably report for work. They also take an active interest in how things might improve, from quality and continuity of care to operational efficiency; a true stakeholder in the success of the organization.

Employee engagement is possible to measure and several frameworks have been developed for doing so. Consider the following in either developing an internal employee engagement monitoring process or evaluating those available from outside partners.

- Audience: All employees or segmented by nonsupervisory or supervisory, licensed professional or non-licensed, department, location, shift, or targeted demographics (e.g., length of service)?
- Anonymity: Participation rate drives both the reliability and validity of the information gathered, and better decisions result from greater participation. Each employee must trust that questions can be answered truthfully without fear of retribution.
  - Reduce the risk of discovery by avoiding hand-written responses and delivering completed surveys directly to an off-site location by mail.

- ▣ The more personal information that is collected, the more suspiciously people tend to view the anonymity of the process—which can erode participation.

- ▣ Design: Length of the survey is a hot topic, with so much to ask about and the risk of dropping the participation rate for a questionnaire that (a) takes too long to complete, (b) is either difficult to understand or so simple it feels demeaning, or (c) asks questions that seem irrelevant or unimportant to the employee. Furthermore, literacy skills vary greatly in our field because we typically have both highly educated people and those who are not. Similarly, language proficiency is becoming increasingly diverse, with a growing number of employees understanding best a language other than English.

- ▣ Time: This parameter has at least two elements: cycle and context. Annual employee surveys were once the norm among organizations that conducted them, but pressure to shorten that cycle has built up in an era when people have greater expectations about immediate gratification and speed. Context relates to timing—when to conduct the assessment to minimize potential distractions caused by an event or other influences, which might temporarily shape the results. Example: Distributing the survey immediately after an announcement about a wage increase (+) or staff reduction (−).

- ▣ Communication: Sharing the survey results with the staff is critical—swiftly, transparently, and focused—to reinforce the organization's commitment to the process. Present opportunities to become involved in developing and implementing plans that address significant concerns that emerged. Also, follow-up by reporting sharing progress made throughout the year.

- ▣ Champion: Any project that owes its birth to the reported results of an employee engagement survey deserves a champion—a person who accepts responsibility for leading the effort to effectively address the core concern or opportunity selected for action. Some organizations apply a synonym to describe this person, such as project owner or team leader. No matter how large the work group that is appointed to work on the solution, the leadership axiom that generally holds true is, "when it is everyone's job, it is nobody's job." Designating a champion puts a face on the project and heightens the probability of not only completion, but success.

- ▣ Celebrate: Improvement is the core purpose of an employee engagement query—in the organization's clinical outcomes, operational performance, and corporate climate. However, avoid the mistake of limiting recognition to those who produce obvious winners. Also celebrate the efforts of those who were bold enough to try something that seemed promising but simply did not produce the results anticipated. Celebrate *trying* when it was not required, so that people learn to trust that engaging is truly valued!

Cultivating employee engagement is about aligning an organization's actions with its values by drawing on their knowledge and ideas to improve operations. It can lead to pride and loyalty that goes beyond great service to producing advocates. The chief benefit of increasing employee engagement is not just a "feel-good" exercise, but it is good business. As employee engagement goes up, organizations typically experience greater productivity and lower rates of turnover, absenteeism, tardiness, work injuries, conflicts, and grievances (Macleod, 2018).

A Net Promoter Score (NPS) provides a useful "snapshot" of an organization's degree of employee engagement. Originally introduced as a method for measuring the satisfaction and loyalty of customers, the NPS has been adopted by progressive employers to learn more about similar issues concerning their employees. This technique has been shown to be predictive of other key indicators of employee engagement.

Sometimes referred to as the "Ultimate Question," employees are simply asked, "How likely are you to recommend working here to a friend or colleague?" Answer options typically range from 0 to 10, and respondents fall into one of at least three NPS categories:

1. Promoter   (9–10)
2. Passive   (7–8)
3. Detractor   (0–6)

To calculate an organization's employee NPS, subtract detractors from promoters (ignoring the passives) and divide the sum by the total number of respondents (Fitoussi, 2019). A positive NPS indicates more people would recommend the organization as an employer of choice; a negative NPS suggests the opposite.

$$\text{Employee NPS} = \frac{(\text{Promoters} - \text{Detractors})}{\text{Total Respondents}}$$

Having a clear understanding of what matters most (and sometimes *least*) to employees can help better understand why an NPS is high or low as well as why it is trending up or down. MyInnerView, Inc., is a company that conducts a high number of staff satisfaction surveys for nursing homes across the nation. Its analysis of responses from over 223,400 long-term care employees identified seven key areas—in descending order of priority—on which long-term care leaders should focus to build staff engagement (Huaiquil, 2019):

1. Management cares about employees
2. Management listens to employees
3. Management helps to reduce job stress
4. Fair evaluations
5. Staff respect for residents
6. Safe workplace
7. Supervisor cares about you as a person

EMPLOYMENT LAWS AND COMPLIANCE

The postacute care continuum is a "people helping people" field, which makes it what economists call "labor intensive." Compliance with all applicable laws and regulations is included in the conditions of participation in Medicare and Medicaid, which adds significant incentives for meeting or exceeding those related to employment.

There are over 180 laws and regulations pertaining to American workplaces and their employees. They include employment issues from pre-employment to retirement, cover companies of all sizes, and address topics from safety and documentation to discrimination and fair labor practices. They affect the workplace activities for about 10 million employers and their estimated 125 million workers (DOL, 2019).

It is a key responsibility of the health services executive to understand the key provisions of major labor laws and regulations and how they apply in their setting and to remain informed concerning changes as they develop. Furthermore, establishing and properly resourcing systems that can ensure compliance protects the interests of staff and the organization. Rather than listing here an exhaustive list of them, significant federal laws that are administered by the DOL and relevant to postacute care are grouped by function in the following. Many states have companion sets of laws and regulations to follow as well. If they are incompatible, the federal version typically prevails.

Wages and Work Hours

The **FLSA** prescribes standards for wages and overtime pay, which affect most private and public employment. The DOL's Wage and Hour Division enforces the rules. The FLSA also restricts the hours that children under age 16 can work and prohibits children under age 18 from working in certain jobs deemed too dangerous (DOL, Wage and Hour Division, 2009).

The **Immigration and Nationality Act (INA)** applies to noncitizen aliens who are authorized to work in the United States under certain visa programs, and its provisions are also enforced by the Wage and Hour Division.

Other employment laws are less well known because they apply only to a postacute care setting operated by a federal agency, such as Veterans Affairs, or they might apply if a federal agency partially funds private construction through a grant or loan, such as the U.S. Department of Housing and Urban Development (HUD) or the U.S. Department of Agriculture (USDA). These laws are administered by the DOL's Wage and Hour Division.

- The Davis-Bacon Act requires payment of prevailing wages and benefits to employees of contractors engaged in federal construction projects.
- The McNamara-O'Hara Service Contract Act sets wage rates and other labor standards for employees of contractors furnishing services to the federal government.
- The Walsh-Healey Public Contracts Act requires payment of minimum wages and other labor standards by contractors providing materials and supplies to the federal government.
- Veterans' Preference: Veterans (and other eligible persons) are provided preference in initial hiring and protection in reductions in force. Claims of violations are investigated by the Veterans' Employment and Training Service (VETS).

Workplace Safety and Health

The **Occupational Safety and Health Act** is administered by the Occupational Safety and Health Administration (OSHA). Safety and health conditions are regulated by OSHA or OSHA-approved state programs. Employers have a general duty to provide their employees with work assignments and a workplace free from serious hazards.

Workers' compensation programs differ by state (see Mandatory Insurance Coverages, p. 80). The DOL's Office of Workers' Compensation Programs does not have a role in the administration or oversight of state workers' compensation programs.

The **Federal Employees' Compensation Act (FECA)** established a comprehensive workers' compensation program that covers the disability or death of a federal employee resulting from an injury sustained while performing their job.

Employee Benefit Security

ERISA regulates employers who offer pension or welfare benefit plans for their employees. The Employee Benefits Security Administration (EBSA) oversees a wide range of fiduciary, disclosure, and reporting requirements on fiduciaries of pension and welfare benefit plans.

COBRA is also administered by the EBSA, ensuring all reporting requirements are met concerning the continuation of healthcare insurance coverage for people who change employers.

The **Health Insurance Portability and Accountability Act (HIPAA)** also includes healthcare insurance plan portability requirements on group plans.

Employee Protection

Most labor and public safety laws and regulations, as well as several regarding protection of the environment, provide whistleblower protections for employees who complain about violations by their employers. Remedies can include job reinstatement, payment of back wages, and even fines. The OSHA typically enforces such whistleblower protections.

The **FMLA** is administered by the DOL's Wage and Hour Division. It requires an employer with 50 or more employees to provide up to 12 weeks of unpaid, job-protected leave to eligible employees for the birth or adoption of a child or for the serious illness of the employee or their spouse, child, or parent.

The **Consumer Credit Protection Act (CCPA)** is administered by the DOL's Wage and Hour Division and regulates the garnishment of employee wages by employers.

Employee Polygraph Protection Act (EPPA) bars most employers from using lie detectors on an employee, permitting polygraph tests only in limited circumstances. It is administered by the Wage and Hour Division.

The **Uniformed Services Employment and Reemployment Rights Act** preserves the reemployment right of any person who serves in the armed forces, including an employee who is called up from the reserves or National Guard. These rights are administered by the VETS.

Unions and Collective Bargaining

In 1935, the **Wagner Act** created the National Labor Relations Board (NLRB), "an independent federal agency that protects the rights of private sector employees to join together, with or without a union, to improve their wages and working conditions" (NLRB, 2019). It gives employees the right to form and join a union, and it requires employers to bargain collectively with a union selected by a majority vote of the employees in an appropriate bargaining unit.

The Wagner Act was been amended several times since its passage. In 1974, coverage and protection expanded to include healthcare workers, with special provisions recognizing the importance of ensuring that the needs of patients would be met during contingencies arising from labor disputes. The rules governing the collective bargaining and certifying employee representation by a union are complex—and strictly enforced. The health services executive must develop a working knowledge of them to avoid a technical violation and negative consequences. For more in-depth information, visit www.nlrb.gov.

The **Labor Management Reporting and Disclosure Act (LMRDA) of 1959**, also known as the Landrum-Griffin Act, protects union funds and promotes union democracy by requiring labor organizations to file annual financial reports, by requiring union officials, employers, and labor consultants to file reports regarding certain labor relations practices, and by establishing standards for the election of union officers. The act is administered by the DOL's Office of Labor Management Standards (OLMS).

Volunteers

While not technically an employee, a volunteer typically performs valuable services that enhance the quality of life for those served by the organization, so we include this category here. A volunteer faces many of the same workplace risks as an employee, such as occasional exposure to infectious diseases, cleaning chemicals, hazardous waste, aggressive behavior by cognitively impaired or mentally ill clients, weather-related or other disasters, and environmental dangers (i.e., stairs or wet floors). They deserve certain protections as well.

Many of the rules and agencies already described have provisions for differentiating volunteer effort from work for which compensation is due. The OSHA and the DOL's Wage and Hour Divisions are chief among them. Generally, if a volunteer is performing a task for which an employee would normally be paid—*in lieu* of the employee's effort (not as an addition to the minimum required)—it bears further examination. A volunteer's work can add value, but it cannot simply save operating costs at the expense of what could reasonably be expected to be paid labor.

There is also a rising interest among postacute care providers in expecting a volunteer to meet other qualifications that an employee does, including a criminal background check, drug test, TB test, or inoculations against flu, pneumonia, shingles, or hepatitis. We serve frail, vulnerable people who often have compromised immune systems—a volunteer meeting the same standards as an employee in these areas constitutes sound risk management.

Academic Affiliations and Students

Clinical training programs desire training sites to put their students in direct contact with real patients. Academic programs in health administration and leadership also need meaningful experiential learning venues. Helping develop the health and human service professionals of tomorrow can pay dividends in several ways. Beyond the satisfaction of knowing hundreds of lives will be served throughout their careers, hosting students from such programs can:

- bolster the organization's public image as a progressive care provider,
- refresh the staff's skills and reaffirm their motivation for joining this field,
- complement the service level and quality of life for the residents,

- restore a sense of purpose among residents as mentors to students preparing for their careers, and

- serve as a recruiting vehicle by providing an "inside track" with students (future applicants) and faculty (referral sources—or *possibly* future applicants).

Although the students are typically more akin to volunteers than employees, it is imperative to formalize such a relationship with an affiliation agreement. Both secondary and postsecondary schools with health professions training programs generally have a template already developed or the organization can prepare one. In either event, it is money well spent to have legal counsel review any affiliation agreement that gets executed. Whether the students are in clinical or nonclinical roles, it is advisable to clearly set forth expectations about the responsibilities of the supervising faculty, students, and hosting staff as well as professional liability insurance coverage. Also, if a student receives any remuneration—a stipend, scholarship, temporary lodging, or meals—it is beneficial to check with the school's financial aid office to verify whether there are any effects on the student's financial assistance status as well as any possible income tax ramifications.

POLICIES AND PROCEDURES

Employee Handbook

For any employee to thrive and flourish, it is imperative for them to have access to—and understand—the rules governing the organization and the rewards of working for the organization. An entire chapter could be devoted to the employee handbook—it is so vital to the success of each employee and to the organization's overall performance. In fact, there are books devoted to constructing an effective employee handbook. There are several options about content, design, and distribution strategies suggested in the "Additional Resources" section of this chapter, but a few are highlighted in the following:

- Content: Each of the topics mentioned earlier concerning orientation and onboarding is important to address. Provide guidance around behaviors that are valued and encouraged, those that are prohibited, and the potential consequences of both. An employee wants—and certainly deserves—to know what is expected. Include explicit instructions about how to offer suggestions for improvement, express concerns or file a grievance, and fulfill attendance and punctuality expectations, as well as describing the organization's progressive disciplinary steps. Consistent, fair, and equal treatment in *applying* the policies and procedures described in the employee handbook is an essential practice in building a corporate culture that fosters confidence and high employee engagement.

- Design: Ease of use serves as the key driver in designing an employee handbook; finding the right information should take little time and answer the question posed. As mentioned concerning employee engagement surveys, literacy skills vary greatly in our field, and the list of languages understood is becoming increasingly diverse.

- Distribution: Employers are increasingly posting the employee handbook online, making it easier to periodically update and to print a targeted portion at a time, as needed. Some progressive organizations complement the written employee handbook with a searchable video version, audio version, or both. The main goal here is accessibility.

- Acknowledgment: Regardless of the distribution method, every employee should sign an acknowledgment form verifying that they received and understand and agree to abide by the contents of the Employee Handbook, and have the form filed in their HR record. If a significant change is made, it is also a good practice to collect signed acknowledgment forms reflecting each employee's renewed pledge.

Operational Policies and Procedures

In addition to the employee handbook, it is standard practice for an organization to also have policies and procedures addressing specific operational matters. They are generally organized by department or professional discipline, such as nursing, dining services, environmental services, business office and administration, social services, and life enrichment and volunteers (aka activities). Some are interdisciplinary and bridge several departments, such as policies and procedures for care planning, staff development, or information technology. Like the employee handbook, it is critical that the people who need to understand the policies, and procedures well enough to competently interpret and apply them *must* have access to them…whether in printed versions stored in conveniently placed binders or online with appropriate security measures installed.

SUMMARY

Human resources is an area where effective leaders need to make sure that all the i's are dotted and t's are crossed. Making sure that the human resources systems are in place is critical. The costs of turnover and impact on the quality of care and service are directly related to how well all the elements of a good human resource program are attended to by an organization. Effective leaders understand the value of attracting and keeping staff members for the long-term success of an organization.

KEY POINTS

1. The human resources domain is multifaceted because postacute care is labor intensive; people are the most important resource for fulfilling an organization's mission, upholding its values, and successfully pursuing its vision.
2. Human resources management starts with assisting departments with recruiting, screening, hiring, orienting and onboarding, training, supporting, and retaining competent, motivated staff members.
3. The health services executive must develop familiarity with and implement systems that effectively:
   a. foster a corporate culture of trust based on consistently fair and equal treatment,
   b. assess employee performance and engagement and lead to improving both,
   c. administer competitive compensation and benefits,
   d. process payroll on a timely basis and accurately,
   e. minimize workplace conflict,

      f.   ensure compliance with applicable employment laws and regulations, and

      g.   communicate expectations among all team members.

4. Policies and procedures only work when the people responsible for following them can easily access and understand them.

LEADERSHIP ROLES

The health services executive should make every effort to be accessible and to establish trust among all key stakeholders—customers and their families, staff members and their families, contract professionals and vendors, regulators, and the community-at-large—that they can be counted on to treat people fairly and consistently. Policies and procedures are the most effective when the organization's leader applies them in ways people believe is just.

HIGH-IMPACT PRACTICES

1. **Recruitment and Retention (R&R) Bonus:** Some claim there is no better ambassador for an organization than one of its own employees. A long-term care provider tested this axiom by offering a three-part bonus to any employee who recruited someone to join the staff full-time, regardless of the position, paying increased amounts the longer the new hire stayed. An applicant had to name the employee as a "sponsor" on the original employment application; if more than one employee was named, they shared the R&R bonuses. The sponsor received $100 at hire, $200 at 90 days $300 at 180 days, and $400 at the 1-year hire date anniversary. The "power ball" feature of this program was that at the close of each calendar year, the names of all the sponsors responsible for new employees who reached the 1-year mark in that year went into a pool for a drawing (as many times as there were qualifying new hires) to win a new compact model car plus a fuel card for one tank of gas per week for a year! The impact on vacant positions was almost immediate, and employee turnover dropped by one half in the first year of the program. After the first grand prize was awarded—with great fanfare and attracting local media attention—turnover dropped by one half again, and the organization was compelled to start a waiting list for some positions. With so many different employees becoming true stakeholders in the outcome, newly hired staff members enjoyed a robust support system as they integrated into their new workplace. The cost of the program, including applicable payroll taxes, was less than the cost of filling one vacant entry-level position per year with temporary agency personnel. The value of the net return on investment not only topped $110,000 in year one, but it also resulted in enhanced continuity of care, staff morale, and resident and family satisfaction scores.

2. **Contemporary Employee Handbook:** After learning through its employee engagement survey that many staff members found its employee handbook difficult to understand and awkward to use, a progressive postacute care organization decided to transform how it communicated with its employees about those policies and procedures. First, the most recent version of the handbook was checked for completeness, verifying that all changes made since it was last published were updated. Second, the local university's English department was consulted to recommend revisions that made it

readable at the eighth grade level (instead of requiring interpretation by an attorney) without sacrificing its meaning. Third, the same school's Spanish department was asked to translate the revised handbook, since an increasing number of employees (and prospective employees) speak Spanish as their first language. Working with the organization's webmaster consultant, the entire new document—in both languages—was posted online in a password-protected section of the website labeled "People Matter."

3. **Employee Engagement:** The study by MyInnerview, Inc., of long-term care workers' expectations identified seven key topics that are sought by them to feel engaged. Here are a few examples of how to address each one.

HSE™ Focus	High-Impact Practice
Management cares about staff	1. Conduct performance evaluations on time, showing the importance to the organization of each employee's success. 2. Ensure work schedules and assignments are clear, well organized, posted in advance, and honored. 3. Know at least one thing about each staff member—family, outside interests, or something you share in common—that you can connect on when you meet.
Management listens to staff	1. Conduct regular and frequent rounds—slow down, linger, and be present. 2. Regularly measure and take action on employee engagement survey results. 3. Create consistent, formal, and structured systems for receiving employee suggestions, insights, and feedback.
Management helps reduce job stress	1. Decrease institutional noise pollution (i.e., excessive use of paging). 2. Support grieving staff when a resident/client passes away. 3. Provide training about effectively dealing with challenging residents or families.
Fair evaluations	1. Ensure job descriptions are current. 2. Include an employee's self-evaluation as an integral part of the process. 3. Ask if the employee thinks the review is fair; probe further if the answer is "no."
Staff respect for residents/clients	1. Consistent assignments build relationship-centered care, bolster efficiency, and enhance satisfaction of care recipients, their families, and employees. 2. Maintain a system for investigating allegations of disrespect and visibly enforce. 3. Celebrate and highlight instances of exemplary displays of resident/client respect.
Safe workplace	1. Sponsor safety contests and provide rewards for working a targeted number of consecutive days without experiencing an injury that results in lost time. 2. Institutional: Ensure there are plenty of well-maintained and appropriately distributed transfer devices. 3. Home health: Include safe driver training to the staff development core.

(continued)

HSE™ Focus	High-Impact Practice
Supervisor cares about you as a person	1. Write a personal note to an employee to express thanks for going beyond the call of duty, congratulate them on a birthday, hire date anniversary, graduation, or wedding of a child, or show concern about a personal tragedy. 2. Publicly recognize individual achievements—work related and personal. 3. Adjust schedule or assignment, if feasible, to accommodate changing needs (i.e., transportation challenges, marital status, or family configuration).

QUESTIONS FOR DISCUSSION

1. Describe the key contributing factors leading to high employee turnover in postacute care organizations.

2. What is the difference between employee retention and staff turnover, and how are they calculated?

3. What is the most effective frequency for discussing performance and why?

4. Discuss whether the relationship between employee engagement and quality of care shows a correlation or demonstrates causality.

5. Name three positions in a postacute care organization that present a challenge in determining whether they should be classified as exempt or nonexempt. Why is each one difficult to classify?

6. What information should appear in an employee acknowledgment form concerning an employee handbook, and why is each element important?

CASE PROBLEMS

1. **Rehab—Keep It in the Family:** An employee was injured in a car accident seriously enough to require time off from work so that he could engage in physical therapy and regain his mobility, strength, and stamina to safely return to the job. The organization negotiated with the insurance carrier a reduced daily rate. Receiving those services through his employer at a discounted rate not only saved him out-of-pocket expenses for his copays (calculated as 20% of a lowered charge) but added reimbursable volume in the therapy department, positively affecting revenues and productivity. It also provided additional encouragement to him from coworkers and residents, reminding him how much his swift and complete recovery—and permanent return—meant to them.

   Questions:

   a. What potential events, circumstances, or interactions might serve as barriers to the success of this arrangement?

   b. Does this approach present a conflict of interest? Why, or why not?

   c. How do you imagine residents, their families, and other staff members might react to this scenario?

2. **Recruitment Labels:** Some organizations have begun *rebranding* their recruiting efforts by utilizing new descriptive terms aimed at getting the attention of the people they want to attract, to be viewed as contemporary and less corporate sounding (Eubanks, 2016). Recruiters are becoming "talent acquisition directors," intending to show that they are interested in providing opportunities for people to apply their talents in ways that meaningfully contribute to advancing the organization's mission (in contrast to merely performing work or earning a paycheck). Another nuanced title, based on the success of the Disney platform in a variety of healthcare and human services settings, is "casting director." The Disney approach treats every day as a performance and guests (aka residents/patients/clients/participants) as the most important audience (Lee, 2004). Of course, one runs the risk of becoming "too cute," and some prospective team members might decide to not take the organization seriously. But for many, the downside risk has been more than offset by the number and quality of applicants they have attracted.

   Questions:

   a. Create an alternate title for each of five positions in a senior living organization that you believe could serve as an attention grabber and describes to the person who hears it for the first time the purpose of each job.

   b. How would you test whether this approach could be effective in your organization?

3. **Transportation in the Gig Economy:** Instead of investing heavily in acquiring, maintaining, and ensuring a fleet of vehicles—and employing drivers with first aid, CPR, and transfer skills training—an increasing number of health care providers (and payers) are contracting with nontraditional mobility companies, such as Lyft and Uber, for nonemergency medical transportation services (Grenoble, 2017). Not only is this reducing expense, but it is reportedly providing better service—eroding wait times and missed medical appointments by double-digit percentages, elevating patient satisfaction scores, and dramatically lowering visits to the ED for nonurgent health episodes. Noninstitutional senior living providers might also explore this model for transporting both caregivers and care recipients.

   Questions:

   a. What other preparation or qualifications would you recommend for drivers providing on-demand transportation services?

   b. What other services could follow a similar path to enhance an elder's autonomy and self-determination?

NAB DOMAINS OF PRACTICE

20 HUMAN RESOURCES
20.01 Ensure that human resource management policies and programs comply with federal and state regulations.
20.02 Establish the planning, development, implementation, monitoring, and evaluation of recruitment, selection, and retention practices.

20.03 Establish the planning, development, implementation, monitoring, and evaluation of employee training and development programs.

20.04 Establish the planning, development, implementation, monitoring, and evaluation of employee evaluation programs.

20.05 Establish the planning, development, implementation, monitoring, and evaluation of compensation and benefit programs.

20.06 Establish the planning, development, implementation, monitoring, and evaluation of employee health and safety programs.

20.07 Establish the planning, development, implementation, monitoring, and evaluation of employee satisfaction and organizational culture.

20.08 Establish the planning, development, implementation, monitoring, and evaluation of employee disciplinary policies and procedures.

20.09 Establish the planning, development, implementation, monitoring, and evaluation of employee grievance policies and procedures.

20.10 Establish the planning, development, implementation, monitoring, and evaluation of leadership development programs.

20.11 Promote a safe work environment (such as safety training and employee risk management).

20.12 Promote a positive work environment (using techniques such as conflict resolution, diversity training, or staff recognition programs).

20.13 Facilitate effective written, oral, and electronic communication among management and staff.

20.14 Ensure employee records and documentation systems are developed and maintained.

20.15 Establish a culture that encourages employees to embrace care recipients' rights.

A summary of the related knowledge, skills, and core expectations across service lines—and unique features of each service line—is available at www. nabweb.org/filebin/pdf/Annotation_of_Tasks_Performed_Across_LOS _in_LTC.pdf.

Source: Reproduced with permission from National Association of Long-Term Care Administrator Boards. (2016). *Annotation of tasks performed and knowledge and skills used across lines of service in long-term care.* Retrieved from https://www.nabweb.org/filebin/pdf/ Annotation_of_Tasks_Performed_Across_LOS_in_LTC.pdf

REFERENCES

Argentum. (2018). *Senior living labor and workforce trends: 2018.* Retrieved from https://erickson .umbc.edu/files/2018/02/Argentum-Senior-Living-Labor-Workforce-Trends-2018.pdf

Bishop, C., Weinberg, D., Leutz, W., Dossa, A. Peefferle, S., & Zincavage, R. (2008). Nursing assistants' job commitment: Effect of nursing home organizational factors and impact on resident well-being. *The Gerontologist, 48*(Suppl. 1), 36–45. doi:10.1093/geront/48 .Supplement_1.36

Blakely-Gray, R. (2017, February 1). *State mandated paid sick leave.* Retrieved from https://www .patriotsoftware.com/payroll/training/blog/state-mandated-paid-sick-leave-laws/

Bossart, M. (2016, September 12). *When can an employee take FMLA parental leave?* Retrieved from https://www.patriotsoftware.com/payroll/training/blog/can-employee-take-parental -leave/

Bowblis, J. (2011). Staffing ratios and quality: An analysis of minimum direct care staffing requirements for nursing homes. *Health Services Research, 46*(5), 1495–1516. doi:10.1111/j.1475-6773.2011.01274.x

Browning, D. (2017, May 1). *How do we balance autonomy and risk for older adults?* Retrieved from https://www.nextavenue.org/older-adults-balance-autonomy-risk/

Capterra. (2019). *Recruiting software tools: Compare product features and ratings to find the right recruiting software for your organization.* Retrieved from https://www.capterra.com/sem-compare/recruiting-software

Cirillo, A. (2018a, March 23). *The advantages of career ladders in long-term care.* Retrieved from https://www.verywellhealth.com/the-advantages-of-career-ladders-197844

Cirillo, A. (2018b, September 11). *Six steps to effective employee retention: Long-term care workforce turnover hampers care.* Retrieved from https://www.verywellhealth.com/employee-retention-197832

Clark, A. (2015). Quality EAPs carry their weight. *Benefit Magazine, 52*(12), 42–47.

Dellefield, M. E., Castle, N. G., McGilton, K. S., & Spilsbury, K. (2015). The relationship between registered nurses and nursing home quality: An integrative review, 2008–2014. *Nursing Economics, 3*(2), 95–108, 116.

Dictionary.com. (2020). *Perquisite.* Retrieved from https://www.dictionary.com/browse/perquisite?s=t

Doyle, A. (2019). *The difference between an exempt and a non-exempt employee.* Retrieved from https://www.thebalancecareers.com/exempt-and-a-non-exempt-employee-2061988

Eubanks, B. (2016). *Human resources job titles: The ultimate guide.* Retrieved from https://upstarthr.com/human-resources-job-titles-the-ultimate-guide/

Fitoussi, V. (2019, March 1). *Four key performance indicators to measure employee engagement.* Retrieved from https://www.saplinghr.com/blog/4-kpis-measure-employee-engagement

Feuerberg, M. (2001). *Appropriateness of minimum nurse staffing ratios in nursing homes report to congress: Phase II Final, December 2001.* Washington, DC: Centers for Medicare and Medicaid Services.

Grenoble, R. (2017, August 30). Lyft, Uber increasingly offering medical transportation services. *Huffington Post.* Retrieved from https://www.huffpost.com/entry/lyft-uber-non-emergency-medical-transport_n_598885c9e4b09a4d1ec68784

Gurston, S. (2019, September 17). *Legal THC limit in Michigan: Is there one that proves marijuana-impaired driving?* Retrieved from https://www.michiganautolaw.com/blog/2019/09/17/legal-thc-limit/

Handrick, L. (2018, June 25). *New employee orientation.* Retrieved from https://fitsmallbusiness.com/new-employee-orientation/

Hopkins, C. (2017, April 26). *Section 125 cafeteria plan—What it is and how it works.* Retrieved from https://fitsmallbusiness.com/section-125-cafeteria-plan/

Huaiquil, A. (2019). *Association executive says connection, metrics to employee engagement.* Provider Long Term and Post-Acute Care. Retrieved from http://www.providermagazine.com/news/Pages/2019/0719/Association-CEO-Says-Connection,-Metrics-Key-to-Employee-Engagement.aspx

Institute of Medicine Committee on Nursing Home Regulation. (1986). *Improving the quality of care in nursing homes.* Washington, DC: National Academies of Science.

Kappel, M. (2017, May 3). *What is compensatory time off?* Retrieved from https://www.patriotsoftware.com/payroll/training/blog/a-look-at-compensatory-time-off/

Kemper, P., Brannon, D., Barry, T., Stott, A., & Heier, B. (2008). Implementation of the better jobs better care demonstration: Lessons for long-term care workforce initiatives. *The Gerontologist, 48*(Suppl. 1), 26–35. doi:10.1093/geront/48.Supplement_1.26

Lee, F. (2004). *If Disney ran your hospital: 9½ things you would do differently.* Bozeman, MT: Second River Healthcare.

Macleod, D. (2018). What is employee engagement? *Engage for Success.* Retrieved from https://engageforsuccess.org/what-is-employee-engagement

Marquand, B. (2019, May 28). *Ordering the combo: Life insurance with long-term care insurance.* Retrieved from https://www.nerdwallet.com/blog/insurance/combine-life-insurance-long-term-care/

McKay, M. (2017, September 26). *Definition of non-exempt employee.* Retrieved from https://bizfluent.com/info-8130435-definition-nonexempt-employee.html

McKnight's Long-Term Care News. (2012, October 16). *Survey assesses turnover and retention rates among assisted living workers.* Retrieved from https://www.mcknights.com/news/survey-assesses-turnover-and-retention-rates-among-assisted-living-workers/

Miller, G. (2019, January 6). *Should you buy supplemental life insurance through your employer?* Retrieved from https://20somethingfinance.com/should-you-buy-supplemental-life-insurance-through-your-employer/

Mozga, M. (2015, April 28). *Survey: Home care worker turnover topped 60% in 2014.* Retrieved from https://phinational.org/survey-home-care-worker-turnover-topped-60-percent-in-2014/

National Labor Relations Board. (2019). *NLRB's history.* Retrieved from https://www.nlrb.gov/about-nlrb/who-we-are/our-history

Peterson, D. (2018, October 20). *A step-by-step guide to resolving conflicts peacefully.* Retrieved from https://www.thoughtco.com/steps-to-conflict-resolution-31710

Pratt, J. (2016). *Long term care: Managing across the continuum* (4th ed.). Burlington, MA: Jones and Bartlett.

Priz, E., & Priz, S. (2010). *Workers' compensation: A field guide for employers.* Riverside, IL: Advanced Insurance Management.

Quilter, D. (2019, June 11). What some nursing homes do to retain quality staff. *Forbes.* Retrieved from https://www.forbes.com/sites/nextavenue/2019/06/11/what-some-nursing-homes-do-to-retain-quality-staff/

Rosen, C. (2014). *How ESOPs, profit sharing plans and stock bonus plans differ as employee ownership vehicles.* Oakland, CA: National Center for Employee Ownership. Retrieved from https://www.nceo.org/articles/esops-profit-sharing-stock-bonus-plans

Scales, K. (2018). *Growing a strong direct care workforce: A recruitment and retention guide for employers.* Bronx, NY: PHI Direct Care Workforce Resource Center.

Senge, P. (2000). *The art of the learning organization.* New York, NY: Doubleday.

Shaw, H. (2013). *Sticking points: How to get four generations working together in the 12 places they come apart.* Carol Stream, IL: Tyndale House Publishers.

Singh, D. (2016). *Effective management of long-term care facilities* (3rd ed.). Burlington, MA: Jones and Bartlett.

Society for Human Resource Management. (2019). *What is an EAP?* Retrieved from https://www.shrm.org/resourcesandtools/tools-and-samples/hr-qa/pages/whatisaneap.aspx

Stott, A., Brannon, S., Vasey, J., Dansky, K., & Kemper, P. (2007). Baseline management practices at providers in better jobs better care. *Gerontology and Geriatrics Education, 28*(2), 17–26.

Sullivan, P. (2016, December 9). Combine long-term care with life insurance? Do the numbers first. *New York Times.* Retrieved from https://www.nytimes.com/2016/12/09/your-money/combine-long-term-care-with-life-insurance-do-the-numbers-first.html

Sundararajan, A. (2015). *The gig economy is coming: What will it mean for work?* Retrieved from https://www.theguardian.com/commentisfree/2015/jul/26/will-we-get-by-gig-economy

Tilley, J., Black, K., & Ormond, B. (2003). *Nursing staff ratios for nursing facilities: Findings from case studies of eight.* Washington, DC: The Urban Institute. Retrieved from https://aspe.hhs.gov/basic-report/state-experiences-minimum-nursing-staff-ratios-nursing-facilities-findings-case-studies-eight-states

TOMO Drug Testing. (2015, November 4). *What are the different panel drug tests?* Retrieved from https://www.yourdrugtesting.com/what-are-the-different-panel-drug-tests/

U.S. Department of Health and Human Services, Centers for Medicare & Medicaid Services. (2019). *Staffing data submission—Payroll based journal (PBJ).* Retrieved from https://www.cms.gov/Medicare/Quality-Initiatives-Patient-Assessment-Instruments/NursingHomeQualityInits/Staffing-Data-Submission-PBJ.html

U.S. Department of Homeland Security, Citizenship and Immigration Service. (2019). *I-9: Employment eligibility verification.* Retrieved from https://www.uscis.gov/i-9

U.S. Department of Labor. (2019). *Summary of the major laws of the Department of Labor.* Retrieved from https://www.dol.gov/general/aboutdol/majorlaws

U.S. Department of Labor, Bureau of Labor Statistics. (2018, July 20). *USDL-18-1182: Employee benefits in the United States—March 2018.* Retrieved from https://www.bls.gov/news.release/pdf/ebs2.pdf

U.S. Department of Labor, Veterans Employment and Training Service. (2019). *About USERRA.* Retrieved from https://www.dol.gov/vets/programs/userra/

U.S. Department of Labor, Wage and Hour Division. (2009). *Fact Sheet #54—The health care industry and calculating overtime pay.* Retrieved from https://www.dol.gov/whd/regs/compliance/whdfs54.pdf

U.S. Department of the Treasury, Internal Revenue Service. (2019a). *About form W-2: Wage and tax statement.* Retrieved from https://www.irs.gov/forms-pubs/about-form-w-2

U.S. Department of the Treasury, Internal Revenue Service. (2019b). *De minimis fringe benefits.* Retrieved from https://www.irs.gov/government-entities/federal-state-local-governments/de-minimis-fringe-benefits

U.S Department of the Treasury, Internal Revenue Service. (2019c). *EP abusive tax transactions—Deductions for excess life insurance in a section 412(i) or other defined benefit plan.* Retrieved from https://www.irs.gov/retirement-plans/ep-abusive-tax-transactions-deductions-for -excess-life-insurance-in-a-section-412i-or-other-defined-benefit-plan

U.S. Department of the Treasury, Internal Revenue Service. (2019d). *Health savings accounts.* Retrieved from https://www.treasury.gov/resource-center/faqs/Taxes/Pages/Health-Savings -Accounts.aspx

U.S. Department of the Treasury, Internal Revenue Service. (2019e). *Retirement plan options.* Retrieved from https://www.irs.gov/retirement-plans

U.S. Department of the Treasury, Internal Revenue Service. (2019f). *Topic #510: Business use of car.* Retrieved from https://www.irs.gov/taxtopics/tc510

Wessels, K. (2018). *2018 employee benefits—The evolution of benefits.* Alexandria, VA: The Society for Human Resource Management. Retrieved from https://www.shrm.org/hr-today/trends -and-forecasting/research-and-surveys/Documents/2018%20Employee%20Benefits%20 Report.pdf

Yee-Melichar, D., Boyle, A., & Flores, C. (2011). *Assisted living administration management: Effective practices and model programs in elder care.* New York, NY: Springer Publishing Company.

ADDITIONAL RESOURCES

Hiring—Onboarding

- Custom promotional products can help attract new staff and foster morale:
  - Deluxe Enterprise Operations, LLC. (2020). Available at https://www .deluxe.com/products/promotional/?sscid=21k3_2zq85&affiliateSource =SAS&SSAID=SS876691#.XFhASPZFxPY

- Attracting, onboarding, and retaining employees within the healthcare industry:
  - American Society for Healthcare Human Resources Administration. Available at http://www.naylornetwork.com/ahh-nwl/articles/index-v2.asp ?aid=134767&issueID=22500
  - Orientation checklist. Available at https://fitsmallbusiness.com/wp -content/uploads/2018/06/New-Hire-Orientation-and-Onboarding -Checklist.pdf

- Streamlining the onboarding process by automating much of it with a simple HR platform, such as Zoho People (easy-to-use HR tool that offers employee onboarding, attendance management, time tracking, appraisals, and secure document storage to help manage new hire paperwork, onboarding checklists, and employee records). Available at https://www.zoho.com/people/?utm_source=fitsmallbusiness&utm_medium=cpc&urm_campaign =People

Employee Handbook

Heathfield, S. (2018, December 11). *Employee manual handbook template*. Retrieved from
    https://www.thebalancecareers.com/need-to-know-what-goes-in-an-employee
    -handbook-1918308
Home health agency employee handbook from 21st Century Health Care Consulting. Retrieved
    from https://homehealthmanuals.com/employee-handbook/
Wellhoefer, J. (2018, April 8). *Best practices for creating an engaging employee handbook*. Retrieved
    from https://blog.mcclone.com/employee-handbook-best-practices

Other

42 C.F.R. Section 483. (2020). *Requirements for states and long-term care facilities*. Retrieved from
    https://ecfr.io/Title-42/cfr483_main
Blakely-Gray, R. (2018, November 5). *10 types of paid time off you can offer employees*. Retrieved
    from https://www.patriotsoftware.com/payroll/training/blog/types-of-paid-time-off/
Migoya, D. (2017, August 25). Are you high? The science of testing for marijuana impairment
    is hazy and evolving. *Denver Post*. Retrieved from https://www.denverpost.com/2017/
    08/25/marijuana-impairment-testing/

CHAPTER 4

Financial Management in Senior Care

INTRODUCTION

The importance of financial performance by senior care organizations is paramount to their success and ultimately their survival. The phrase "No margin, no mission" is a popular message in administrative circles and underscores the necessary focus of both key leadership and management staff of organizations to this critical area. The responsibility of financial management may not be the reason someone chose this profession, yet it is required of everyone who chooses this career path. One of the first key things for anyone in a leadership position to know is the basics of healthcare financial management, including basic accounting approaches and reports. Leaders also need a capable support staff based on the ongoing needs and complexity of financial management responsibilities in the senior care continuum. Another step is to gain an awareness of the complexity of reimbursement structures, key cost drivers, and the changing market. An individual also must understand their financial role in the organization and how to use the necessary tools to effectively manage the organization's financial position.

BASIC ACCOUNTING PRINCIPLES

A basic accounting course or background experience is a prerequisite skill set and provides a foundation for any leader or administrator of an organization to build from. An awareness of generally accepted accounting principles (GAAP) and how debits and credits flow through an organization's business office is a good starting point. It is the responsibility of leaders to make sure that they have accurate financial information and records with a good system of checks and balances in place. A few of the key reports that are imperative when assessing the financial information of your organization that individuals will be exposed to include the following:

- **Income Statement:** An income statement reflects the monthly and annual (year-to-date) information derived from revenues and expenses. The report is a historical reflection of decisions made every day and week by the key management team members.

- **Balance Sheet:** The balance sheet is a profile of the assets and liabilities of the organization at a point in time. This report is often described as the measure of the fiscal health or stability of an organization.

- **Cash Flow Statement:** The cash flow statement is tracked on a regular basis and is sometimes associated with a "spend down sheet" used by leaders to assist their team members in paying attention to their ongoing expenses, both expected and unexpected.

- **Financial Ratios:** Financial ratios are also available on a regular basis and used by a variety of individuals within corporations and communities or services sites. These ratios include three broad categories:

  - **Profitability** or **margin ratios** reflect the organization's surplus or deficit of revenues after expenses. A few of the key profitability ratios and their respective formulas are shared here:

    - **Operating margin ratio** is calculated by subtracting your overall expenses from your overall revenues and then dividing by your overall revenue.

    - **Net operating margin ratio** is calculated the same way and also considers other revenues and expenses. This ratio includes the addition of interest income and any change in current asset utilization less interest, depreciation, and amortization expense divided by your total revenue.

    - **Occupancy percentages** in residential care and utilization rates in home- and community-based services (HCBS) are also key indicators to pay attention to.

  - **Liquidity ratios** reflect the ability of an organization to pay off or cover their current liabilities. A few of the key liquidity ratios and their respective formulas are shared in the following:

    - **Current ratio** is calculated by dividing the current assets by the current liabilities.

    - **Days cash on hand** is arrived at by dividing your cash and cash equivalents by your operating expenses less your depreciation divided by 365 days.

    - **Accounts receivable days** are calculated by dividing your total revenue by your resident or client revenues divided by 365 days.

  - **Capital** or **debt ratios** calculate a company's ability to financially leverage itself by comparing its total obligations to total capital available. The focus of these ratios is to give lenders a sense of an organization:

    - **Debt service coverage** measures the ability of an organization to meet its annual debt service needs by dividing its annual income available for making payments by its annual principal and interest payments.

    - **Debt to capitalization ratio** is calculated by dividing the total debt by the debt and current equity combined.

    - **Capital spending ratio** is also used as a measure of reinvestment and is arrived at by dividing the annual capital spending by total revenues.

These key ratios are extremely useful in understanding the financial picture of the organization. The individuals who use these ratios largely depend on the amount of influence or control they have on each of the respective ratios. A couple of good examples would be the current ratio and days in accounts receivable. The current ratio is linked to broader organizational financial goals and may be more in the wheelhouse of the chief financial officer, whereas the days in accounts receivable measure is often driven more by the relationships with both payers and customers and require more site-specific energy and actions by an administrator. An effective leader will have policies and procedures in place for managing the payment collection process and have steps and assigned responsibility for different payer sources and acceptable or unacceptable time frames identified for staff to use as a guide for effective payment collection approaches.

STAFF SUPPORT AND INVOLVEMENT

One of the necessary elements of financial success for senior care and services leaders is the ability to depend on their staff. A key hire or existing working relationship is their point person for all accounting and office functions of the organization. This role may be referred to as the CFO, business office director, or office manager and is usually directly responsible for financial functions. Administrative trust in this person to be on top of all the processes of the office—for example, accounts payable, accounts receivable, payroll, and management of resident funds—can make or break the organizational financial performance. At another level, depending on the size and scope of the senior care and service offerings, each of these processes may have a designated staff member focused on each of these respective business-related processes. Each of the department or service line managers within the organization also depends on this core group of office-related staff. It is imperative for all managers to work with the CFO so they can get the necessary information that will assist them with the operation of each of their areas.

BUDGETING

The need for a good budgeting approach and system with all senior care organizations is critical to their annual financial health and performance. Knowing how to effectively prepare and utilize a budget is a necessary skill for all leaders and managers in this field. Budgeting should also be viewed as an extension of a strategic plan and operating goals expressed in numbers.

A good operating budget is a best estimate of the expected revenues and expenses over a defined period, which in most cases is a year. A good budget is a tool for monitoring the flow of revenues and expenses of an organization and in senior care. A couple of the key drivers are utilization projections in HCBS and projected occupancy in the residential care settings. One of the biggest expenses in all senior care services is the key cost driver of labor or staffing, which includes all the extra expenses of overtime, the associated fringe benefits, and potential temporary pool utilization.

Another key feature that needs to be understood is that a budget should serve as a financial guide and allow for adjustments or flexibility depending on internal changes or changes in the marketplace. A budget is both fixed and variable expenses and, depending on care and service needs or demand (occupancy or utilization levels), variable expenses, such as staffing or supplies, may need to be adjusted. A proactive leader is always paying attention to both the budget and actual performance, is cognizant of the needs within the organization, and is attentive to the resources of the organization.

One last factor to consider is the level of involvement of the multiple levels of persons responsible for the budget or their accountability for their respective areas or departments, for example, department heads. Clearly, the more involved people are in the development of a budget, the more buy-in, and acceptance they will have for any required accountability for a specific area, service line, or organization.

Think of financial management as goal setting (budgeting) and goal attainment (adherence to the financial plan). Financial management is, at its core, managing assets to achieve your goals and objectives. Lastly, always remember your mission when you allocate resources, whether financial or other. Are you making decisions that ultimately improve the lives of those you serve?

Bob Seibel,
President, Carriage Health Care

Capital Budgeting

Capital budgeting is another component that is important for any organization serving the current and changing needs of seniors. Generally, this process involves larger purchases or expenses that are characterized as assets that would have a life expectancy of over a year. A few examples of capital budget items include major equipment, remodeling or expansion projects, or investment in new programs or services. Once again, involvement in the process generally results in a better, more accepted final product.

An example of steps to develop a capital budget is as follows:

1. Decide on the amount of money set aside for the next year.
2. Request ideas, including actual descriptions and costs from the management team.
3. Consolidate and share the list.
4. Agree on some key values that are important for making decisions, such as improvement of customer care or satisfaction, mitigating risk or enhancing safety, employee productivity, new product or revenue growth, market position, and return on investment.
5. Have each person representing departments or service lines share their needs.
6. Use a nominal group process to vote.
7. Share the results of the vote and what might be included in the capital budget of the next year.

This is just an example of one process, which involves a lot of confidence and trust in the management team of an organization. A leader who uses this type of process may still want to maintain final authority for making any necessary revisions based on their broader perspective of the needs of the organization, market, and any other organizational considerations. This final decision authority is usually accepted well by the department or service line–related managers if stated up front at the beginning of the process.

FINANCING AND SOURCES OF CAPITAL

Before discussing the various arrangements used for financing by organizations, it makes sense for one to understand the ownership structure of the broader continuum. This is important because the ownership type does make a difference in the type of financing and source of capital an organization may use. Table 4.1 gives a snapshot of the environment in place in a given year (Harris-Kojetin et al., 2019).

Administrators must be aware of the sources of capital that can support the property and upkeep costs of their building or operation. There are a variety of ways to arrange financing and capital debt structure, such as for-profit, nonprofit, or government guaranteed financing arrangements.

TABLE 4.1 Ownership Type by Senior Service Area in a Given Year

		Service Type				
Ownership %		Adult Day Center	Home Care	Hospice	Skilled Nursing Facility	Residential Care Facility
	For-profit	44.7	80.6	63	69.3	81
	Nonprofit	50.8	14.8	22.8	23.5	17.7
	Government	4.6	4.6	14.1	7.2	1.3

The following are short descriptions of each of these approaches.

For-Profit Sources of Capital

There are different sources of capital each with its own requirements and investment goals. They fall into two general categories: debt financing, which involves borrowing money and paying it back with interest; and equity financing, where resources are invested in the organization in exchange for part ownership. Some of the more common arrangements are described in the following:

- Lending institutions comprise a variety of alternatives for acquiring capital for a new development, remodeling project, or new company. Commercial banks are one traditional source of capital with a set mortgage term and interest rate. An investment bank is in the business of raising capital, and often, it may be in the form of bonds. Bonds can be issued using a fixed or variable rate, and bond investors receive a promise from the borrower to repay the principal and a percentage of the par value as interest at a specified date. The investment banker structures the project's financing, and an underwriter distributes the bonds to the investing public (including institutional and retail investors). There are also tax-exempt bonds available, which may be particularly attractive to nonprofit groups.

■ There are also a multitude of for-profit ownership arrangements in place with various organizations. These can range from an independently financed owner (sole proprietor) all the way to a publicly traded S corporation, with a plethora of options in between. A few arrangements that are noteworthy include the following:

■ Limited liability corporation (LLC), whereby the owners are not personally liable for the company's debts or liabilities. LLCs are hybrid entities that combine the characteristics of a corporation with those of a partnership or sole proprietorship and are common within the assisted living world and regional skilled nursing facilities (SNFs).

■ A real estate investment trust (REIT) is essentially a pool of investor dollars used to acquire healthcare real estate assets. These are typically large companies that have a portfolio of products and are involved in acquiring mortgages and in some cases mortgage-related assets.

■ Employee-owned companies (or employee stock ownership plan [ESOP]). Lastly, there also appears to be a growing number of organizations that are becoming employee owned across the continuum. For example, in the home healthcare arena, there are a large number of organizations that are independently owned and have individuals looking for an exit strategy, and this appears to be an attractive strategy for the noncorporation entities.

Nonprofit Sources of Capital

In the nonprofit space, there are also some fund development or "fundraising" efforts that work well for these organizations. They use major development campaigns to help fund projects or build endowments for both their current and future needs. With the majority of giving in this country being largely from individuals, it is important for progressive boards and leaders to be in a relationship with their constituencies. Customers and families are appreciative of the services they receive and are generally open to hearing about the needs of the organization. Leaders need to be personally involved in development efforts, committed to the needs of the organization, and both visible and visionary in their actions. Leaders also need to be comfortable and willing to ask prospective supporters for their financial backing. An organized and board-supported effort is much more likely to succeed, and nonprofit leaders as well as others should be appropriately trained to guide this activity for both annual fundraising and major campaign or development efforts.

Government Sources of Capital

In the senior care field, there are also several entities that are supported by government-related structures, such as city-, county-, or state-owned properties. This is more common in the SNF field with these government-affiliated organizations sponsored by taxes and their corresponding revenues, with elected officials serving as the ownership group. The financing arrangements may include a number of the previously mentioned sources, but they also may benefit from other government-backed programs These government-affiliated sites will often have separate board or oversight committees established to work with the administrator to provide oversight for these properties. In the home- and community-based service arena, a number of home health entities are affiliated with government-sponsored public health service programs. There is also the presence of veteran's senior care communities and services sponsored by the military branches of the government.

Traditional sources of debt capital include the following:

- Government-sponsored sources, such as the Federal National Mortgage Association (FNMA), commonly known as Fannie Mae, or the Department of Housing and Urban Development (HUD)
- Lending institutions, such as commercial banks or finance companies
- Federal Housing Administration (FHA) and tax-exempt bonds
- The U.S. Department of Agriculture (USDA) is also involved in rural housing development projects

Leverage typically ranges from 60% to 80% for secured debt instruments.

Equity financing can be arranged with either public or private real estate investment companies that have equity ownership positions. Organizational operators may also own a significant portion of their communities. Private equity firms also may have a role in the capital structure and tend to seek shorter-term investments.

Lease financing is typically provided by investment companies such as public and private REITs. Because lease financing is normally capitalized at the corporate level through the capital markets, properties financed with leases are often considered as having 100% financing often with longer-term expectations.

Recently, some REITs are using a partnership structure under the REIT Investment and Diversification and Empowerment Act (RIDEA) of 2007, which allows REITs to keep a share of the building's operating income and not just the lease payments (National Investment Center [NIC], 2019).

All these arrangements are significantly influenced by the operating incomes (or losses) generated by the revenue sources and projections that are influenced by government programs, insurance revenues, and the private out-of-pocket payments from consumers. In summary, the capital structure for senior care and service properties comes from a few primary sources: debt, equity, lease capital, government programs, and donations.

Successful people I have known have depended on good mentorship from and with others with experience in this broad field. You also need to always remember that financial decisions are fundamentally an evaluation of risk and reward. For new leaders, find a mentor that understands that concept and listen carefully to their advice.

Don Husi,
Managing Director, Ziegler

PAYMENT SOURCES AND REIMBURSEMENT

The field of senior care has a wide range of services, and each of those services has a distinct set of revenue streams. It is important for the leader of any of the senior care organizations to have a fundamental understanding of the foundation of payment sources, which includes Medicaid, Medicare, insurance programs, private funding, and other alternative sources of payments.

Medicaid

Medicaid is a program that was put into place in 1965 to serve as a safety net for the poor and disabled poor in the country. This program is a means-tested program, and beyond those elderly patients, it is also available for both disabled persons and children with disabilities. The Children's Health Insurance Program (CHIP; formerly SCHIP) eligibility is coordinated today under state agencies and part of the health insurance exchanges in the Patient Protection and Affordable Care Act (ACA). Medicaid waivers under Section 1915(c) of the Social Security Act support HCBS based on the *Olmstead v. L.C.* (527 U.S. 581) court decision. Medicaid is also available for HCBS or managed care (under Section 1915(b)). This is often used to provide a hospital/skilled level of care in the community. Each state has its own approach and set of waivers available that can be found on the Centers for Medicare & Medicaid Services (CMS) website (Medicaid.gov, 2019). These waiver programs also apply to assisted living facilities based on means testing requirements.

The more traditional use of Medicaid dollars in senior care applies to SNFs. Under this program, individuals of any age can qualify for Medicaid (means-tested) resources. Individuals can have up to 133% of the federal poverty level (FPL) under terms in the ACA. A few other Medicaid funding factors include the following:

- They must also satisfy residency/citizenship requirements.
- Eligibility can be determined based upon qualification for and receipt of monies under Supplemental Security Income rules, which is also a means-tested program; eligibility can be governed by states.
- States participating in Medicaid *must* cover certain populations and can elect to cover more than what is required.

The Medicaid program is funded 50% by the federal government and 50% by each state, although some states have a larger federal contribution (e.g., 60%/40%, based on population).

Medicare

Medicare is a federally funded program established in 1965 for those 65 and older requiring the use of healthcare services. The Medicare program has four parts that are summarized as follows:

Part A covers hospital care (inpatient), SNF care, nursing home (NH) care, hospice, and home health services.

Part B covers medically necessary services on an outpatient basis (diagnose/treat medical condition), preventive services (healthcare to prevent illness/early detection), and ambulance services, medical equipment, and some mental healthcare.

Part C covers voluntary supplemental insurance known as Medicare Advantage plans (formerly "Medicare + Choice") usually organized as health maintenance organizations (HMOs)/preferred provider organizations (PPOs). These are private insurance plans that manage benefits under Parts A, B, and D. Each plan must be approved by the CMS under the Medicare program rules and can also cover other services such as vision and dental care.

Part D covers prescription drug plans (PDPs), which provide insurance for the costs of prescription drugs, which can be a significant cost for many seniors. These plans are often managed by pharmaceutical benefit managers, which serve as the intermediaries between the drug companies and the insurance company.

Medicare criteria, eligibility, and approaches are as follows:

- Age 65 or older
- Eligible for Social Security Disability Insurance (SSDI) or Railroad Retirement Board (RRB) benefits
- Traditionally, those who are blind or disabled in some way
- Anyone with end-stage renal disease (ESRD), including regular dialysis treatments or kidney transplant, and eUnidentifiedligible for other benefits
- Must also satisfy residency/citizenship requirements

Medicare is funded 100% by the federal government (via tax dollars), and individuals are automatically enrolled in Medicare Part A, the same way they are eligible for Social Security. Participation is voluntary for Parts B and D, and in some cases, private benefits may provide better coverage than Parts B and D. Penalties can also be assessed if enrolling late or outside enrollment periods (and sometimes cannot enroll outside of the designated time frames). As mentioned, Part C is also voluntary and is considered a supplemental plan that can vary depending on insurance program (although this still needs to be approved by the CMS).

Medigap Plans

There are also coverage options frequently called "Medigap plans," which are private insurance plans that are purchased to fill in the "gaps" provided under Medicare Parts A and B. These plans must be identified as "Medicare Supplement Insurance" plans to be valid and can cover all of a particular benefit or only a certain percentage. This product is also state dependent, whereas some states have implemented standardization of plan guidelines that other states have not advanced or implemented. Some of the examples of benefits covered include the following:

- Covering deductibles and coinsurance payments under Parts A and B
- Costs of blood transfusion (e.g., first 3 pints)
- SNF care coinsurance
- Excess charges over Medicare covered rates

The difference between a Medicap plan and Medicare Advantage plan is that although both are private insurance plans, the Medigap plan is supplemental and covers most if not all the noncovered other costs, for example, copayments and deductibles, of the Medicare program.

Private Health Insurance

General health insurance may have limited coverage for long-term care (LTC) services, but often these plans are focused on the typical approach to insurance for the general public. The market for specific LTC coverage has evolved a bit, and LTC plans have a range of choices and prices. Some of the considerations include the following:

- Whether home- and community-based care/services are included
- Dollar amount of benefits
- Cost of premiums, copayments, and deductibles
- Length of coverage
- Elimination period, which is the time from use to payment

The amount of LTC insurance covering specific services has grown incrementally over the years but still is a small portion of revenue for most services.

Skilled Nursing Facilities

One of the models of reimbursement that has replaced the fee for service approach in skilled nursing is the prospective payment system. This methodology is basically a per diem, all-inclusive rate based on case mix (a reflection of acuity level). The base rate is determined by the mean costs of various SNFs adjusted for inflation and wages and then using a case mix adjuster for each resident to reflect resource costs. More recently, Medicare has advanced a new patient-driven payment model (discussed later in this chapter) that also incorporates therapy needs and expenses of short stay skilled nursing in a bundled payment model.

The pie chart in Figure 4.1 illustrates the various payment sources comprising the skilled nursing environment including those affiliated with Continuing

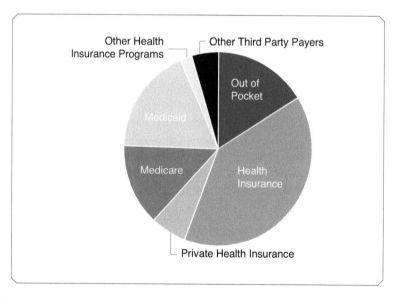

Figure 4.1 Nursing Care Facilities and Continuing Care Retirement Communities Expenditures by Source of Funds: 2018

Source: Data from Centers for Medicare & Medicaid Services. (2018b). *Office of the actuary. National health care expenditures.* Retrieved from https://www.cms.gov/Research-Statistics-Data-and-Systems/Statistics-Trends-and-Reports/NationalHealthExpendData/NHE-Fact-Sheet

Care Retirement Communities, which reflect most dollars accounted for being reimbursed by Medicaid, Medicare, and health insurance (which may be a government-contracted insurance). It is reported by the National Investment Center (2018) that skilled nursing centers are depending on approximately 50% of their revenues from Medicaid. Private reimbursement for SNFs is usually at a higher rate to allow providers to cross-subsidize the rates historically set at a lower rate than even expenses in many cases. There are still some states that have an equal pay rate law, which does not allow organizations to charge a differential.

Assisted Living Facilities

Financing for assisted living facilities comes from multiple sources, yet most people still pay out-of-pocket for room and board and the services they receive. Payment methodologies range from all-inclusive rates to the other side of the spectrum, which has a basic rate for rental with most other services billed a la carte based on the tenant's need and use of services. In some cases, private LTC insurance policies can support assisted living residence, especially the care-related features. For those with limited income and assets (at the option of each state), Medicaid can finance the cost of the services provided to eligible individuals, excluding room and board. The HHS survey (National Health Policy Forum, 2013) found that 43% of residential care facilities had at least one resident whose services were paid by Medicaid. However, of all these facility residents, only 19% had their care financed by Medicaid. State Medicaid agencies can provide services, including the section 1915(c) HCBS waiver program and other Medicaid state plan options. The most frequently used Medicaid option for financing services, such as home health aide, personal care, and homemaker services, for Medicaid-eligible residents is found in Section

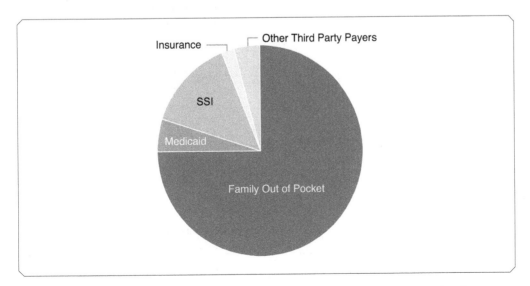

Figure 4.2 Assisted Living Expenditures Percentage Distribution by Source of Funds

SSI, supplemental security income.

Source: Data from National Care Planning Council. (2002). *Guide to long term care planning.* https://www.longtermcarelink.net/eldercare/assisted_living.htm

1915(c) of the HCBS waiver program. A recent report by the Department of Health and Human Services (DHHS) Office of the Inspector General (OIG) found that, in 2009, 35 state Medicaid programs covered services for more than 54,000 Medicaid beneficiaries in 12,000 facilities under 40 waiver programs of Section 1915(c). The total annual cost to the Medicaid program was estimated at $1.7 billion at the time, with an average annual cost of $31,000 per resident. The recent data would probably suggest that Figure 4.2 would likely have a greater percentage of Medicaid utilization than when the assessment was originally done, and less supplemental security income.

Home Care and Hospice Services

The home care and hospice reimbursement formulas are quite different with Medicare accounting for over 40% and the remaining portion being a combination of other state/local government contributions, private insurance, and out-of-pocket expenses paid by the client or family (Figure 4.3). The reimbursement methodology varies once again but does use some of the Medicare approaches used by other settings with a prospective payment system in place. The Outcome and Assessment Information Set (OASIS) is the quality reporting system for home care that also drives the Medicare A reimbursement based on condition and needs.

The Balanced Budget Act of 1997, as amended by the Omnibus Consolidated and Emergency Supplemental Appropriations Act (OCESAA) of 1999, called for the development and implementation of a prospective payment system (PPS) for Medicare home health services. Under the prospective payment, Medicare pays home health agencies (HHAs) a predetermined base payment. The home health PPS is composed of some key features, including the following:

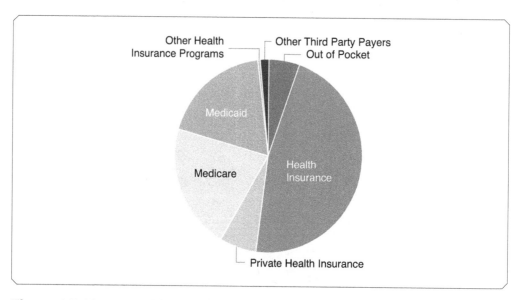

Figure 4.3 Home Healthcare Expenditures Percentage Distribution by Source of Funds: 2018

Source: Data from Centers for Medicare & Medicaid Services. (2018b). *Office of the actuary. National health care expenditures.* Retrieved from https://www.cms.gov/Research-Statistics-Data-and-Systems/Statistics-Trends-and-Reports/NationalHealthExpendData/NHE-Fact-Sheet

- Payment for the 60-day episode, which can be renewed based on condition
- Case mix adjustment, which adjusts payment for a beneficiary's condition and needs using the OASIS categories
- Adjustments for beneficiaries who change locations or are discharged and readmitted within a 60-day episode
- Consolidated billing requires all services to be in a bundled rate, except for durable medical equipment

Medicare pays providers an initial payment of approximately 50% of the expected expenses and then adjusts the final payment based on a review and actual costs.

Costs of Care

The approximate median monthly costs of care for each of these service lines vary across the states and depend a great deal on the type of services required by an individual resident, tenant, or client. The median monthly costs for a private room in a skilled care facility is $8,500, assisted living care and service is $4,000, and in-home care is $4,300 (based on 44 hours/week) were reported in a recent study done by Genworth (2018) over the past 14 years. As discussed, there also are a variety of payment types, which also drive reimbursement rates depending on the source and type of payment.

General Insurance Trends Across LTC Service Lines

On a broader level in terms of commercial LTC insurance across the senior service continuum, recent data focused on LTC revenue sources indicates that individuals are paying for over a quarter of the services, and that private insurance contributes to a quarter of that portion.

LTC insurance policies remain a relatively modest portion of revenue based on slow growth and even a declining rate of purchasing of these products. The key factors associated with this challenge appear to be high costs of premiums, the inability of individuals likely to use services to be eligible based on a condition, and the societal tendency to not view the services offered as attractive options (Stevenson, Cohen, Tell, & Burwell, 2010). One current trend is the formation of LTC insurance partnership programs with states to allow a benefit described as "dollar-for-dollar" asset disregard or "spend down" protection. Individuals who purchase a policy in a state with this program "earn" one dollar of Medicaid asset disregard for every dollar of insurance coverage paid on their behalf. This type of program may help raise the value of purchasing a policy if the insurance premiums can be set an affordable rate (American Association for Long-Term Care Insurance, 2019).

Private out-of-pocket payment is a major source of revenue, especially in the assisted living and senior housing fields. The private rate setting approaches for each of these lines of service follow the methodology highlighted as follows.

The skilled care market historically charged on a nonbundled rate, which means that ancillary services are extra; for example, private rooms and rehabilitation. The other extra amenities generally fetch a premium rate. For certified facilities, rates are often higher than Medicare and Medicaid rates on an all-inclusive basis. This is set up to help the facilities offset lower Medicaid rates and is called cross-subsidization, which is important to consider. In some states, they have rate equalization (e.g., Minnesota), which means that the private pay rate cannot be greater than the daily Medicaid reimbursement rate set by the state. The other element that needs consideration is that organizations must also look at the competitive marketplace. There is also the provision of managed care that set its rates on a negotiated basis considering the acuity needs and the quality of the facility. Metrics are increasingly becoming important to organizations, so they are in network with groups or managed care organizations.

Accountable care organizations (ACOs) are now being advanced, and there is a system that defines these ACOs based on their inception date. ACOs are organizations that have voluntarily decided to participate, accept, and pool risk with a set of other providers with the intention that a coordinated care approach will provide better quality and ultimately save dollars. The senior care field has started to more aggressively move to not just being a contractor with ACO systems but rather to have entered more intentional and advanced strategic partnerships with other providers; for example, hospitals, physician groups, and major insurance groups (which may still offset the risk levels of provider partners).

The most recent model of payment is the patient-driven payment model implemented in October 2019. It comprises two primary factors: base rates that correspond to each component of payment illustrated in Figure 4.4, and the case-mix

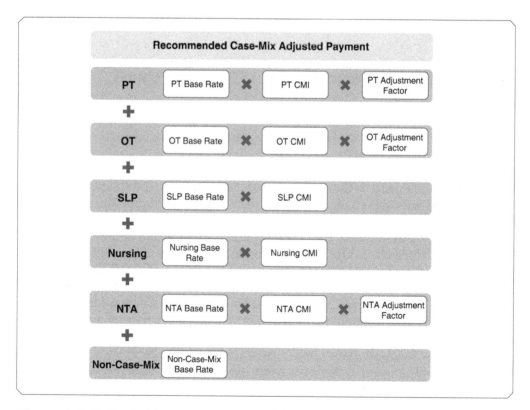

Figure 4.4 Patient-driven payment model

CMI, case-mix index; NTA, nontherapy ancillary; OT, occupational therapy; PT, physical therapy; SLP, speech-language pathology.

Source: Centers for Medicare & Medicaid Services. (2018a). *Skilled nursing facilities patient-driven payment model technical report.* Retrieved from https://www.cms.gov/Medicare/Medicare-Fee -for-Service-Payment/SNFPPS/Downloads/PDPM_Technical_Report_508.pdf

index (CMI) that corresponds to each payment group. The focus of the model is to focus on a resident's condition and care needs, rather than the amount of care provided, to determine reimbursement levels.

The big change in this new model is that therapy costs are included in the overall payment rate. This new approach has been recently implemented, and the expectation is that the success of the program will be evaluated in the years ahead.

In the home care arena, the model is slightly different and is called the patient-driven grouping model (PDGM). Beginning January 1, 2020, the PDGM relies more on clinical characteristics and other patient information to place home health periods of care into meaningful payment categories and eliminates the use of therapy service thresholds. These categories include admission source, timing, clinical grouping, functional impairment, and an adjustment for comorbidity. In conjunction with the implementation of the PDGM, there will be a change in the unit of home health payment from a 60-day episode to a 30-day period. This is another attempt of the CMS to move toward a value-based payment model across the spectrum.

The future of payment models can be summarized by the following key areas and trends and innovations in the industry.

1. The role of two-sided risk arrangements, including ACOs, alternative payment model (APMs), and bundles
2. Medicare's changing reimbursement system as evidenced by PDGM
3. Continued growth and new flexibilities for Medicare advantage plans, including special needs plans (SNPs) and other demonstration projects
4. Initiatives that continue to push for collaboration and coordination across network efforts

The conclusion is that quality approaches and payment models will continue to evolve and change as we face the changing demographics and corresponding care and service demands for this country. The leader of an organization in the senior care continuum must stay both current and well versed in the payment model landscape to anticipate how any changes will impact the fiscal health of their organization.

OTHER IMPORTANT FINANCIAL CONSIDERATIONS FOR SENIOR LIVING ORGANIZATIONS

Antifraud Programs

Fraud and abuse are concerns of the public for any program that has government funding, but it needs even more scrutiny in the field of senior care because of the complexity of reimbursement and volume of dollars associated with Medicare and Medicaid programs. The integrity of organizations is paramount for the practice of fiscally responsible approaches. Fraud and abuse can fall into six general categories:

1. Billing for unnecessary services or unauthorized services
2. Billing for service not rendered by the organization
3. Upcoding or billing for services at a level of complexity higher than required
4. Unbundling or billing for services separately when they should be reported in an overall rate

5. Kickback or receiving gifts or renumeration in exchange for services or preferential treatment

6. Medical identity theft or inappropriate use of a patient's medical or other information

The Office of the Inspector General in concert with the DHHS has both antifraud programs and an approach to both investigation and sanctions or penalties.

Risk Management

The concept of risk management encompasses a few different areas. Programs that reduce risk factors that may lead to action that damages the facility's reputation or results in economic loss.

Risk management programs are designed to identify and solve problems before they get out of hand and to prevent lawsuits. The focus of risk management is assessing the following risk factors:

- Inadequate training and supervision of employees
- Inadequate policies and procedures
- Use of restraints or other resident care procedures
- Inadequate safety and security measures
- Failure to comply with applicable regulations

Functions of a strong risk management program include the following:

- Identification of methods to mitigate risk exposure in a healthcare setting
- Recognition of environmental and occupational risk exposures
- Application of risk control techniques to reduce errors and increase resident safety
- Utilization of quality improvement techniques and tools

The typical program components for the continuum of care with a few common examples are illustrated in Table 4.2

Cybersecurity is also a current risk management concern with the shift to the electronic use, management, and transfer of both patient and employee data. A data security breach occurs when there is a loss or theft of, or other unauthorized access to, sensitive, personally identifiable information that could result in the compromise of the confidentiality or integrity of data. Most states have laws requiring notification of security breaches involving personal information. It is imperative that a leader has a proactive approach to keeping data polices up-to-date and working well for their information needs.

Liability

Regarding liability, senior care and service leaders are subject to two types:

Professional liability for administrators or directors is for injuries to a resident or patient caused by breach of duty on the part of a healthcare professional in their employ.

TABLE 4.2 Common Risk Management Items for Different Care and Service Settings

Components\ Service Examples	Skilled Nursing Facility	Assisted Living	Home Care
Clinical	Timely and accurate minimum data set	Preadmission screening to handle medical complexity	Fall-related evaluation
Operational	Workplace safety and health hazards	Safe environment should be provided for all residents	Abuse in an independent environment
Business	Contracts and antikickback provisions	Resident contracts should contain all the facility's commitments and actual practices	Travel-related autorisks

General liability involves all other claims that do not involve the standards or quality of care or service provided by licensed practitioners—claims citing the failure of the organization as a whole to provide safe, appropriate care and service.

For most people involved in organizational leadership, the general insurance policy should have coverage for the individual acting as an agent of the organization in good faith. The organization should also have a good property and casualty insurance plan in place.

Leaders should also have a good relationship with designated legal counsel for the organization and use it as a resource for administrative legal areas, including needs of an individual or themselves, a situation or organizational issue. Legal assistance should also be used for the development and review of agreements and contracts, application of any federal and state laws that may require interpretation, and any pertinent or particularly sensitive policies and procedures. One of the innovative ways that some organizations have attempted to be proactive and avoid any type of litigation with either customer or employee issues is to create a corporate compliance "hot line." The purpose of these "hot lines" is to create another more independent sounding board and vehicle for addressing issues.

Another significant element of financial health is the effective management of a worker's compensation program. Each of the lines of service in the senior care field is labor intensive and often in a very demanding work environment. The keys to a strong program include working in partnership with a progressive insurance carrier or agent; evaluating both your workforce and your work environment for risk and proactively making any positive changes; and promptly responding to any worker's compensation claims and having an effective back-to-work program.

REPORTS

A successful administrator will understand the different types of reports and their use in making sure the organization is headed in the right direction financially. Key reports that all senior care leaders will rely on include the following.

- **Dashboards** inspired by the balanced scorecard (Kaplan & Norton, 1996) are data that provide a means of monitoring, measuring, and analyzing relevant data sets in several key performance areas while displaying aggregated information in a way that is both intuitive and visual. They offer a comprehensive overview of their company's various internal departments, goals, initiatives, processes, or projects. These are measured with key performance indicators (KPIs), which provide insights that help to foster improvement. Senior living CEOs point largely to three key areas they are measuring: occupancy and census, revenue, and staffing. They are also looking closely at resident satisfaction, sales and marketing activity, and any care or service changes that are taking place in their communities or organizations. There is also a trend to take full advantage of today's technology platforms with this product.

- **Cost reports** are financial reports that identify the cost and charges related to healthcare activities. Medicare-certified institutional providers are required to submit an annual cost report to a Medicare Administrative Contractor (MAC). The cost report contains provider information such as facility characteristics, utilization data, cost and charges by cost center (in total and for Medicare), Medicare settlement data, and financial statement data.

- An **audit** is an official inspection of an individual's or organization's accounts, typically by an independent body. This should also be dependable and fairly presented financials that help organizations and their ownership or governing body groups make some quality decisions. The key to the audit is that the information is accurate, unbiased, objective financial information that can be used with a variety of stakeholders.

- **Tax returns** are also critically important to the senior care continuum of services, especially considering the variety of ownership structures. It is essential that the leadership feels comfortable with the accounting firm or organization preparing the returns, and a key is to make sure that there is a good understanding of the necessary information and the timing exchange.

These reports are rather common practice yet are essential for maintaining the financial health of the organization. An effective leader will have proactive policies and procedures in place within the healthcare financial management arenas.

SUMMARY

It is critically important that an administrator or director is comfortable with the financial management responsibilities of their role, including the basic foundational skills of accounting and budgeting. A leader also must understand financial management strategies and the nuances of different payment sources in the senior care continuum of services. There are also a variety of applications and approaches that support the financial health of the organization and are necessary to have in place. The effective administrator or director of the senior care organization also has to commit to staying abreast and current with the changing environment of the healthcare financial system being driven by the move from a volume to value-based payment model and philosophy.

KEY POINTS

1. Foundational financial skills are a prerequisite to be a healthcare manager.
2. Key financial indicators and reports can serve as effective tools.
3. The diversity of ownership in senior care drives a variety of financing approaches.
4. Senior care and services have a complex payment and reimbursement system.
5. Several related functions are critical to solid financial performance, including paying attention to the ongoing changes.

LEADERSHIP ROLES

1. Guide the organization financially: "The buck stops here"
2. Know how to budget and employ financial strategies
3. Support the accountability of key management personnel
4. Understand the variety of related tools and reports
5. Grasp the complex health and service payment models

HIGH-IMPACT PRACTICES

1. Developing a strong financial management team with continued investment in ongoing education and making resources available to stay current with changes
2. Making sure there are proactive approaches and policies in place so that the organization is supporting managers with information and staying ahead of the necessary functions
3. Practicing appropriate transparency with the leaders within and affiliated with the organization, so that there are fewer surprises when navigating the road map of financial improvement and success

QUESTIONS FOR DISCUSSION

1. How does a leader know if they are financially fit when it comes to knowledge level?
2. What are the resources an emerging leader would want to use to make sure they are up to date with both current and proposed reimbursement systems?
3. How much does a leader need to be in the loop with the financial interests of the ownership of the senior care organization?
4. Where can someone find resources for all the related financial applications and needs of the organization?

CASE PROBLEMS

1. Some SNFs are facing the challenge of decreased occupancy due to outdated physical plants. The decision to invest in an older building is a big one and needs to be navigated wisely so that resources are used well. How would you get the right people and organizations involved in an early discussion about the future? List all the necessary stakeholders and how their role might be helpful. Conversely discuss the risks of moving forward.

2. Assisted living approaches vary when it comes to extra services and how they charge for them based on both their operational and financial performance, along with their position in their marketplace. Consider the pros and cons of bundled services and alternatively an a la carte approach. What are the factors that one would need to consider before advancing any recommendations?

3. A senior care continuing care organization is considering expanding their home care services. What are the different internal and external ways this could be done and how would capacity, expertise, and funding streams factor into the decision? Discuss the pros and cons of each of your approaches.

NAB DOMAINS OF PRACTICE

30.01 Ensure that financial management policies, procedures, and practices comply with applicable federal and state regulations.

30.02 Develop, implement, and evaluate the service provider's budget.

30.03 Oversee the billing and collections process and monitor the accuracy of charges and timely collection of accounts.

30.04 Negotiate, interpret, and implement contractual agreements to optimize financial viability.

30.05 Develop, implement, monitor, and evaluate financial policies and procedures that comply with Generally Accepted Accounting Principles (GAAP).

30.06 Monitor and evaluate the integrity of financial reporting systems and audit programs.

30.07 Establish safeguards for the protection of the service provider's assets (such as insurance coverage, risk management).

30.08 Develop, implement, monitor, and evaluate systems to improve financial performance.

30.09 Manage and adjust expenses with fluctuations in census/occupancy/ care recipient levels (such as staffing rations).

30.10 Monitor and address changes in the industry that may affect financial viability.

Source: Reproduced with permission from the National Association of Long-Term Care Administrator Boards. (2016). *Annotation of tasks performed and knowledge and skills used across lines of service in long term care.* Retrieved from https://www.nabweb.org/filebin/pdf/Annotation_of_Tasks_Performed_Across_LOS_in_LTC.pdf

REFERENCES

American Association for Long-Term Care Insurance. (2019). *Long term care insurance partnership plans.* Retrieved from https://www.aaltci.org/long-term-care-insurance/learning-center/long-term-care-insurance-partnership-plans.php

Centers for Medicare & Medicaid Services. (2018a). *Skilled nursing facilities patient-driven payment model technical report.* Retrieved from https://www.cms.gov/Medicare/Medicare-Fee-for-Service-Payment/SNFPPS/Downloads/PDPM_Technical_Report_508.pdf

Centers for Medicare & Medicaid Services. (2018b). *Office of the actuary. National health care expenditures.* Retrieved from https://www.cms.gov/Research-Statistics-Data-and-Systems/Statistics-Trends-and-Reports/NationalHealthExpendData/NHE-Fact-Sheet

Genworth. (2018). *Cost of care study.* Retrieved from https://www.genworth.com/aging-and-you/finances/cost-of-care/cost-of-care-trends-and-insights.html

Harris-Kojetin, L., Sengupta, M., Lendon, J. P., Rome, V., Valverde, R., & Caffrey, C. (2019). Long-term care providers and services users in the United States, 2015–2016. National Center for Health Statistics. *Vital and Health Statistics, 3*(43).

Kaplan, R. S., & Norton, D. (1996). Using the balanced scorecard as a strategic management system. *Harvard Business Review, 74*(1), 75–85.

Medicaid.gov. (2019). *Statewide transition plan for home and community based services.* Retrieved from https://www.medicaid.gov/medicaid/home-community-based-services/statewide-transition-plans/index.html

National Care Planning Council. (2002). *Guide to long term care planning.* https://www.longtermcarelink.net/eldercare/assisted_living.htm

National Health Policy Forum. (2013). *The basics of assisted living: Facilities, financing, and oversight.* Washington, DC: George Washington University. Retrieved from http://www.nhpf.org/library/the-basics/Basics_AssistedLiving_01-29-13.pdf

National Investment Center. (2018). *Skilled nursing data report.* Retrieved from https://info.nic.org/hubfs/Skilled%20Nursing/4Q17%20SNF%20Release/Skilled%20Nursing%20Report%20-%204Q17%20SNF.pdf

National Investment Center. (2019). *Industry participants in the seniors housing & care property market and their business models.* Retrieved from https://www.nic.org/industry-resources/industry-faqs/industry-participants-seniors-housing-care-property-market-business-models/

Stevenson, D., Cohen, M., Tell, E., & Burwell, B. (2010). The complementarity of public and private long-term care coverage. *Health Affairs, 29*(1), 96–101. doi:10.1377/hlthaff.2009.0920

ADDITIONAL RESOURCES

AARP: http://www.aarp.org/health/health-insurance/info-06-2012/understanding-long-term-care-insurance.html

American Health Care Association: https://www.ahcancal.org/facility_operations/privacysecurity/Pages/RiskAssessmentSecurityTools.aspx

Occupational Safety and Health Administration: https://www.osha.gov/SLTC/nursinghome/hazards_solutions.html

U.S. Centers for Medicare & Medicaid: https://www.cms.gov/Medicare-Medicaid-Coordination/Fraud-Prevention/Medicaid-Integrity-Education/Downloads/nursinghome-provider-booklet.pdf; https://www.cms.gov/Medicare/Quality-Initiatives-Patient-Assessment-Instruments/HomeHealthQualityInits/index.html

There are also a variety of accounting and capital management firms focused in the senior care field that will serve as great resources for emerging leaders.

Other

Indiana University Lilly Family School of Philanthropy at IUPUI. (2019). *Giving USA 2019: The annual report on philanthropy for the year 2018.* Special report by the Giving USA Foundation.

Environment

INTRODUCTION

Providing effective leadership around all aspects of the postacute care (PAC) "environment" encompasses a wide variety of responsibilities, from establishing and monitoring systems that ensure consistent regulatory compliance to exercising sound stewardship of the organization's physical plant; from executing good governance to proactively managing risk; and from protecting people's safety, dignity, and privacy to maintaining a clean and comfortable atmosphere. Although the underlying concepts apply across all the lines of service, this domain of professional practice is one of the most diverse because the circumstances vary so extensively among settings.

PHYSICAL PLANT OPERATIONS

The design of a building is typically shaped by the needs, capabilities, and preferences of its intended occupants, as well as the anticipated uses for each area. It is essential to balance the goals of safety and comfort with having the flexibility to meet people's changing needs. Older facilities and houses can present some limitations and challenges, but modifications can often effectively enhance their functionality for aging in place.

Most states, and even some local governments, have established building and construction codes with the fundamental purpose of public protection. The National Fire Protection Association (NFPA) is the most widely accepted authority on standards for buildings—commercial or residential—to minimize the risk of harm to anyone who enters. Its "Life Safety Code" (NFPA, 2019) is the premier source for strategies to ensure people's safety based on building construction, protection, and occupancy features that minimize the effects of fire and related hazards.

The NFPA-101 covers life safety in both new and existing structures. For determining compliance, the date of construction generally drives which version of the code applies. However, renovations and contiguous additions trigger the expectation to follow the most current code edition. Also, the NFPA-101 is either referenced or incorporated into federal, state, and local regulations governing construction, healthcare facility licensing, or certification for participation in Medicare or Medicaid.

The NFPA's National Electrical Code (NEC), a separate but closely related set of standards, sets the foundation for electrical safety in residential, commercial, and industrial occupancies, including requirements for electrical wiring, overcurrent protection, grounding, and installation of equipment.

Keeping Current

The NFPA periodically makes evidence-based adjustments to both the Life Safety Code and the NEC. Knowing which rules to apply is essential for effective environmental planning and management. Whether exploring the feasibility of modernizing or repurposing an existing structure, of constructing an addition, or of introducing a new facility, it is sound practice to consult its site early in the design phase to have the most current information about the NFPA's relevant codes (NFPA, 2020).

Maintenance

Maintaining the physical plant, grounds, and equipment in "as-new" operating condition is simply exercising good stewardship. Not only are they all valuable assets of the organization (or the homeowner), but their functionality directly affects the quality of life experienced by those who live, work, and visit the site.

Preventive Maintenance

Preventive or preventative maintenance (PM) is a planned activity designed to improve the performance and life of building systems or equipment, as well as to avoid unplanned interventions. It is a nonclinical subset of QAPI (quality assurance and performance improvement; discussed in greater detail in Chapter 2, Customer Care, Supports, and Services).

The PM program commonly includes (a) systematic inspection, (b) detection of irregularities or signs of wear and tear, and (c) correction of identified problems all with the common goal of reducing the risk of failures. Unless the PM program is effective, all subsequent maintenance strategies tend to take longer to implement, incur higher costs, have a higher probability of failure, or some combination of all three.

Depending on the complexity and size of the operation, organizing a PM program can be done manually or by utilizing software specifically designed for this purpose. The PM program might focus on building systems (heating, ventilation, and air conditioning [HVAC], lighting, plumbing, windows and doors, etc.) or equipment (for direct care, cooking, cleaning, communication, or laundry; furniture, business office equipment, or the medical records system; etc.). Regardless, the key information needed for appropriately setting up scheduled inspections and responding with effective interventions includes the following:

- Description of item (manufacturer, model, and serial numbers)
- Location
- Purchase/install date
- Warranty: Terms and expiration date

- ▣ Authorized inspector
  - ▣ Internal (qualified)
  - ▣ External: Third-party service contact info; business affiliation agreement (if applicable)
- ▣ Inspection schedule (monthly, quarterly, semiannually, or annually)
- ▣ Inspection history and repair record
- ▣ Estimated replacement date (updated with each inspection for capital budgeting purposes)

One of the biggest challenges to operating an effective PM program is appropriately assigning resources—specifically, staff *time*—to accomplishing this charge. It is not uncommon for urgent tasks to outrank the importance of routine PM activities. Unfortunately, this can have the unintended, ironic consequence of growing the list of urgent tasks when things either unexpectedly break or stop running properly.

Workflow

One common practice for keeping the environment safe, clean, and comfortable is to invite everyone's observations about it—those who reside, work, or visit there. Setting up a simple and accessible method for people to alert the organization about situations that pose a risk essentially "deputizes" them as unofficial inspectors and empowered advocates.

Once a potential problem is identified, it is important to track the speed and effectiveness of the organization's response. This typically begins with a designated team leader assigning a priority level to the referral, based on its potential impact on safety, sanitation, comfort, or regulatory compliance. Establishing priority levels informs staff assignments, but the tension between "important" and "urgent" rarely disappears. Executive judgment must be applied to resource allocation decisions.

Once completed, there is an opportunity for stakeholder development, thanking and informing the originator of the referral about the outcome. This often is overlooked or falls prey to time constraints, but it can be a practical, effective contributor to building a truly "person-centered" organizational culture.

Recordkeeping

An often-cited axiom throughout healthcare and human services is "If it is not documented, it didn't happen." Of course, failing to write down and store descriptions of events, observations, or verifications does not really erase them from history. However, when it comes to government regulatory agencies or third-party payers, they rely on information that can be retrieved in print.

The types of records, who has access to them and for what purpose, and how long they must be retained (or retrievable), vary by discipline or record category (see Table 5.1).

Security levels and ease of access are influenced by where and how information is stored. In order to foster efficiency, it is important for those who rely on stored records to retrieve them as easily as possible while protecting the same information from unauthorized people. Whether the records are printed (also referred to as "hard copies") or electronic (scanned versions of hard copies or data stored by proprietary software), establishing and enforcing policies and procedures for

TABLE 5.1 Recordkeeping Guidelines

Record	Access By	Access Purpose	Example(s)	Retention
Medical/care	Recipient or designee Care professional Payer Regulator	Informed Care coordination Reimbursement Compliance	Chart/Electronic medical record (All)	At least 6 years*
Employment	Human resources and administration Employee regulator	Fair and equal treatment Informed compliance	Employee file Training and licenses	3–5 years**
Business contracts	Administration Regulator Contracted party	Operations Compliance Performance	Resident/client Goods, services, affiliations, warranties (any of those listed)	5 years*** after expiration
Other compliance	Regulator public	Compliance transparency	Inspection reports	5 years***

* The Health Insurance Portability and Accountability Act (HIPAA) administrative simplification rules require retaining a medical record for 6 years from the date of its creation or the date when it last was in effect, whichever is later; HIPAA requirements preempt any state law that requires a shorter period.

** Most federal requirements for employee record retention fall within this time frame; individual states may have additional obligations.

*** It's good practice to mirror the medical records retention guideline, but not required in most jurisdictions.

Source: 45 CFR 164.316(b)(2).

effectively safeguarding protected health information (PHI) and related business records are paramount.

Storing hard copies, no matter how meticulously organized or cataloged, requires physical space—which is typically in short supply in most PAC settings. Furthermore, doing so on-site adds to the volume of combustible materials in the event of a fire emergency. It is best to minimize the amount of paper records kept in the building by storing off-site or scanning those records for which the probability of needing is relatively low before the applicable retention standard is met.

Similarly, routinely backing up electronic records in a remote location—either with an off-site server or in the cloud—enhances an organization's ability to operate during a disaster. Maintaining parallel sets of the same data for this purpose is commonly referred to as "redundancy."

Grounds

The land on which the building(s) sit is also a key asset. Maintaining its appearance affects the daily experience of those served, as well as their families, employees, volunteers, and visitors. It also impacts the surrounding community's image of the organization, including that of prospective clients and their families. It is important to neither overlook nor underestimate the value of this function.

The scale and complexity of landscaping can make a difference in whether it is more advisable to maintain the grounds internally or to outsource any portion of it. Mowing and trimming the lawn is typically the most routine groundskeeping task, which places seasonal demands on personnel and requires maintaining and storing lawn equipment (as well as fuel) and perhaps treating the yard to prevent weeds, pests, or disease. Similarly, snow removal and keeping sidewalks and parking areas safe during winter months can be challenging in many locations because of inconsistent demands. Finding the optimal blend of internal effort and purchased services for groundskeeping requires ongoing evaluation.

Note (In-Home Services): When the grounds belong to the client, such as someone who is receiving home health or hospice services, opportunities to collaborate with organizations outside of healthcare and human services emerge. Such activities are almost exclusively funded privately, by either the client or their family, but some other sources may emerge that recognize the advantages—cost and life satisfaction—of keeping elders at home.

Transportation

Not every PAC organization owns or operates either a vehicle or fleet of them, but it is not at all uncommon. Do *not* assume that because the members of the maintenance staff have tools and other skills that they are also proficient vehicle mechanics. That is like assuming your father knows how to carve the Thanksgiving turkey just because of his title in your family! Develop vehicle maintenance affiliations in advance of need, either with the purchase source or with a reputable shop recommended by the manufacturer. Vehicle fleet management is a key risk avoidance and safety responsibility, and it should be considered an investment rather than a cost.

In addition to the mechanical performance and safety of each vehicle, it delivers a message about the organization to anyone who sees it on the road or rides in it. A truck, van, or car that looks neglected or worn out and has the organization's logo or name on its door may give rise to suspicion about the quality of services one can expect to receive. A resident who boards a bus that appears not to have been cleaned out since the last outing might wonder what *else* has been ignored about the bus and about how valued a customer they are considered.

Policies governing who may drive a company-owned or leased vehicle and for what purpose are also essential to establish in advance. Insurance carriers typically adjust premiums based on the driving record of those drivers—and may disqualify a driver who exceeds the stated safety limits. Driving with passengers can require additional training and licensing in many states, so be sure to check state and local regulations.

Safety and Security

One of the top reasons for elders and their families to seek supportive services is the desire to keep people both safe and secure, to minimize their risk of harm, and to bolster their confidence about the protection and comfort provided by their living environment. Although the two terms are related and commonly used interchange-ably, there are some subtle differences.

Proactively ensuring a *safe* setting for people to live, work, and visit involves both mindful, safety-conscious facility design and ongoing attention to maintaining those safety features in working order. The NFPA's Life Safety Code and its enforce-ment illustrate this concept wonderfully.

Security typically addresses perimeter protection or containment (Box 5.1). The goal is to minimize the risk of harm by outside forces, from allowing entry by an intruder or a wandering resident leaving the property undetected to preventing the theft of valuable items, such as the personal belongings of residents or staff, medi-cations, or HIPAA-Personal Health Information.

BOX 5.1 Security Versus Shackles

Keeping a resident *secure* has some unique challenges associated with it. Balancing the need to prevent harm with preserving one's protected rights of autonomy and self-determination is often difficult to reduce to a set of rules that apply in all instances. For instance, physical and chemical restraints were widely applied interventions until the past decade but now require much greater scrutiny and justification. A person who has not been declared legal-ly incompetent by a court with appropriate jurisdiction cannot be contained against their will, even if the intent of doing so is for their own protection. This can be considered "false imprisonment" and can trigger some severe legal and reputation consequences for the organization. This has emerged as a particularly challenging dilemma for organizations serving people diag-nosed with dementia or other behavior-altering cognitive disorders.

Emergency Preparedness

Achieving both safety and security is particularly demanding when the routine of daily life and operations are disrupted by a natural disaster or another emergency. Although right now not every PAC service line is *required* to develop an emergency preparedness plan, it is prudent to do so. After all, it is much better to have one and not need it than to need one and not have it!

Along with hospitals, skilled nursing facilities (SNFs) and home health agencies now have, as a requirement of participation in the Medicare or Medicaid programs, the expectation to develop a plan for meeting the health, safety, and security needs of both those in their care and their staff during an emergency or natural disas-ter. The plan must consider all plausible hazards (natural or human-made), define operations during the disaster (including communication and coordination with other healthcare providers and the community), include extensive training and drilling, and undergo internal review at least once annually. Although intended for Medicare- and Medicaid-certified providers, senior living organizations that either do not participate in those programs or operate noneligible service lines should also engage in similar planning activities.

Standardizing emergency preparedness guidelines to facilitate smoother col-laboration across the healthcare continuum is a primary objective of the Centers for Medicare & Medicaid Services (CMS). Referenced throughout the specific rules governing emergency and disaster preparedness are protocols developed by the Federal Emergency Management Agency, the National Incident Management System, and the Incident Command System. The CMS also requires that providers coordinate their emergency preparedness plan with local, state, and federal agencies (Todd, 2017).

Hazard Vulnerability Analysis   Determine which hazards are the most likely to present a risk, the potential impact on the operation at varying levels of severity, and the capacity for effective response (internally and with community support).

- Common hazards for consideration:
    - Fire
    - Utility interruption (electric, gas, water, and communication)
    - Mechanical or equipment failure (HVAC, elevators, or lifts)
    - Internal pipe burst (sprinklers, supply line, or sewer)
    - Epidemic* or care-related emergency
    - Threats: Bomb, homeland security, or active aggressor

- Common hazards related to specific locations or regions (if applicable):
    - Severe weather (tornado, hurricane, wind or ice storm, or drought)
    - Flood
    - Wild fire
    - Earthquake
    - Industrial accident
    - Explosion (propane or other gas tanks)

Incident Command   Describe each assignment, delegation of authority, and organizational structure to preserve continuity of operations throughout the event.

Response   Plan for providing subsistence—food, water, shelter (in place and evacuation scenarios, including transportation), medication, and access to medication and treatment records.

Communication   Develop tactics for keeping stakeholders informed: families, regulatory agencies and emergency responders, receiving providers (if evacuating), as well as backup plans for communication methods (such as HAM radio or satellite phones).

---

* In early 2020, the COVID-19 (or Novel Corona-19) virus first caused an *epi*demic—an abnormal, rapid increase in the number of cases of a disease within a geographic area—in many communities. It then expanded at break-neck speed into a true *pan*demic—when a disease, typically caused by a previously unknown pathogen, spreads across many countries and affects large populations (Caceres, 2020). Although preparation for responding to an epidemic certainly helped, the magnificent scale and unprecedented speed of transmission was simply unimaginable beforehand.

Training and Testing All employees are to receive training on emergency procedures, including full-scale drills and exercises. Fire drills are expected to be performed at least quarterly on each shift. Home health agencies are also expected by the CMS to participate in community emergency preparation planning.

Evacuation

Under NFPA-101, SNFs are built to have sprinkler systems and at least two areas that are separated by special fire-resistant building materials and fire-rated doors to allow relocation away from an affected area to a safe one while firefighters extinguish the fire. Other institutional PAC settings have less consistent sprinkler system and fire separation requirements. When a fire is discovered or an alarm triggered, there is typically very little time to decide whether to evacuate—partially or completely.

Partial Evacuation An emergency or disaster that affects only one part of a building may just require transferring residents to another section of the same building or to an adjacent structure in order to preserve their safety. For example, a fire in a resident's room should result in all people moving to at least another designated fire-separation section of the building.

- Most single-family homes and many apartment buildings are not designed with multiple NFPA-compliant fire sections, so partial evacuation is extremely rare for home health providers to consider.

Complete Evacuation When an emergency or disaster affects more than one part of the building, it may become necessary for everyone to leave in order to remain safe. This may also require transportation to another location to provide adequate shelter and to preserve continuity of care, as well as implementing the plan's tracking system for monitoring each resident's location until returned.

- Institutional example: A tornado blows the roof off a substantial part of an SNF, including the service core with the kitchen, resulting in relocation of the residents to the sites listed in the emergency preparedness plan.

- Home- and community-based services (HCBS) example: A chimney fire, caused by the ignition of built-up creosote in the flue of a home health patient's fireplace, results in significant roof damage. The staff member on duty at the time facilitates evacuation of the premises and relocation of the patient to a site listed in the emergency preparedness plan.

    In either event, familiarity with the emergency preparedness plan is the key factor in implementing it successfully. Involving the community in its development—and periodically in drills—can save not only time, effort, and money but people's lives. Do not wait to meet the local Fire Chief or emergency medical services team on the day they are needed.

In-Place Sheltering or Isolation

A precursor to some of the same disasters that prompt an evacuation can be sheltering in place. For instance, the safest locations during a tornado are in a below-surface space, under a staircase, in an interior bathroom, or near a weight-bearing interior wall. According to the National Weather Service (2020), staying put—in the right place—is likely the best short-term strategy for survival in such an event.

However, the danger presented by certain other disasters, such as a public health pandemic, may not be from directly altering the physical surrounding of the care recipient. In such a circumstance, the best protective measure may be isolating the person from others in order to reduce the risk of exposure and possible transmission of a disease. It can be important to provide for physical separation and even to consider air exchange rates and routes.

Such isolation requires closely following "Standard Precautions," as defined by the Centers for Disease Control and Prevention (Siegel et al., 2019). That includes hand hygiene, use of personal protective equipment (such as gloves, masks, and eyewear), safe injection practices and sharps handling, respiratory hygiene and cough etiquette, using sterile instruments and devices, and aggressively cleaning and disinfecting environmental surfaces (doors, hardware and frames, counters, and high-touch surfaces).

Elopement

When people hear this term in relation to senior living settings, they often express surprise because this term more commonly prompts an image of a couple who secretly leaves town to marry in favor of participating in a traditional, public wedding. However, in this context, it pertains to a resident or patient who is incapable of adequately protecting themselves and departs the premises unsupervised and undetected (Kosieradzki & Smith, 2003). The CMS conditions of participation in Medicare and Medicaid, state licensure regulations, and third-party accrediting body standards, such as those of The Joint Commission, expect providers to proactively address this risk by having appropriate measures in place for both prevention and response.

Assessing whether someone presents an elopement *risk* can be multifaceted—some contributing factors might relate to the person and others to the environment. This takes professional judgment and awareness of changes in people's disposition, capacity, and circumstances. Safety emerges as the chief concern, and it should guide decisions about both prevention and response. Conditions that significantly correlate with elopement risk include whether an individual

- has a court-appointed legal guardian;
- has previously escaped or eloped;
- either consistently or intermittently:
    - lacks the cognitive function to reliably make reasonable and relevant decisions; or
    - exhibits behaviors that pose a danger to self or others.

Complicating the challenge of estimating this risk is the potential for other influential factors coming into play.

1. *The well-meaning (or unaware) visitor or volunteer,* who may allow the resident to follow them through the exit door without realizing that doing so might pose a threat (maybe even politely open the door for the resident to pass through first!).

2. *The convincingly compensating resident,* who looks, sounds, and seems perfectly "normal," which can contribute to the previous item happening. With so

many providers adopting a core philosophy of "person-centered care," this phenomenon is increasingly widespread.

3. *The "no guardianship" resident,* where the absence of a guardian *technically* makes containing a person without their consent "false imprisonment."

4. *The person diagnosed with dementia,* who might exhibit one of the hallmark behaviors of this condition—an intense focus on "going home" and seeking the familiarity afforded by getting there.

5. *NFPA-required fire exits,* which purposely have bold and highly visible signage indicating the way to leave. Depending on the designed layout, there could be several options for departure.

6. *Windows that open fully,* regardless of height; if a resident wants to leave intensely enough, they may not exercise sound judgment in calculating the dangers associated with passing through an opened window.

7. *Compromised sight lines* that result from a design approach aimed at protecting an individual's privacy but that sometimes produce the unintended consequence of losing sight of the person who wishes to leave undetected.

None of the questions raised by the items on the preceding list has a clear-cut answer or single best solution. Additional reflection and consideration regarding the last three items in the list is imperative, however. The codes and standards designed to keep people safe presume that all people affected have the cognitive capacity to recognize a dangerous situation and to understand how to respond. Some do not, so how can we find new ways to balance the competing levels of comprehension without eroding the ultimate goal of safety?

Some organizations establish time limits concerning the frequency of observed resident presence. Exceeding that limit triggers a search initiative. Others launch their elopement response when it becomes reasonably certain the patient is missing without authorization (MedLeague, 2019). To prevent unnecessary searches (or unrest), it is wise to have procedures in place for residents to sign out and sign back in upon return. This is also useful information to have during a disaster event to confirm who should be there. The key is to do what is reasonably necessary to return the patient to a safe environment.

SUPPLY CHAIN MANAGEMENT

Purchasing and Procurement

Quality specifications, that is, describing an item as completely as possible so that the pricing offered by competing vendors informs a meaningful comparison, are beneficial. Products such as food and paper goods are often available in a wide variety of quality grades, composition, weights, and sizes. The more narrowly defined the request, the more reliable the pricing comparison. People who regularly use or consume a given product—caregivers or recipients—can serve as a valuable resource in developing and refining quality specifications.

Pricing comparisons are important to perform periodically to ensure fiscal responsibility. Some providers do so continuously, and others follow a schedule for reviewing prices—quarterly, semiannually, or annually. It is common for suppliers to offer financial incentives for consistently buying their products, rewarding purchase volume, percentage of spending on an item or group of items, or some combination of both. This is typically achieved through rebates or reduced pricing for a future period. During periods of fuel price volatility, many vendors have found it necessary to add supplemental "surcharges" for delivering their goods. A thorough price analysis process includes all of these factors, not merely the list price for a particular supply item.

Group purchasing organizations (GPOs) pool the purchasing power of their members in order to obtain more favorable pricing for goods and services than they would likely be offered by vendors and suppliers if the members bought them separately. The concept of a GPO is modeled after a farming cooperative. Sales volume and market share matter enough to many manufacturers and distributors of goods that they adjust pricing as an enticement for people to select their products. This can include either a narrowly targeted menu or a broad range of items, from food and nutritional supplements, medical supplies, and adult briefs to chemicals for laundry and cleaning, paper and office supplies, and even building supplies.

Some GPOs also branch into negotiating lower costs for services, such as contract therapists, professional clinical consultants (pharmacists, dentists, podiatrists, vision care professionals, or mental health professionals), insurance protection, or employee benefits.

How a GPO is corporately organized varies. Its members might be customers, or they might also serve as stockholders or co-owners, benefiting not only from lower prices for goods and services obtained through the GPO, but sharing in any profit generated by the GPO through successfully achieving its operating purpose. Additionally, a GPO might have different levels of membership that offer benefit-sharing commensurate with either a member's financial investment in the GPO, commitment of market share to it (percentage of the member's purchases of covered products or services), or both. Many vendors offer rebates to customers achieving targeted sales thresholds; pooling purchasing activities provides GPO members the opportunity to share in higher tier rebates, as well.

"Receiving" is the term applied to describe the procedures surrounding where to physically accept delivery of the goods that were ordered, stocking the inventory, and verifying that the invoice matches the packing sheet with respect to units delivered and product specifications and that prices charged reflect the current contract. Some products—such as pharmaceuticals and biologicals, or durable medical equipment—also call for additional attention to the "chain of custody" to ensure that the same items that were shipped by the vendor arrive intact and ready for their intended use. It is increasingly common for vendors to rely on third-party, commercial transport companies than deploying and maintaining their own delivery fleets and drivers.

An effective and smooth receiving process starts with providing ease of access for the delivery driver or team, minimizing the length and complexity of entry to the site and pathway to the unloading point. Another consideration is how to establish delivery routes that avoid disrupting the lives of residents and workflow of staff members—not only preventing the interruption of caregiving or other services but preserving the safety and comfort of those who live, work, or visit there.

"Inventory control" means regularly accounting for the arrival, storage, internal distribution, and reordering of supplies to ensure that there is enough of every product on hand when needed and that any items with published expiration dates or shelf life are either used within the prescribed time or removed from inventory. An accounting principle applies here—first-in-first-out (FIFO)—achieved by rotating stocked items in such a fashion that the newest arrivals are stored for last retrieval. A grocery store serves as a good example of FIFO rotation—just observe how newly arriving products are placed on the shelf by the stores' stock staff. This is particularly challenging to manage in a home health setting, where there is less likely to be multiple containers of the same food, medicine, or medical supplies. However, keeping track of expiration dates is equally important in all PAC environments.

When a golfer shoots "par" for a particular hole, that means they took the number of strokes to sink the ball in the hole on the green that the course designer intended. Similarly, the amount of a given product that is typically needed to meet the residents' collective needs for any restocking cycle—per shift, day, week, or month—is known as a *par level*. With the exception of high-acuity SNFs and home health agencies engaged in providing postacute rehabilitation, par levels tend to stabilize over time. It is generally a good practice to include some reserve capacity, however, to minimize the risk of actually running out of any supply before the next regularly scheduled delivery date.

> **Example**: If an assisted living community's memory care neighborhood routinely goes through 10 cases of toilet paper per week and has a weekly delivery schedule with the supplier, it might be wise to set the neighborhood's par level for toilet paper at 11 (10% over routine use). When placing the next order, request the number of cases that will bring the inventory back up to 11.

Ideally, the volume of each product received and used equals the number needed to replenish the inventory back to the "par" level. If there is a negative difference—some items that are unaccounted for—that is sometimes referred to as "shrinkage." This can happen through ineffective controls, inconsistently tracking charges or distribution, or even pilferage (internal theft). In any event, shrinkage proves expensive, and preventing it should always be a risk management target.

Another related matter is properly labeling containers that have been opened and stored, as well as food that has been prepared and saved for future serving. Information that should be prominently and *legibly* displayed on such a container includes at least:

- Date stored (month/day/year)
- Time stored (24-hour military time recommended: 1:30 p.m. = 13:30)
- Person completing label

One of the most consistently cited regulatory violations among licensed PAC communities is incomplete labels on food containers. Although less regulated in a person's home, it is considered good practice to follow the same protocol for storing any opened container retained for future use.

Charging customers accurately for consuming direct care items that are not included in the normal daily rate is important. Some organizations apply labels with barcodes printed on them to be scanned and entered into the accounting system as supplies are used. Many rely on the manufacturer's Uniform Bar Code (UBC) for the same purpose. Whether the item is reimbursable by Medicare, Medicaid, or other third-party payers may also influence the decision about whether to capture the information for billing purposes.

LEGAL AND REGULATORY ENVIRONMENT

Corporate Structure

There are a variety of options for how to corporately organize a PAC provider entity, depending on its primary purpose and ownership structure. Each model has distinct requirements, advantages, and limitations. The three broad categories of ownership are proprietary (for-profit), tax-exempt (not-for-profit), and public. Their duties and responsibilities are consistent, but their composition and mode of operation can vary considerably.

Sponsorship: Proprietary Sponsorship

A "proprietary" service provider organization is typically owned by an individual, partnership, or corporation and strives to generate an operational profit that benefits the owner. The governing board of a smaller proprietary organization commonly includes all of the owners. However, stockholders typically elect board members for a larger, corporate ownership structure. The chief benefit of this arrangement for investors is that they share personally in the financial success of the organization.

Note: It is becoming increasingly popular for a financial investor—such as a real estate investment trust, insurance company, or pension fund—to purchase the major assets of an operation (building and land) and contract with a provider organization to deliver PAC services at the site. This infusion of capital into the business environment of PAC has fostered the much-needed modernization and upgrading of many older facilities. However, it has also posed some new challenges for balancing financial performance return on investment expectations with achieving quality care indicators and regulatory compliance.

Sponsorship: Tax-Exempt

A "tax-exempt" service provider organization—sometimes referred to as "not-for-profit" or "nonprofit"—serves a community or members of a religious group or fraternal order. Any profit (operating margin) generated by the enterprise is reinvested in the organization, not distributed to any individual. This arrangement qualifies the organization to become designated by the U.S. Department of the Treasury's Internal Revenue Service (IRS) as exempt from taxation by the federal government, and many state and local authorities honor that designation by also exempting the organization from taxation—ranging from corporate income to property or sales tax. The section of the IRS Code that addresses this exemption is 501(c)(3), so often a tax-exempt provider is referred to as a "501(c)(3) organization." This qualification also permits donors to deduct contributions to the organization from their taxable income on their individual income tax returns.

Sponsorship: Public

A "public" service provider is government-owned, at the federal, state, or local level. The ownership is comprised of voters in the jurisdiction, and its governing body commonly includes elected or appointed government officials—sometimes complemented by interested community leaders. The Department of Veterans Affairs operates a national network of hospitals and healthcare services for eligible U.S. military veterans; some states also operate SNFs and senior housing aimed at assisting veterans; and many counties and municipalities own PAC communities and services.

Governing Body

It is customary for any service organization—regardless of ownership design—to have a governing body, a group of people who accept legal responsibility for how the organization operates and who oversee its performance. This is most commonly referred to as the organization's board of directors or board of trustees. Most states expect a provider organization to have a governing body; the Medicare and Medicaid programs require it. Some state licensing regulations include extensive details concerning the requirements for a governing body, ranging from registering its articles of incorporation and bylaws with the Secretary of State to rules for holding its meetings. A governing board's roles and responsibilities typically include at least the following (Pratt, 2016):

1. **Mission, Values, and Vision:** Developing the core purpose, strategic priorities, and goals of the organization

2. **Program and Service Performance:** Monitoring the organization's quality outcomes and indicators, legal and regulatory compliance, ethical integrity, and financial outcomes

3. **Executive Leadership:** Hiring a qualified chief executive officer, evaluating their performance in the role, and providing relevant and helpful advice

4. **Succession Plan:** Developing and following policies and procedures designed to ensure that sound board and executive leadership both continue beyond the terms of incumbents

I firmly believe that a culture of trust among members of the governing board body, executive leadership, staff, residents and related stakeholders is a prerequisite for true strategic thinking to bear fruit.

Michael P. Cicchese, FACHCA, FACHE,
Board Member, Atlantic Shores Cooperative
Association

Contract Services: Authority and Responsibility

Former U.S. Senator from North Dakota, Byron Dorgan, was known for reminding his colleagues in Congress that "You can delegate authority, but you cannot delegate responsibility" (BrainyQuote, 2019). We agree. While there may be operational advantages to contracting with an outside service company for clinical, support, or business functions, giving them the *authority* to carry out certain activities, the *responsibility* for performance ultimately remains with the provider organization. If a contracted therapy company, environmental services firm, or electronic health record vendor makes some costly mistake, the health services executive (HSE™) does not have the option of assigning blame externally. Contracted services are typically viewed by regulators and customers (sometimes even in court) as an extension of the organization.

Leader's Role: Working With the Governing Body

In order for the governing body to fulfill its duties, its members need accurate, timely, and relevant information about the operation, as well as about external factors that might affect the organization. The highly effective HSE™ equips the governing board by regularly supplying and interpreting such information. *Internal* reports typically include updated information on the following:

- **QAPI:** Highlights regarding clinical metrics and efforts toward continuously enhancing quality
- **Financial Performance:** From operating and capital budgets to financial statements, balance sheets, cash flow analyses; reports on occupancy and client volume and invested reserve funds; and financing options for working capital or projects
- **Regulatory Compliance:** Inspection reports (federal, state, and local agencies) and associated plans of correction, if applicable
- **Risk Management:** Status of legal liabilities outstanding (or resolved since the previous report) arising from incidents relating to a client's care, a staff member's injury on the job or disciplinary action, or injury sustained by a visitor
- **Client Satisfaction:** Survey feedback from resident and family members about their experience with the organization
- **Employee Engagement:** Survey feedback from staff members about their experience working for the organization
- **Strategic Plan Progress:** Achievement of the goals and objectives articulated in the organization's strategic plan
- **Fundraising (Tax-Exempt):** Resources secured, in the pipeline or prospective sources for requests of support

Reports on *external* forces that have the potential to affect the operation, positively or negatively, commonly include the following:

- **Competition:** Challenges and opportunities related to decisions made by competing providers, from wages, staffing patterns, and service lines to capital improvements, mergers and acquisitions, or changing a primary vendor
- **Legislation or Regulation:** Proposed, under consideration or soon-to-be implemented new laws and regulations (or changes in enforcement of either)
- **Economic Condition:** Economic developments that impact the operation, from weather-related crop damages driving up the price of certain commodities to fluctuations in the Consumer Price Index and anticipated workforce development needs for senior living organizations

- ■ **Innovations and Professional Trends:** Promising new developments in the field that improve caregiving outcomes, efficiency, or staff recruitment and retention

The volume of information available to share can become overwhelming for a member of the governing board to receive. It is the responsibility of the HSE™ to discern which information would serve the board best and to provide an element of analysis and interpretation, as needed. Most governing boards are comprised of highly talented community leaders, but not all of them are necessarily deeply familiar with the world of PAC or senior services.

A growing "high-impact practice" is for the HSE™ to develop with the board a "dashboard" of performance indicators that shows less detail, summarizing the overall operational health of the organization—not merely financial outcomes. Such a dashboard has been embraced and popularized in several other industries since David Norton and Robert Kaplan introduced in the early 1990s the notion of a "balanced scorecard" (Kaplan & Norton, 1992). However, this is still relatively new in senior living. They suggested that relying on traditional financial metrics as the primary indicators of performance can provide misleading signals concerning either innovation or continuous improvement efforts—two things that an increasingly competitive environment demands. Now, a simple Internet search using keywords such as "balanced scorecard, dashboard, or key performance indicators" will provide numerous examples, templates, and even software for developing a relevant and effective operations dashboard that can prove useful to both governing boards and staff leadership. Exhibit 5.1 illustrates how this approach could apply to senior living lines of service.

Regulations, Standards, and Laws

PAC service lines collectively comprise one of the most heavily regulated fields in America. Some attribute this to the relatively frail nature of the people served: predominantly older and/or disabled adults. Therefore, there is arguably a societal expectation that people who have some marked disadvantage deserve advocacy and protection. Others point to the fact that the number one payer for such services is the government—from the CMS and the Administration on Community Living (ACL) to the federal Departments of Housing and Urban Development (HUD), Agriculture (USDA), and Veterans Affairs (VA). It certainly has a keen interest in ensuring that the quality of care delivered is commensurate with the cost, as well as having a duty to protect the interests of its most vulnerable citizens. Consumers and their families are rarely equipped to evaluate, monitor, and respond effectively to poor quality of services.

Regulation has the potential for addressing market failures and upholding at least minimal standards for quality. This orientation has been the hallmark of laws and regulations governing PAC, especially for SNFs, home health, hospice, adult day care, and affordable housing. The chief limitation of this approach is that it emphasizes minimal compliance as the standard to meet and lacks incentives for achieving *excellence.*

For instance, it is plausible for an SNF's executive leader to announce, perhaps with a great air of pride, that the Inspector General's survey team just completed a "deficiency-free" annual inspection. Statistically, that places the organization in an exclusive group toward the top of its peers. However, that means the organization

EXHIBIT 5.1 Sample Balanced Scorecard for Senior Living

FINANCIAL PERSPECTIVE	
Stakeholder/Stockholder View	
Goals	**Metrics**
Survive	Cash Flow & Debt Ratio
Succeed	Operating Income & Days Cash on Hand
Prosper	Market Share

CUSTOMER PERSPECTIVE		INTERNAL OPERATIONS PERSPECTIVE	
Care Recipient/Advocate View		*Strategic Aspirations*	
Goals	**Metrics**	**Goals**	**Metrics**
Person-Centered Experience	Satisfaction Rating	Provider of Choice	Referrals
Quality	Reg Compliance, Accreditation & 5-Star Rating (SNF/IRF/HHA)	Alignment	Staff Engagement Rating & Attendance
Care Continuity	Staff Retention	Risk Management	Legal/Insurance Costs

INNOVATION & LEARNING PERSPECTIVE	
QAPI & Value	
Goals	**Metrics**
Staff Development	Scholarship/CE Investment
Technology	HL7 & ROI
Mission Focus	New Services Contribution

CE, continuing education; IRF, inpatient rehabilitation facility; HHA, home health agency; QAPI, quality assurance and performance improvement; ROI, return on investment; SNF, skilled nursing facility.

Source: Adapted from Kaplan, R., & Norton, D. (1992). The balanced scorecard: Measures that drive performance. *Harvard Business Review, 70*(1), 71–79.

merely satisfied all the *minimum requirements* for licensure renewal, Medicare, or Medicaid recertification, or all three in a snapshot review on the date of the survey. Unfortunately, there is not an opportunity in the current format to recognize efforts that resulted in *exceeding* the minimum standards, so this is literally the best one can do!

As much as possible, efforts to ensure service quality should be guided by evidence, should value the perspectives of key stakeholders, and should recognize the limitations of both regulatory enforcement and market forces. The introduction of QAPI expectations, value-based purchasing, and refinements to the CMS five-star rating system are all positive steps. However, there remain abundant opportunities for incentivizing innovation and exceeding minimum standards, rewarding sustained high performance, and recognizing the relevance of both consumer satisfaction and employee engagement.

Federal Programs

Our discussion here is focused on the provider's compliance with the rules and regulations set forth for participation in each program described. Key federal programs (not an exhaustive list of available benefit programs) that serve older and disabled adults across the PAC continuum are presented in alphabetical order of the agencies charged with administering them.

Administration on Community Living (ACL)   The Older Americans Act (OAA) was enacted in 1965 in response to public concerns about a lack of community social services for older persons. It established authority for grants to states for community planning and social services, research and development projects, and training in the field of aging services. The law also established the Administration on Aging (AoA)—now the ACL —to serve as the federal focal point on matters concerning older persons.

The agency oversees a wide array of HCBS programs through a national network of state Area Agencies on Aging (AAA) and tribal organizations. The OAA also includes provisions for multipurpose senior centers, nutrition programs, transportation assistance, community service employment for low-income older Americans, family caregiving training, and vulnerable elder rights protection activities (such as the Long-Term Care Ombudsman program and elder abuse screening and prevention initiatives).

The Long-Term Care Ombudsman program was purposely placed outside of the CMS to provide an independent consumer advocacy option for residents of long-term care communities and their families or representatives. Ombudspersons visit more frequently than state survey teams and typically develop a less formal relationship with residents, families, and staff. They are trained to moderate the resolution of complaints by residents or families who have not been satisfied by the response of management. Although ombudspersons do not carry the same level of authority as state surveyors with regard to imposing punitive sanctions, working closely and cooperatively with them as an additional resource is generally in the best interest of the organization and the people it serves. Compliance with regulations governed by the ACL is expected when the organization receives funding for any of the agency's programs, as stipulated in a services agreement.

Centers for Medicare & Medicaid Services   The CMS, an administrative agency of the U.S. Department of Health and Human Services (DHHS), has overall responsibility for regulating PAC providers accepting payment from Medicare or Medicaid. It promulgates regulations that must be followed in order to participate in either program, referred to as "certification." It also publishes a set of "Interpretive Guidelines" (also known as the State Operations Manual) for inspectors and providers to fully understand what is expected—how compliance with the regulations is determined. For SNFs, there are over 400 distinct standards (also referred to as "F-Tags") classified under 21 categories (CMS, 2018). They are listed in the following with the corresponding section in which they appear as part of the Code of Federal Regulations, Title 42):

1. 483.10 Resident Rights
2. 483.12 Freedom from Abuse, Neglect, and Exploitation
3. 483.15 Admission Transfer and Discharge Rights
4. 483.20 Resident Assessment
5. 483.21 Comprehensive Person-Centered Care Plans
6. 483.24 Quality of Life
7. 483.25 Quality of Care
8. 483.30 Physician Services
9. 483.35 Nursing Services
10. 483.40 Behavioral Health Services
11. 483.45 Pharmacy Services
12. 483.50 Laboratory Radiology and Other Diagnostic Services
13. 483.55 Dental Services
14. 483.60 Food and Nutrition Services
15. 483.65 Specialized Rehabilitative Services
16. 483.70 Administration
17. 483.75 Quality Assurance and Performance Improvement
18. 483.80 Infection Control
19. 483.85 Compliance and Ethics Program
20. 483.90 Physical Environment
21. 483.95 Training Requirements

The "Interpretive Guidelines" published by the CMS are periodically updated with clarifications about how to apply the standards. It is best to rely on the most recent version of the document, which can be accessed at www.cms.gov. The requirements for participation were revised in 2016 to reflect advances made over the past several years in the service delivery and practice. One of the significant shifts was to make these requirements more readily available to both surveyors and providers (the most current set of survey protocols and interpretive guidelines can be found in the additional resources at the end of this chapter). It is imperative that any senior care leader has access and reviews the most current information available from the CMS prior to any inspection or survey process. Also, national trade associations and their state affiliates typically serve as an information clearinghouse concerning changes in the rules (or their interpretation by the CMS) and trends concerning the most commonly cited deficiencies.

The actual site visit and certification for Medicare and Medicaid participation is generally performed by a state agency under a contract with the CMS. That visit—whether for an SNF, home health agency, or hospice provider—is typically referred to as a "survey" and is discussed in greater detail later in this chapter (under the section "Enforcement"). A provider is not supposed to know in advance when the survey team is coming, so that the visit gives a true indication of how the organization operates on any given day. The CMS also makes the survey results available for the public to view and utilize in evaluating options, providing a scorecard at www.medicare.gov/nursinghomecompare.

Surveys must be performed periodically (between 9 and 15 months apart) or in response to a complaint filed by a resident, family member, or employee. When the 12-month anniversary of the most recent annual survey is approaching, the organization is said to be entering its calendar "window" for a return visit by the survey team. A chief criticism of the current system by consumer advocates is that this relatively predictable calendar window offsets the value of unannounced inspections because it allows providers to prepare for the event, giving less of a true picture about daily operations during the rest of the year.

There are similar processes in place for certifying home health and hospice providers to participate in Medicare (CMS, 2014). Many states also include adult day care in their Medicaid plans.

Housing and Urban Development

HUD has several programs aimed at providing safe, clean, comfortable, and affordable housing for older and disabled adults—primarily those who are frail and/or have modest to very low incomes. Over one-half million older or disabled Americans benefit from its array of housing programs. HUD's most widely developed program aimed at this population is the "Supportive Housing for the Elderly Program," found in section 202 of the Housing and Urban Development Act. It provides very low-income elderly with options that allow them to live independently, but with available supportive services, such as cleaning, meals, community activities, or transportation. Section 811 of the law describes similar accommodations for adults who are permanently disabled.

Under the 202 program, HUD provides capital advances to eligible sponsors to finance the construction, rehabilitation, or acquisition of residential buildings that will serve as supportive housing for very low-income elderly persons and provides rent subsidies for the projects to enhance affordability. Project rental assistance is provided (up to two thirds of the HUD-approved "fair market rent") to cover the difference between the HUD-approved operating cost for the project and the tenants' contribution toward rent. Project rental assistance contracts are approved initially for 3 years and are renewable based on the availability of funds (HUD, 2019a).

The Low Income Housing Tax Credit (LIHTC) program takes another approach to achieving affordability by matching investors with sponsors to finance senior housing at very low interest rates, making it possible to offer significantly lower rents to low-income elders (rather than providing rent subsidies).

Each of HUD's programs have codified minimum standards for maintaining a financed property and its ongoing operation, with periodic (at least annual) inspections to ensure compliance. Inspections are conducted by the Real Estate Assessment Center (REAC), which has the mission of providing and promoting "the effective use of accurate, timely, and reliable information assessing the condition of HUD's portfolio, to provide information to help ensure safe, decent, and affordable housing and to restore the public trust by identifying fraud, abuse, and waste of HUD resources" (HUD, 2019b). Upholding the prescribed standards for both the physical plant and operations is a condition for renewing any rent subsidies, if applicable. However, civil monetary penalties are not an available remedy, as they are concerning Medicare and Medicaid recertification.

HUD's Office of Fair Housing and Equal Opportunity (FHEO) strives to eliminate housing discrimination, promote economic opportunity, and achieve diverse, inclusive communities. Laws implemented and enforced by FHEO include the following:

- The Fair Housing Act
- Title VI of the Civil Rights Act of 1964
- Section 109 of the Housing and Community Development Act of 1974
- Section 504 of the Rehabilitation Act of 1973
- Titles II and III of the Americans with Disabilities Act of 1990
- The Architectural Barriers Act of 1968
- The Age Discrimination Act of 1975
- Title IX of the Education Amendments Act of 1972
- Section 3 of the Housing and Urban Development Act of 1968

The Fair Housing Act was originally enacted in 1964 and has undergone periodic revisions that have expanded the range of people it protects (U.S. Department of Justice, 2019). It prohibits discrimination in making housing available—by owners or sponsors, as well as by other stakeholder entities, such as municipalities, lenders, or insurance companies—based on someone's race or color, religion, gender, national origin, familial status, or disability. Although it prohibits a housing provider from refusing to rent or sell to families with children, there is an exception for facilities designated as "senior housing" (typically 55 years and older, but some funding programs have an even higher qualifying minimum age).

Someone who believes they have been the victim of an illegal housing practice may file a complaint with HUD or initiate a lawsuit in federal or state court. If force (or the threat of force) is applied to deny or interfere with someone's fair housing rights, the Department of Justice can represent the person in pursuing criminal proceedings.

Note: While it is expected of organizations participating in any of HUD's programs to publicly display an organization's adherence to the Fair Housing Act, it is simply good practice to prominently proclaim the organization's status as an "Equal Housing Opportunity" provider on its signage, marketing materials, and website.

Veterans Affairs The Administration for Veterans Affairs offers benefits for certain PAC services, most of which are limited to conditions directly related to a veteran's service. Many states sponsor SNFs and/or assisted living facilities for qualified veterans—and sometimes for spouses or widows, as well. Such an SNF might be certified for Medicare, Medicaid, both, or neither.

The VA directly operates over 100 "community living centers" across the country (VA, 2019a). Recent additions to this network have embraced in the design of their physical plant and programs many of the principles of resident-centered care espoused by organizations such as the Pioneer Network, Eden Alternative, and the Green House Project. Eligibility is based on service-connected clinical need, level of disability, enrollment in the VA health system, income, and availability.

The VA's "Community Nursing Home Program" partners with licensed SNFs to offer needed services to eligible veterans near their homes and families. While similar in design and purpose, the VA has its own set of standards for a provider to participate in this program that supersede requirements for state licensure or certification by Medicare or Medicaid (VA, 2019b).

A veteran who can no longer live alone due to their physical or mental status, has no support person who can provide monitoring or assistance with activities of daily living (ADLs), and does not need nursing home care might qualify to participate in the VA's "Community Residential Care (CRC) Program" (VA, 2019c). More than 550 assisted living facilities, personal care homes, family care homes, group living homes, and psychiatric community residential care homes contract with the VA to provide such supportive housing and services. While they are inspected and approved by VA medical center staff, the veteran chooses the provider.

Wartime veterans and their surviving spouses who are 65 years and older may be entitled to a tax-free benefit called "Aid and Attendance," which is designed to provide financial aid to help offset the cost of long-term care for those who need assistance with ADLs.

Each of these VA programs has compliance expectations for the beneficiary, the provider, or both. Understanding those expectations and establishing procedures to internally monitor compliance can enhance the success of the relationship with your organization. In addition to providing a much-needed community service, participating in any of the VA's programs bolsters the organization's public image.

Key State Programs

Each state develops its own State Health Plan (SHP) to determine its priorities for achieving public wellness, allocation of financial and human resources, and synchronizing with federal programs that might support its efforts. If a state wishes to offer health services that go beyond the minimum required by Medicaid, it may request special permission (called a "waiver") from the CMS to do so under section 1115 of the Social Security Act's Title 19. Many states have successfully advanced innovative programs to enhance the lives of previously underserved citizens by this approach.

Individual states also reserve the right to govern the practice of health professionals through discipline-specific professional practice acts, which typically set up licensure requirements for entry and renewal, as well as independent boards to oversee compliance. The primary purpose of such rules and oversight is public protection—that minimum standards for qualification to practice are upheld. Due to a federal mandate, all states license nursing home administrators. An increasing number are also licensing administrators in related settings, such as assisted living and residential care communities or HCBS.

Some professions have advocated for states to recognize a common set of professional practice standards, reducing the need for acquiring separate licenses in each state to perform the same duties. The Nurse Licensure Compact (NLC), an initiative of the National Council of State Boards of Nursing (NCSBN), has been the most successful of those efforts, thus far. The NLC enables licensed nursing professionals to have greater geographic mobility among over 30 states that have come together around uniform licensure standards (NCSBN, 2019). The HSE™ qualification introduced by the National Association of Long-Term Care Administrator Boards (NAB) is patterned after the NLC and includes aspects to also broaden the scope of practice to other settings across the PAC continuum.

Other state programs that interpret statutes by promulgating regulations and enforcing them typically address the following:

- **Safe Workplace Environment:** In addition to Occupational Safety and Health Administration (OSHA), many states operate a workplace safety agency that enforces state regulations aimed at protecting employees while on duty.

- **Licensure:** Licensure sets standards for operating an organization providing certain healthcare services, typically including hospitals, long-term acute care (LTAC) hospitals, SNF, outpatient and ambulatory care clinics, and some HCBS, such as adult and child day care programs, home health agencies, and hospice. Many states either license or certify assisted living facilities as well.

- **Building and Construction Codes:** Complementing the NFPA's Life Safety Code, many states have additional requirements that address conditions or risks that may be unique to the area and merit specific attention, such as weather (hurricane, tornado, severe temperatures, or snow), natural disaster (earthquake or volcano) or other emergencies (power outage or chemical spill), or proximity to an airport, nuclear power plant, railroad or interstate highway, petroleum refinery, or other plant handling hazardous materials. Such codes call for special design features that enhance the probability a building can safely house those who live and work there throughout each targeted circumstance.

Key Local Programs

It is common for local municipalities to regulate certain operational activities of PAC providers. The size of the community's local government and its capacity for committing resources to fund such efforts contribute to the rigor and sophistication with which such efforts are executed.

- **Health and Sanitation:** The local (city or county) public health department generally accepts responsibility for ensuring that potable (safe to drink) water is delivered at every consumption portal (faucet, spigot, or drinking fountain), and, in institutional settings, that food preparation and storage procedures comply with established standards, hazardous waste is disposed of properly, and air circulation is adequate to serve the needs of the persons served. In many jurisdictions, the local health department might participate in or coordinate vaccination programs concerning flu, pneumonia, or hepatitis.

- **Planning and Zoning:** In addition to the NFPA's Life Safety Code and state-specific building and construction codes, local governments often have requirements restricting property use aimed at clustering similar enterprises in a community. Typical categories for such separation include residential (from single-family homes to multifamily housing), commercial (from retail stores to other businesses) and industrial (from light manufacturing to power plant), and public use (parks and other green spaces). Some planning and zoning commissions have developed very specific rules governing a building's characteristics beyond safety regulations, such as height, appearance (materials or architectural style), position on the property (set back from each boundary), or fencing. In communities with such an agency, building permits are generally issued *only* with its approval.

■ **Human Rights:** It is increasingly common for local governments to organize an enforcement unit to address discrimination in the workplace, housing, or commerce locations against people who are not specifically named as part of a federally protected class. Under current federal laws, individuals are protected against discrimination based on race or skin color, national origin, genetic information (such as family medical history), gender or pregnancy, religion, disability, or age. Some local jurisdictions have also added protections against discrimination based on marital status, political affiliation, and sexual orientation or gender identity.

Private Quality Standards

There are nongovernmental organizations (NGOs) that were formed with the express purpose of fostering quality among business enterprises, in general, and more specifically acute and postacute healthcare providers. Some of the most widely recognized ones are listed in the following (in alphabetical order.)

Accreditation Commission for Health Care   The Accreditation Commission for Health Care (ACHC) is another tax-exempt NGO that accredits home health and hospice providers, as well as an array of other healthcare organizations. The ACHC has CMS Deeming Authority for Home Health and Hospice (and for renal dialysis and durable medical equipment, prosthetics, orthotics, and supplies) and a quality management system that is ISO 9001-certified. The qualifications for ACHC accreditation are described in more detail at www.achc.org.

Baldrige Award   One of the most widely recognized quality standards for conducting business is the Malcolm Baldrige National Quality Award, according to the National Institute of Standards and Technology. Relatively new to the fields of healthcare and human services, the award is not given for specific services or products. To receive the Baldrige Award, an organization must demonstrate having systems in place that ensure continuous improvement in overall performance and providing an approach for consistently satisfying and responding to customers and stakeholders. Its criteria center on five key areas of outcome: (a) product/service and process, (b) customer, (c) workforce, (d) leadership and governance, and (e) financial and market. More information about the Baldrige Award requirements and process for qualifying for it can be found at www.nist.gov/baldrige/baldrige-award.

Better Business Bureau   Founded in 1912, the Better Business Bureau (BBB.org) is a private, tax-exempt NGO with the stated mission of advancing marketplace trust in the United States and Canada. It aims to foster trust, innovation, and competition through the development and delivery of cost-effective, third-party self-regulation, consumer dispute resolution, and other programs.

The more than 400,000 businesses that affiliate with the BBB and adhere to its operating standards do so voluntarily. To avoid potential conflicts of interest, the organization refrains from either recommending or endorsing any specific business. Instead, the BBB administers a rating system—awarding letter grades from A+ to F—reflecting its confidence level that a business is operating in a trustworthy manner and will make a good faith effort to resolve any customer concerns filed with the BBB.

Commission on Accreditation of Rehabilitation Facilities   The Commission on Accreditation of Rehabilitation Facilities (CARF International) is a nonprofit accrediting body for health and human services providers, including a variety of aging services in the PAC arena. Originally formed to set standards for medical rehabilitation facilities, sheltered workshops, and homebound programs, it has grown in scope to now also offer quality assessment programs for SNFs and assisted living facilities, continuing care retirement communities (CCRCs), and life plan communities, as well as HCBS, such as adult day centers. Over 7,800 providers are CARF accredited throughout North and South America, Europe, and Asia. To learn more about CARF International, visit www.carf.org.

Community Health Accreditation Partner   The Community Health Accreditation Partner (CHAP) is an independent, nonprofit accrediting body for home- and community-based healthcare organizations. Created in 1965 as a joint venture between the American Public Health Association and the National League for Nursing, CHAP was the first accrediting body for HCBS organizations in the United States and now offers quality verification programs for home health agencies and hospice providers (and home medical equipment, private duty services, pharmacy, infusion therapy nursing, and public health). The CMS selected CHAP as one if its contract Deeming Authority organizations (meeting CHAP accreditation standards to fulfill the conditions of participation in Medicare and/or Medicaid). More information about CHAP is available at https://chapinc.org.

International Standards Organization   Another NGO with a growing influence in healthcare and human services is the International Standards Organization (ISO), whose members are 164 national standards bodies. By coordinating the efforts of quality experts from around the world, it maintains "voluntary, consensus-based, market-relevant international standards that support innovation and provide solutions to global challenges." The ISO-9000 family of quality standards is designed to ensure consumers that a company meets or exceeds internationally recognized performance criteria concerning safety, reliability, and quality. These standards also serve as strategic tools that can help increase productivity, minimize waste and errors, and improve customer outcomes. Unlike the Baldrige Award, ISO offers targeted *certification* for providers of healthcare and senior living services. The most current information about ISO and its quality standards is available at www.iso.org.

The Joint Commission   The Joint Commission (formerly know as The Joint Commission on Accreditation of Healthcare Organizations) is the nation's oldest and largest healthcare standards setting and accrediting body. It evaluates and accredits over 21,000 health providers, from hospitals to SNFs, home health agencies, and hospices. It also offers certification of service lines, such as disease-specific care, palliative care, and healthcare staffing services. Earning The Joint Commission's

"Gold Seal of Approval," which remains active for 3 years, demonstrates to the public an organization's commitment to quality beyond what is minimally required for licensure. Policy makers continue to debate whether to assign The Joint Commission-accredited providers "deemed status" for participating in the Medicare and Medicaid programs, thereby exempting them from the CMS's annual surveys. More information about The Joint Commission's range of accreditation voluntary programs can be found at www.jointcommission.org.

Postacute Care Trade Associations Organizations representing the interests of providers with similar lines of service, corporate structure, or sponsorship are referred to as "trade associations." As part of their efforts to promote quality improvement among their members, they each offer programs to foster quality services beyond standards minimally required by state or federal regulations.

■   The American Health Care Association (AHCA) and the National Center for Assisted Living (NCAL) jointly administer the National Quality Award Program, which is based on the Baldrige Performance Excellence Program's core values criteria applied to the PAC settings of skilled nursing care and assisted living. According to the AHCA website, members may apply for three award levels with progressively rigorous requirements for quality and performance. For the most current information on this program, visit www.ahcancal.org/quality_improvement/quality_award/Pages/default.aspx.

■   LeadingAge (formerly known as the American Association of Homes and Services for the Aging, or AAHSA) created in 1985 the Continuing Care Accreditation Commission to develop aspirational quality standards for CCRCs and evaluate organizations' performance in meeting or exceeding them. The CARF International acquired the program in 2003.

Third-Party Reviews

Indirect assessments of quality performed by independent investigators typically rely on some blend of direct evaluations completed by regulatory agencies (survey and inspection results and related plans of correction), accrediting bodies, and/or consumer feedback. *U.S. News and World Report*'s series of "Best Rankings" is perhaps the most widely recognized one by the general public (*USNWR*, 2019). Since the 1980s, the organization has expanded its scope of comparisons to provide advice about what it considers "life's toughest decisions," from where to live, work, go to school, or travel, to selecting a healthcare provider, realtor, attorney, car, or investment. Although the SNF service line is the only PAC segment currently ranked, the organization has begun separately reporting on short-term rehabilitation and long-term stays. It is important to maintain an awareness about what its website reports about a facility and to report any inaccuracies or errors to its sponsor. To check a facility's current ranking, go to https://health.usnews.com/best-nursing-homes.

A veritable cottage industry has emerged centered on offering advice to consumers about selecting the best option for someone who might benefit from available senior living options—either residential or from HCBS providers. Some of them are incorporated as tax-exempt, not-for-profit organizations (look for the .org suffix in the website address) to either reflect the purity of their mission or to appear more trustworthy to consumers. Some have managed better than others to avoid the potential conflicts of interest associated with providing more favorable recommendations to providers who pay them advertising fees or "partnership" dues than those who do not. It is difficult to create an exhaustive list because new ones emerge routinely, but here are some of the most visited sites (in descending order as listed on Google, October 6, 2019):

- A Place for Mom   https://i.aplaceformom.com
- Senior Advisor   https://www.senioradvisor.com
- Caring.com   https://www.caring.com/senior-living
- Dibbern & Dibbern, Ltd   https://www.dibbern.com
- SkilledNursingFacilities.org   https://www.skillednursingfacilities.org
- MatchNursingHomes.org   http://matchnursinghomes.org
- AssistedSeniorLiving.net   https://www.assistedseniorliving.net
- CaregiverList   https://www.caregiverlist.com/find-senior -care
- Care Pathways   https://www.carepathways.com
- SeniorHousing.net   https://www.seniorhousingnet.com

Additionally, several popular websites created as resources for people searching for their next employer also provide valuable information to consumers about an organization's workplace culture and environment. An increasing body of evidence suggests that an atmosphere with engaged staff members produces better quality outcomes—clinically and experientially (Healthcare Source, 2019). Critics of such websites allege they tend to attract contributors with either the most positive or the most negative comments, rather than a meaningful array of feedback. Nonetheless, incorporating such information into a family's strategy for finding an eldercare service solution can be expected to continue growing. Some of the most frequented sites include the following:

- Great Places to Work   https://www.greatplacetowork.com
- Glass Door   https://www.glassdoor.com
- Fortune   https://fortune.com

Individual Practitioners

All states currently license the administrators of SNFs, and an increasing number also license administrators of assisted living communities and certain HCBS lines of service. A professional licensing board typically maintains records of any disciplinary actions imposed on its licensees, and rules vary as to how much of the details are subject to public access via open record laws and regulations.

Enforcement

Government agencies charged with responsibility for enforcing statutes and regulations, as well as NGO accrediting bodies evaluating adherence to their performance standards, rely on at least some element of on-site assessment by trained inspectors.

TABLE 5.2 Centers for Medicare & Medicaid Services' Regions

Region	Location	States Served by the Region
1	Boston	Connecticut, Maine, Massachusetts, New Hampshire, Rhode Island, Vermont
2	New York	New Jersey, New York, Puerto Rico, Virgin Islands
3	Philadelphia	Delaware, District of Columbia, Maryland, Pennsylvania, Virginia, West Virginia
4	Atlanta	Alabama, Florida, Georgia, Kentucky, Mississippi, North Carolina, South Carolina, Tennessee
5	Chicago	Illinois, Indiana, Michigan, Minnesota, Ohio, Wisconsin
6	Dallas	Arkansas, Louisiana, New Mexico, Oklahoma, Texas
7	Kansas City	Iowa, Kansas, Missouri, Nebraska
8	Denver	Colorado, Montana, North Dakota, South Dakota, Utah, Wyoming
9	San Francisco	Arizona, California, Hawaii, Nevada, Pacific Territories
10	Seattle	Alaska, Idaho, Oregon, Washington

Source: U.S. Centers for Medicare and Medicaid Services. (n.d.). *We're putting patients first.* Retrieved from https://www.cms.gov

Surveys for state licensure and Medicare/Medicaid certification, recertification, and complaint investigations occur without advance notice, with the underlying expectation that the operation is consistent on any given day. The default period for such surveys is annually, with a margin of plus-or-minus 6 months. A complaint can trigger an interim investigation, but the scope can expand if the survey team discovers other issues of noncompliance unrelated to the complaint.

The CMS has 10 regional offices overseeing Medicare and Medicaid provider compliance, shown in Table 5.2. In addition to the initial, annual and complaint surveys performed by state survey agencies, the CMS periodically selects a sample of providers to evaluate for a quality assurance validation of the state survey results. Commonly referred to as a "federal look-behind survey," this inspection's results carry the same duties for response by the provider.

Accreditation inspections typically occur by appointment, which makes preparing for the evaluation team's visit more feasible. Critics of allowing private accreditation to qualify for Medicare/Medicaid "deemed status" point to this feature as a weakness, even though the applicable standards may exceed the minimum requirements for Medicare/Medicaid certification.

Inspection Process

Preparing for inspections should be an integral part of the provider's QAPI program. The feedback gained from an independent snapshot of the operation can inform the strategy and tactics for performance improvement that transcends compliance with minimal standards. Rather than viewing it as a burden of regulatory compliance, leverage the results to set new operational goals that should improve care quality. The cycle of activities is very similar for each of the processes mentioned.

1. An interdisciplinary inspection team observes the operation in person and records its findings, guided by published regulations, related interpretive guidelines, and applicable standards of professional practice. This typically includes reviewing policies and procedures, staff adherence to them, care recipient records, and employee files, observing the physical plant and a variety of operational activities, and interviewing with stakeholders.

2. The inspection team:

   a. Shares its findings informally with the staff leadership and then formally in an "exit conference" with additional stakeholders present.

   b. Prepares and sends a written report of its findings, including any citations for noncompliance with applicable regulations or standards.

3. The provider's leadership team:

   a. Develops a "Plan of Correction" that describes how the organization proposes to remediate any deficiencies cited in the inspection report and by when.

   b. Submits its plan within the prescribed time frame for review and approval by the inspection entity.

   c. Implements the plan and monitors ongoing compliance to prevent recurrence of the cited deficient practices.

4. The inspection entity:

   a. Reviews the plan of correction submitted by the provider, and

      i. If approved, may revisit to verify that the provider has implemented the submitted plan appropriately and effectively.

      ii. If not approved, request modifications to the plan for resubmission and subsequent review.

      iii. (Medicare/Medicaid only)

         1. Determines whether to impose any civil monetary penalties, based on the scope and/or severity of cited deficiencies (up to $10,000/ day, and in some instances, retroactively).

         2. Posts on the relevant Medicare.gov page the most recent findings.

         3. Refers to the state administrator licensing board for further investigation any citation for a "sub-standard level of care."

   b. Notifies the provider when "credible compliance" (Medicare/Medicaid term) has been achieved, meaning the applicable standards have been substantially met.

5. The provider:

   a. Communicates with internal stakeholders the results of the process:

      i. Displays for public view the most recent survey results and plan of correction (mandatory for Medicare, Medicaid, and most state licensure survey findings.

      ii. Displays for public view the certificate of award (optional—and *beneficial*—for accreditation credentials).

    b. May appeal unfavorable inspection findings, either through informal dispute resolution, if available, or through a formal process established by the inspection entity.

Critics of the current approach employed by the CMS contend relatively little evidence exists that supports its underlying assumption that penalties effectively deter poor-quality care or incentivize performance improvement (Goozner, 2019). The CMS's long-standing reliance on punitive measures for providers that fall short of complying with minimal regulatory standards as conditions of participation in Medicare or Medicaid favors its focus on enforcement—perhaps at the expense of true quality enhancement. This will predictably remain a key public policy debate of significant importance, addressing whether we can achieve better public protection through penalizing low compliance or rewarding consistently high performance. Maybe we should move toward some hybrid of the two, as a few of the private accrediting bodies have adopted.

Risk Management

Risk simply refers to any situation or set of circumstances that poses a potential for damaging property or injuring a person. *Managing* risk involves developing and implementing policies and procedures that mitigate—reduce the probability of—a risk resulting in actual harm. It starts with identifying and analyzing an organization's exposure to risk, from the potential for natural disasters or a fire, as discussed earlier, to the dangers posed by the caregiving environment to both caregivers and recipients, such as infectious diseases, hazardous waste, sharps, treatment or documentation errors, privacy compromises, fair labor or safety violations, or even breeches of contract.

PAC settings certainly present a wide range of risks, given the fragile nature of the clients served and the number of people typically involved in making decisions about and delivering services. A contemporary cultural shift toward resolving conflict through litigation amplifies the stakes, manifested in a rising incidence of litigation against providers in response to undesired outcomes (Folk & Haciski, 2013).

Legal Environment

Of course, attorneys prepare for their careers with several years of graduate education and training, so this brief primer is intended only to introduce and highlight some key legal concepts that apply in the context of risk management (Cornell University Law School Legal Information Institute, 2019).

Criminal Law   Criminal laws deal with crime and the legal punishment of criminal offenses, such as theft, assault, trafficking in controlled substances, or murder—behavior that is an offense against the public, society, or the state, even if the immediate victim is an individual. Crimes are typically divided into two broad classes: felonies (most egregious) and misdemeanors. The burden of proof on the state for conviction is "beyond a reasonable doubt," and penalties include incarceration, fines, or both.

Civil Law   Disputes between individuals, organizations, or between the two, such as personal injury, landlord/tenant, or property disputes fall into the category of civil law. The entity initiating the action is called the **plaintiff**, and the entity charged with harming the plaintiff is called the **defendant**. The plaintiff's burden of proof is a "preponderance of the evidence." If successful, some form of compensation is awarded to the plaintiff. Civil law includes several subsets, two of which most frequently apply in the senior living arena: torts and contracts.

Tort Law   Tort laws address situations when one party's behavior causes injury, suffering, or harm to another. Its two main purposes are (a) to compensate the victim for any losses caused by the defendant's violations and (b) to discourage recurrence of the violation. The three categories of tort law are as follows:

- Intentional: Common examples are assault, battery, false imprisonment, trespassing, and intentional infliction of emotional distress.

- Strict liability: The plaintiff must show (a) that the defendant did something that was inherently dangerous, (b) that act caused something bad to happen to the plaintiff, and (c) that the plaintiff suffered actual harm. (Interpretation varies considerably by state.)

- Unintentional or negligence: When harm occurs because the defendant ignored or failed to take reasonable measures to prevent it from happening, considered "carelessly caused" harm. The central characteristics of negligence include the following (Owen, 2007):

  - **Duty:** Obligation of one person/entity to another

  - **Breach:** Acting without *reasonable* care to meet duty

  - **Causality:** The alleged negligence actually caused the harm claimed

  - **Proximate Cause:** Degree of predictability, in logic, fairness, policy, or practicality

  - **Harm:** The extent of damage suffered by the victim (plaintiff in a lawsuit)

Contract Law   Agreements between private parties that create mutual obligations—promises that the law will enforce—are governed by contract laws. While overall contract law is common throughout the country, some specific court interpretations of a contract element may vary between the states. For such an agreement to be legally enforceable, it typically must include the following components:

- **Mutual assent** expressed by a valid offer and acceptance

- **Consideration** so that the parties are exchanging what they have agreed to, usually of commensurate value

- **Capacity** means a person's competence to enter into a valid contract and the ability to perform some act included in the contract

- **Legality** refers to the absence of any contract element that violates the law

If a promise is breached, the law provides remedies to the harmed party, often in form of monetary damages, or in limited circumstances, in the form of specific performance of the promise made (or an agreed upon substitute).

Service agreements are contracts, ranging from resident admission agreements for various congregate senior living settings to patient and participant agreements for HCBS relationships. In addition to the minimum requirements listed earlier, an increasingly widespread practice among senior living organizations is to include some provision describing and requiring an attempt to informally resolve a dispute, perhaps through mediation or arbitration, before filing a potentially costly lawsuit to satisfy a claim. In **mediation**, the disputing parties decide whether to agree to a settlement; the **mediator** they jointly select has no power to impose a binding resolution. In **arbitration**, the parties assign authority to decide the dispute to a jointly selected **arbitrator**. Much attention has been given by the courts to whether such clauses are permissible or enforceable, with no consistent outcomes yet.

Consumer awareness has risen about high-profile lawsuits alleging personal injury—even wrongful death—that resulted in very large plaintiff awards. It has become nearly impossible in many markets to watch television for any length of time without viewing at least one personal injury attorney advertisement focused on this issue. Some states have responded by modifying their tort laws with the goal of reducing the volume of frivolous malpractice and personal injury actions and allow their courts to focus on those that meet some standard for medical merit. Others have favored protecting consumer rights, but often with the unintended consequence of adding significant legal costs to the healthcare delivery system.

Related Legal Concept: Liability According to the International Risk Management Institute (2019), "liability" refers to the legal concept of responsibility for one's actions (or inaction), the duty one has toward another to perform in a way that meets or exceeds an implicit obligation (by law, regulation, or professional standard of practice), or by explicit agreement (by contract).

- **Corporate Liability:** Although it is possible to delegate *authority* for making decisions about how a provider fulfills such duties, *responsibility* for such decisions ultimately belongs to the organization.

- **Professional Liability:** Responsibility for errors or omissions in performing professional duties that result in harming someone.

- **Personal Liability:** When an individual (rather than an organization) is held responsible for someone's harm.

Related Legal Concept: Damages

Financial compensation awarded by a court in a civil action to an individual whose injury resulted from the wrongful conduct of another party is known as "damages" (Cornell University Law School Legal Information Institute, 2019) The three major categories of legal damages are as follows:

- **Compensatory Damages:** Intended to restore what a plaintiff lost as a result of a defendant's wrongful conduct.

- **Nominal Damages:** Awarded to a plaintiff who has experienced an invasion of rights, but who suffered no substantial loss or injury.

- **Punitive Damages:** Awarded to penalize a defendant for particularly egregious, wrongful conduct. In specific situations, two other forms of damages may be awarded: treble and liquidated.

Insurance protection is commercially available for each of the liabilities described, and the lines of coverage have become increasingly subdivided. Consulting with an insurance broker familiar with senior living, in general, and particularly the provider's service lines, is imperative. Our field presents a unique set of risks to manage—complex operating circumstances, vulnerable customer base, intense regulatory oversight, and resource scarcity.

POLICIES AND PROCEDURES

Developing policies and procedures that address the topics covered in this chapter is very challenging because of the fluid nature of the practice domain: environment. Embedding in procedures the most relevant source documents or Internet site hyperlinks is the most efficient strategy for remaining current with external changes among regulatory agencies with oversight responsibilities. Proactively scheduling periodic reviews for possible updating of policies and procedures (at least annually) and conducting targeted in-service education programming for personnel with related responsibilities also serve to keep everyone "on the same page in the hymnal."

SUMMARY

The complexity and volume of information required of an effective leader in these environment areas (as well as others) can be overwhelming. Yet, the key to being successful is to make sure that you have all of the expertise and resources available to you when needed. Nobody expects anyone in a leadership position to remember every last detail or regulation; rather what they admire is the person who knows when they don't know and knows what questions to ask or where to go for answers. An effective leader does understand the approaches and systems required to be in place to run an efficient, safe organization.

KEY POINTS

1. This domain encompasses a wide variety of responsibilities aimed at protecting safety, dignity, comfort, and privacy for all who interact with the organization—consumers, staff and contractors, volunteers, and the general public.
2. Although the underlying concepts apply across all the lines of service, this domain of professional practice is one of the most diverse because the circumstances vary so extensively among settings.
3. Although specific building codes and construction regulations vary by location, most reference adhering to guidelines published by the NFPA.
4. Organized preventive maintenance is more of an investment than an expense.
5. Efficient, thorough, and effective recordkeeping (including redundancy/and backup) is vital.
6. Planning for disasters—and practicing responses by drilling—saves lives.
7. Coordinated procurement and inventory control systems represent sound stewardship.
8. Good governance—regardless of corporate structure or sponsorship—requires *fiduciary* QAPI.
9. Licensure, certification, and accreditation processes expect compliance with minimal standards—the "deficiency-free" inspection should be the HSE™'s floor, not the ceiling.
10. The legal environment for senior living is complex, dynamic, and demanding. Managing the unique risks presented by serving an inherently vulnerable population carries huge responsibilities and comes with high consumer expectations.

LEADERSHIP ROLES

The HSE™ cultivates an organizational culture that considers exceeding compliance with minimum standards and consumer expectations as the norm. This starts with insisting on key stakeholders maintaining a current, working knowledge of all applicable laws, regulations, and standards of practice and continues with establishing systems for ongoing assessment and improvement of relevant policies and procedures. Transparency, consistency, and accountability are paramount. Proactively managing operational risks, including preparing adequately for emergencies and disasters, requires diligence and attention to detail. Allocating resources—financial and time—to all of the aforementioned is a key responsibility of HSE™ leadership.

> *My experience in LTC has demonstrated over and over that the knowledge of the Domains established by NAB will be needed to understand the complexities of any organization – it is a deep well of knowledge that never ends.*
>
> *Steven A. Nash, LNHA President/CEO*
> *Stoddard Baptist Foundation & Stoddard*
> *Baptist Services*

HIGH-IMPACT PRACTICES

1. A home health agency offers value-added services to its patients by partnering with a local homebuilder to design and install supportive home modifications (from entrance ramps to bathroom grab bars and other universal design features) and to coordinate preventive maintenance services for their homes (from HVAC and appliances to smoke detectors and alarm systems).

2. A CCRC contracts with a local funeral home livery service to provide its residents with transportation—to medical appointments or social engagements—in *limousines*.

3. The Director of Maintenance at an SNF sends a brief acknowledgment note to the person who submitted a work order request when the project is completed, thanking them for helping to make it a better place for the residents to live (if a staff member, copied to the department manager and administrator).

4. Texas caps the amount of noneconomic damages a plaintiff can try to recover from the defendant at $250,000, and its long-term care providers experience premiums and claim costs of less than one fourth the national average.

    - 2019 Aon Professional and General Liability Benchmark for Long-Term Care Providers

    - www.aon.com/getmedia/69de85a2-5aad-40af-9dc1-0296f09137f1/2019-LTC-Report_Executive-Summary.aspx

QUESTIONS FOR DISCUSSION

1. A comprehensive disaster preparedness plan should address the organization's response to what events?

2. What are the key determinants of who should have authorized access to the organization's records?

3. Discuss the variables that are important to consider in evaluating a resident's risk for elopement.

4. Describe the key elements of an inventory control system.

5. Compare and contrast corporate sponsorship models found in senior living—proprietary, not-for-profit, and public.

6. Discuss the primary duties of a senior living organization's governing board.

7. Describe how you would design and apply a "balanced scorecard" for communicating with your governing board about organizational performance as the executive leader.

8. Whether for demonstrating compliance with government regulations or private accreditation standards, inspections and site surveys are a central part of operating a senior living organization. Describe the general sequence of activities that occur during and following an inspection by an outside entity for one of these purposes.

9. Select a senior living line of service. Provide examples of events for which a different one of the three categories of tort law apply and why.

10. According to the 2018 Aon Professional and General Liability Benchmark for Long-Term Care Providers, resident agreements that provide for arbitration as a means for resolving disputes close claims more swiftly and at lowers costs. Is this approach consistent with a philosophy of person-centered care? Why or why not?

CASE PROBLEMS

1. Conducting drills for responding to a fire event is a common practice in congregate senior living settings (even required in most). However, a home health agency decided to apply the same safety preparedness principles as an activity for its patients and their supporters, whether family members, neighbors, or both. This included expanding its existing physical plant safety assessment by scheduling actual fire drills using a variety of role-play scenarios. The fire drill log became a new section of the patient's clinical record. In addition to reducing the risk of negative outcomes in the event of a home fire, this approach bolstered the confidence of patients and their advocates.

   Questions:

   a. What key challenges could be expected in implementing a program such as this one?

   b. What three events would be your top priority for an at-home disaster plan and drill, and why?

2. Mrs. Eichert was a petite, pleasantly confused, midstage dementia resident of an assisted living community who had an affinity for walking. She was on the move nearly constantly during waking hours and sometimes during the night. The layout of the campus facilitated continuous pedestrian mobility—indoors and outdoors—without exiting altogether. One afternoon, she turned up missing. Staff members coordinated a search of the property according to procedure, but without the intended result. Local law enforcement was contacted and provided with a photo and description of what she was last seen wearing. Local authorities initiated a "silver alert" for broadcast on the emergency notification network. The immediately surrounding neighborhood was thoroughly searched, using increasingly wider circles of distance from the assisted living campus. With great relief, the turmoil came to a screeching halt when a member of the housekeeping staff discovered Mrs. Eichert taking a nap, curled up with the resident cat under the baby grand piano in the parlor. Her position and size had escaped the sight line of everyone who had checked that room—perhaps in too much rush. Moral: Check everywhere even a child might hide.

    Questions:

    a. What recommendations would you offer to the staff for conducting an elopement event response?

    b. At what point should the resident's family be notified? Why?

3. The governing board of a not-for-profit, faith-based, stand-alone CCRC with over 400 residents decided that in order to most effectively fulfill its duties, two changes must occur: (a) the composition of the board should move toward people with qualifying skill sets and knowledge identified as relevant, and (b) an ongoing board education program should be initiated focused on contemporary governance high-impact practices. An inventory of current board members' background, experience, and interests revealed either a current or imminent (due to term limits) shortage of representation by three desired metrics—healthcare technology, medicine, and human resources. Developing the list of nominees for the next three vacancies on the board incorporated that discovery as priorities, and all three were successfully added. Each board member elected to receive at least one subscription to a senior living trade or professional journal from a list provided by the executive leadership. The CCRC also contracted with a third-party governance consulting firm to facilitate a hybrid learning program—some content delivered online in interactive modules and some in a classroom setting as part of the board meeting agendas. The governing board's self-assessment of its own performance, as well as the organization's key performance metrics (quality, financial, resident and family satisfaction, and employee engagement) steadily and measurably increased.

    Questions:

    a. What skill sets and expertise would be most beneficial to include in the mix for recruiting members to serve on a senior living organization's board of directors?

    b. How can a governing board's performance be effectively measured?

4. Place yourself in a position as an administrator of a nonprofit community–supported senior care campus that has 30 skilled care beds with 10 of them designated as rehab suites, an attached 50 bed assisted living residence, and 100 units of senior housing. You are the only senior living provider in a rural setting in a state that has not had widespread cases of COVID-19. You have just been informed that one of your recently admitted rehabilitation residents has symptoms that are representative of COVID-19.

    Questions:

    a. What are your immediate steps over the next 24 hours?

        1. Who would you reach out to and why?

        2. What initial actions would you take within your senior care community?

        3. What resources would you use?

        4. Develop a stakeholder communication plan that balances who needs to know what, why, and when while protecting privacy.

NAB DOMAINS OF PRACTICE

40 ENVIRONMENT

40.01 Ensure that physical environmental policies and practices comply with applicable federal, state, and local laws, rules, and regulations.

40.02 Ensure the planning, development, implementation, monitoring, and evaluation of a safe and secure environment.

40.03 Ensure the planning, development, implementation, monitoring, and evaluation of infection control and sanitation.

40.04 Ensure the planning, development, implementation, monitoring, and evaluation of emergency and disaster preparedness program, including linkage to outside emergency agencies.

40.05 Ensure the planning, development, implementation, monitoring, and evaluation of environmental services, housekeeping, and laundry.

40.06 Ensure the planning, development, implementation, monitoring, and evaluation of maintenance services for property, plant, and all equipment, including preventive maintenance.

40.07 Ensure the planning, development, implementation, monitoring, and evaluation of appropriate HIPAA compliant technology infrastructure.

40.08 Establish, maintain, and monitor a physical environment that provides clean safe and secure home-like surroundings for care recipients, staff, and visitors.

40.09 Identify opportunities to enhance the physical environment to meet changing market demands.

40.10 Establish, maintain, and monitor an environment that promotes choice, comfort, and dignity for care recipients.

40.11 Assess care recipients' environment for safety, security, and accessibility and make recommendations for referral or modification.

---

50 MANAGEMENT AND LEADERSHIP

50.03 Develop, implement, monitor, and evaluate policies and procedures that comply with directives of the governing body.

50.04 Develop, communicate, and champion the service provider's mission, vision, and values to stakeholders.

50.05 Develop, implement, and evaluate the strategic plan with governing body's endorsement.

50.10 Manage the service provider's role throughout any survey/inspection process.

50.11 Develop and implement an intervention(s) or risk management program(s) to minimize or eliminate exposure.

50.12 Identify and respond to areas of potential legal liability.

50.16 Develop, implement, and evaluate the organization's quality assurance and performance improvement programs.

A summary of the related knowledge, skills, and core expectations across service lines—and unique features of each service line—is available at www.nabweb.org/filebin/pdf/Annotation_of_Tasks_Performed_Across_LOS_in_LTC.pdf.

Source: Reproduced with permission from the National Association of Long-Term Care Administrator Boards. (2016). *Annotation of tasks performed and knowledge and skills used across lines of service in long term care.* Retrieved from https://www.nabweb.org/filebin/pdf/Annotation_of_Tasks_Performed_Across_LOS_in_LTC.pdf

---

REFERENCES

BrainyQuote.com. (2019, August 17). *Byron Dorgan quotes.* Retrieved from https://www.brainyquote.com/quotes/byron_dorgan_167846

Caceres, V. (2020, March 13). What's the difference between an epidemic and a pandemic? *U.S. News and World Report.* Retrieved from https://health.usnews.com/conditions/articles/whats-the-difference-between-an-epidemic-and-a-pandemic

Cornell University Law School Legal Information Institute. (2019). *Wex.* Retrieved from https://www.law.cornell.edu/wex

Folk, T., & Haciski, R. (2013). Legality reality: Litigation on the rise in LTC industry. *Long-Term Living: For the Continuing Care Professional, 62*(9), 27–29.

Goozner, M. (2019, January 3). Are CMS' quality incentive programs working? *Modern Healthcare.* Retrieved from https://www.modernhealthcare.com/article/20190103/NEWS/190109984/editorial-are-cms-quality-incentive-programs-working.

Healthcare Source. (2019). *Employee engagement drives patient care.* Retrieved from http://education.healthcaresource.com/employee-engagement-drives-quality-patient-care/

International Risk Management Institute. (2019). *Professional liability.* Retrieved from https://www.irmi.com/term/insurance-definitions/professional-liability

Kaplan, R., & Norton, D. (1992). The balanced scorecard: Measures that drive performance. *Harvard Business Review, 70*(1), 71–79.

Kosieradzki, M., & Smith, J. (2003). Common injuries—Elopement and wandering. In R. Conlin & G. S. Cusimano (Eds.), *ATLA's litigating tort cases* (Vol. 5). Washington, DC: American Association for Justice Press.

MedLeague. (2019). *Elopement from a long-term care facility.* Retrieved from https://www.medleague.com/elopement-from-a-long-term-care-facility-expert-witness/

National Council of State Boards of Nursing. (2019). *The nurse licensure compact*. Retrieved from https://www.ncsbn.org/nurse-licensure-compact.htm

National Fire Protection Association. (2019). *NFPA-101: Life safety codes and standards*. Retrieved from https://www.nfpa.org/codes-and-standards/all-codes-and-standards/list-of-codes-and-standards/detail?code=101

National Fire Protection Association. (2020). *NFPA-70: National electrical code*. Retrieved from https://www.nfpa.org/Codes-and-Standards

National Weather Service, National Oceanic and Atmospheric Administration. (2020). *Severe weather safety and survival*. Retrieved from https://www.weather.gov/oun/safety-severe-homesafety

Owen, D. G. (2007). The five elements of negligence. *Hofstra Law Review, 35*(4). Retrieved from http://scholarlycommons.law.hofstra.edu/hlr/vol35/iss4/1

Pratt, J. (2016). *Long-term care: Managing across the continuum* (4th ed.). Burlington, MA: Jones and Bartlett Learning.

Siegel, J., Rhinehart, E., Jackson, M., Chiarello, L., and the Centers for Disease Control and Prevention Healthcare Infection Control Practices Advisory Committee. (2019). *2007 guideline for isolation precautions: Preventing transmission of infectious agents in healthcare settings*. Retrieved from https://www.cdc.gov/infectioncontrol/guidelines/isolation/index.html

Todd, J. (2017, April 24). How to prepare for the new CMS rule for emergency preparedness. *Provider Long-Term and Post-Acute Care*. Retrieved from http://www.providermagazine.com/columns/Pages/2017/How-to-Prepare-for-the-New-CMS-Rule-for-Emergency-Preparedness.aspx#magazine-article

U.S. Centers for Medicare & Medicaid Services. (2014). *State operations manual chapter 10: Survey and enforcement process for home health agencies*. Retrieved from https://www.cms.gov/Regulations-and-Guidance/Guidance/Manuals/Downloads/som107c10.pdf

U.S. Centers for Medicare & Medicaid Services. (2016). *Final CMS emergency preparedness rule*. Retrieved from https://www.cms.gov/Medicare/Provider-Enrollment-and-Certification/SurveyCertEmergPrep/Emergency-Prep-Rule.html

U.S. Centers for Medicare & Medicaid Services. (2018). *State operations manual chapter 7: Survey and enforcement process for skilled nursing facilities and nursing facilities*. Retrieved from https://www.cms.gov/Regulations-and-Guidance/Guidance/Manuals/Downloads/som107c07.pdf

U.S. Centers for Medicare & Medicaid Services. (2014). *State operations manual chapter 10: Survey and enforcement process for home health agencies*. Available at: https://www.cms.gov/Regulations-and-Guidance/Guidance/Manuals/Downloads/som107c10.pdf

U.S. Code of Federal Regulations. (2020). *Policies and procedures and documentation requirements*. 45 CFR 164.316(b)(2).

U.S. Department for Housing and Urban Development. (2019a). *Section 202 supportive housing for the elderly program*. Retrieved from https://www.hud.gov/program_offices/housing/mfh/progdesc/eld202

U.S. Department for Housing and Urban Development. (2019b). *Uniform physical condition standards and physical inspection requirements for certain HUD housing; Administrative process for assessment of insured and assisted properties*. Retrieved from https://www.hud.gov/sites/documents/UNIFORM_STDS.PDF

U.S. Department of Justice. (2019). *The Fair Housing Act*. Retrieved from https://www.justice.gov/crt/fair-housing-act-1

U.S. Department for Veterans Affairs. (2019a). *VA community living centers*. Retrieved from https://www.va.gov/GERIATRICS/pages/VA_Community_Living_Centers.asp

U.S. Department for Veterans Affairs. (2019b). *VA community nursing homes*. Retrieved from https://www.va.gov/GERIATRICS/pages/Community_Nursing_Homes.asp

U.S. Department for Veterans Affairs. (2019c). *VA community residential care*. Retrieved from https://www.va.gov/GERIATRICS/pages/community_residential_care.asp

U.S. News and World Report. (2019). *Best rankings*. Retrieved from https://www.usnews.com/rankings

ADDITIONAL RESOURCES

Building and Environment

Regardless of location, an elder's immediate surroundings contribute greatly to their comfort, security, and life satisfaction.

- *Aging in Place:* Golant, S. (2015). *Aging in the right place.* Baltimore, MD: Health Professions Press.

- *Design:* Regnier, V. (2018). *Housing design for an increasingly older population: Redefining assisted living for the mentally and physically frail.* Hoboken, NJ: Wiley.

- *Safety:* The National Fire Protection Association Codes and Standards. Retrieved from https://www.nfpa.org/Codes-and-Standards

Legal Environment

There is no substitute for establishing a trusted relationship with legal counsel, but it is helpful for an HSE™ to have at least an introductory reference text in their personal library.

- Grant, P. D., & Ballard, D. (2013). *Fast facts for nursing and the law: Law for nurses in a Nutshell.* New York, NY: Springer Publishing Company.

- Polzgar, G. D. (2016). *Legal aspects of health care administration* (12th ed.). Burlington, MA: Jones and Bartlett Learning.

- Showalter, J. S. (2020). *The law of healthcare administration* (9th ed.). Chicago, IL: Health Administration Press; Washington, DC: Association of University Programs in Health Administration.

Risk Management

Aon, Inc., is a global risk consulting firm that each year conducts an actuarial analysis of general liability and professional liability claim costs for the long-term care profession in the United States. It provides a set of evidence-based benchmarks for senior living providers to gauge the resources devoted to their risk management and insurance programs.

- *2018 Aon General and Professional Liability Benchmark for Long Term Care Providers* Retrieved from https://www.aon.com/getmedia/c4af82af-61a0-4121-99d2 -dec3ee900044/Long-Term-Care-Benchmark-Report-Executive-Summary.aspx

- *2019 Aon General and Professional Liability Benchmark for Long Term Care Providers* Retrieved from https://www.aon.com/getmedia/69de85a2-5aad-40af -9dc1-0296f09137f1/2019-LTC-Report_Executive-Summary.aspx

Survey and Compliance

It is important for any leader to have the most current version of these protocols:

- Adult Day Care State-Specific Rules and Regulations: https://www.nadsa .org/providers/state-regulations/

- Assisted Living State-Specific Rules and Regulation: https://www.argentum .org/advocacy/state-advocacy/regulatory-resources/

- Home Health Survey Information: https://www.cms.gov/Medicare/Provi der-Enrollment-and-Certification/GuidanceforLawsAndRegulations/HHAs

- Nursing Home Survey Information: https://www.cms.gov/Medicare/Pro vider-Enrollment-and-Certification/GuidanceforLawsAndRegulations/ Nursing-Homes

Other

McKonely and Asbury, CPAs. (2019). *Federal record retention requirements and relevant laws by number of employees.* Retrieved from https://www.macpas.com/wp-content/ uploads/2019/02/Federal-Record-Retention-Requirements.pdf

Zysk, T. (2019). CMS home health emergency preparedness. *Live Process.* Retrieved from https://www.liveprocess.com/blog-cms-home-health-emergency-preparedness-plan -requirements-healthcare

Leadership and Management

The final set of chapters comprising Section III provides a framework for leadership followed by a more specific coverage of both leadership skills and technical areas of competence. The approach involves laying out a set of practices that follow a logical sequence of consideration and perspective.

Chapter 6, Providing a Context for Leadership, provides a senior care context with a general overview of leadership and management. The importance of both distinct yet necessary practices is defined and considered within the context of the senior care continuum. Several models of leadership are explored with the ultimate adoption of a philosophy and an applied approach left up to the individual. The proposition that one size does not necessarily fit all is an underlying sentiment of the chapter.

Chapter 7, Strategic Thinking and Innovation: Positioning for the Future, and Chapter 8, Marketing and Public Relations for Senior Living Organizations, orient the leader for positioning their organization for the future by instilling strategic thinking and an awareness of market relationships. The influence of leadership and the necessity of both competency and engagement in these related-but-separate processes serves as a precursor to success as an organization.

Chapter 9, Critical Thinking and Operational Practice for the Health Services Leader: Pulling It Together, lifts the importance of critical thinking and operational practice; pulling one's team and organization together to foster both effective and efficient operations. The relationship with quality management principles and how an organization gets things done is reinforced in the content of the material and associated resources.

Chapter 10, People: Human Resources and Relationships, highlights the importance of human resources and relationships. People are and should be considered assets throughout the senior care facility and from support staff to C-Suite professionals. Core to this topic is the connection between an exceptional leader and an exceptional workplace culture that values staff effectively.

Chapter 11, Customer Service: How Are We Different?, brings us back to the core of what we do for the individuals we serve as patients, residents, clients, participants, and tenants. We also explore how senior services are different from other industries and embrace that responsibility. Good leaders must understand customer perspectives and embrace the opportunity to listen and understand the needs of the individuals we serve. We explore the customer perspective along with numerous high-impact practices.

Chapter 12, Personal Development: Investing in Yourself, outlines the need for ongoing personal development by investing in oneself. The professional education, competency, and responsibility required to practice as a leader in the senior living care field is addressed. The ongoing approach and resources needed to keep an individual growing at a consistent, healthy pace in developing their career in this noble profession are also shared.

CHAPTER 6

Providing a Context for Leadership

INTRODUCTION

You probably have heard the phrase "It all starts at the top." Well in senior care, the top is not too far away from anybody who works in the organization. Based on a generally flat organizational structure, we believe this statement to be very true in this profession. Unlike the more traditional hierarchical hospital structures with additional levels of management, senior care organizations have fewer layers between the on-site service leaders and the actual residential care and support services staff who interact with and provide services for customers every day. Good senior care leaders use this as an advantage—they can be more aware of their organization's service provision and can use their relationships with staff to set a tone of care and service excellence across the organization. The most effective leaders also understand they are not any more important than anybody else in the organization.

> *One of the notions that make a great deal of sense for an executive administrator to understand is that they can be gone for a week and generally not be missed too much, whereas the housekeeper can't be gone for a day and the care and service system has major problems or shuts down.*
>
> *Tom Goeritz, MBA, NHA, Administrator/ Consultant, St. John's Lutheran Home*

A variety of different types of senior services creates many varying demands and opportunities for leadership and management. Service settings range from the more formal to informal types of services. Services of the traditional skilled nursing facility have increasingly become medically complex based on greater resident acuity needs and specialized with a greater subacute and rehabilitation focus. Assisted living has emerged as an alternative to the nursing home, offering care and services in a less institutional setting with an emphasis on greater privacy and flexibility. Senior housing services continue to serve a less frail population, but many are making health and support services more readily available to their tenants. Community-based services, including home care, are often the preferred choice of frail older adults who desire to stay in their own homes.

Without credible empirical research, one can only conjecture how much the different long-term care (LTC) settings impact leadership style, focus, and approach. Practical observations and some limited research in the senior service field reveal some of the unique challenges that effective leaders in each line of service can address. Leaders across lines of services must be aware of industry demands that inform a different approach or focus including the following:

- Nursing facility administrators and management staff should be able to proactively understand, plan, and execute person-centered change. Administrators should learn to overcome the barriers that drive them to focus on regulatory compliance and personal control to evaluate their effectiveness.

- Assisted living administrators and management staff should balance their focus on marketing and customer service with the need to develop and institutionalize effective quality management systems that consistently meet and exceed the expectations of the customers. This is essential to minimize the need for more regulatory requirements. The current pattern of public disclosure and reporting of operational challenges impacting care and service reflects what happened with additional regulations advanced for nursing homes more than 30 years ago because of leadership gaps.

- Both senior housing and community-based service administrators should create and communicate a shared vision that is supported by effective systems and training. These are essential to effectively lead a complexity of services with more empowered staff in a community rather than single building.

Everyone in an organization has a role including executives. One of the elements that make an executive's role interesting is that every senior care executive practices their craft in a way that leverages their individual interests and strengths. While putting their mark and leadership style in place, they also need to ensure that it works for the organization they are leading and evolves over time and with situations. Some established models and key tenets frame both leadership and management and assist executives with a greater understanding of how they can understand their role, including how they can work with their management teams. One must first understand leadership and management in order to be an effective senior care executive

FOUNDATIONS OF LEADERSHIP AND MANAGEMENT

In common vocabulary, "leadership" describes the traits and behaviors of people whom we admire because of their ability to bring people together to achieve a shared objective. Leadership is also used to identify formal positions of authority (specialized role view) and the informal influence that seems to naturally occur in any kind of social group by any one at any time (shared influence view). Attempts to create a more technical definition have created as many definitions as there are approaches used to research this subject. These various approaches include traits such as personality and values, behaviors and patterns of activities, the amount and type of power used to influence others, and how the situation and context impact leadership effectiveness. A common link found in most research is that leadership involves purposeful influence in a group or organization.

In *Leadership in Organizations*, Yukl (2006) defines leadership as "the process of influencing others to understand and agree about what needs to be done and how to do it, and the process of facilitating individual and collective efforts to accomplish shared objectives" (p. 8). This definition is useful because it provides for both direct and indirect influences on the preparation for future challenges as well as the current work of the group or organization. Yukl describes leadership as going well beyond the ability to direct the completion of tasks or to achieve a particular result through sheer will and determination. His text recognizes that effective leaders achieve results by inspiring followers and by training and coaching them to develop the necessary skills to perform their jobs well.

Much of the literature on leadership over the past few decades tries to distinguish between a leader and a manager. Some suggest these roles are qualitatively different and mutually exclusive. This literature has brought us maxims like, "Managers do things right, but leaders do the right things" (Bennis & Nanus, 1985, p. 21). The manager is often described as the dependable operational workhorse and the leader as the great organizational visionary. Unfortunately, this stereotypical approach has been accepted in popular literature and creates the misconception that the "manager" is less able and less valuable than the "leader" in the organization. This is the furthest thing from the truth in the health administration and aging services field.

Kotter (1990) and others conclude that it is the *processes* rather than the roles of leadership and management that are distinct and that the processes do not necessarily require different types of people. This approach says that management processes seek to produce predictability and order, whereas leadership processes seek to produce organizational change. Kotter found that the processes of leadership and management need to be compatible and are both necessary for an organization to be successful. Strong leadership processes alone can disrupt order and efficiency and create unrealistic demands for change. An unbalanced focus on management processes may discourage innovation and risk-taking while producing a bureaucracy without clear purpose.

Extensive research by the Gallup organization found that "the most important difference between a great manager and a great leader is one of focus" (Buckingham & Coffman, 1999, p. 63). Effective managers look inside the company to see how to develop the talents and strengths of its people based on their individual differences in style, goals, needs, and motivation. The core activities of an effective leader tend to be different. Leaders look outward at the competition, at the future, and at strategies. While leadership is a critical role, it will not produce a great organization unless effective managers are there to help channel individual talents into performance. In essence, different talents will more naturally support the different processes of leadership and management. Some are blessed with the talent to be both. Even so, managers should not be criticized if they do not have the natural inclination to look outward. The focus on developing effective leaders should not be greater than the focus on developing effective managers. "Great vision without great people is irrelevant" (Collins, 2001, p. 42). One cautionary note to add; in this highly regulated service area, we must not become too inward-looking, reactive, and management oriented in our efforts within a senior care organization. Leadership and outward thinking are needed as well.

The description of the administrator's role by the Association of University Programs in Health Administration (AUPHA) is an exception to this management emphasis. The AUPHA states, in part, "The administrator must have a firm commitment to a philosophy of care and service to the patient/resident population. Their primary professional role is as a shaper and designer of an institutional or service environment, the ultimate purpose of which is quality patient care" (AUPHA,

2000). It is imperative that leaders also understand how to work with governing boards, owners, and corporate level managers who often lack an understanding or sensitivity to the complexity of daily operations and the changing environment.

The definitions of management and leadership have some overlap, yet their focus is what stands out as a key difference. Management is focused on today, and leadership is focused on tomorrow, both critically necessary for the survival of the organization. One also needs to understand that people are generally not one or the other but rather have orientation tendencies toward one or the other based on the requirements of their role or their own personality. Leadership in health and aging services requires that LTC leaders are considering the needs and wants of the future elders that we will serve while management makes sure that the everyday care and service delivered are exceptional.

> You are faced with hiring a new director of housekeeping, and it has come down to two final candidates. You ask the same question of each, what do you consider the most important function of this role? Candidate A says she feels like making sure that the facility and resident rooms are clean every day, and Candidate B says he feels like making sure that he is aware of what the facility housekeeping needs are over the next year. Who would you hire and why?

Both management and leadership are necessary for an organization to thrive, and you need a team that has some balance with both perspectives. One must understand the phases of development of leadership professionals in this field and should allocate resources to develop a systematic and objective leadership development process. The best way to start is by identifying what skills are most needed by managers. In a broad sense, the importance of three basic types of skills will shift, as a manager assumes greater responsibilities in an organization and takes on more leadership roles (Figure 6.1; Dana, 2005).

Technical skills are important for the beginning manager but less important for the senior leader. The need for effective relational skills (human resource and communication) becomes more important, as the manager assumes more people responsibilities and should effectively negotiate for resources and influence results

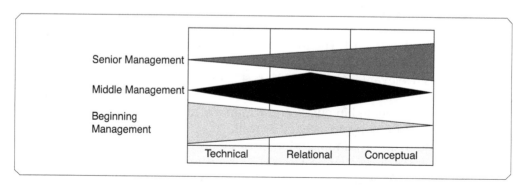

Figure 6.1 Shift in Importance of Management Skills

Source: Reproduced with permission from Dana, J. D. (2005). Strategic differentiation and strategic emulation in games with uncertainty. *Journal of industrial Economics, 53*(3), 16.

working across departments or service lines. Conceptual skills are essential for senior managers. Conceptual skills include good judgment, foresight, intuition, creativity, effective planning, problem-solving, and coordination of the various organizational functions (Yukl, 2006, pp. 198–199).

This developmental shift in management skills is a very important concept for LTC providers to understand as they look at the development of department, unit, and shift supervisors. Many senior care organizations promote people to management from their own ranks. They are often promoted because they are loyal, perform their job well, and never cause any problems. As a result, many managers are not as effective because they have never received management or leadership training and cope by simply imitating what someone else did before them (Dana, 2005).

Basic management skills should be developed if not already present. Training for health services executives (HSEs™) and managers should include work design, conflict resolution, performance evaluation, communication styles, problem-solving methodologies, and coaching. Leaders and managers should also learn to use idea-generating tools, consensus-building tools, effective meeting techniques, and quality improvement tools (Dana, 2005).

While not everyone may be able to lead an organization, department, or work unit, every willing member of the organization should have the opportunity to prepare and be ready to lead in a particular circumstance or at a particular time. Some people have no idea that they are capable of leading until they learn how or have the opportunity. Many individuals can develop the traits of effective leadership by (a) developing new habits to guide their behavior; (b) learning the principles, skills, and techniques related to leadership; and (c) translating the attributes and knowledge into meaningful activities and actions.

LEADERSHIP THEORY

Understanding the approach to leadership models is very helpful for executives, not for doing research, but rather for framing organizational context. Jago (1982) put together a matrix that does one of the better jobs of classifying and simplifying these concepts (Table 6.1). On the vertical axis, traits and behaviors are listed, and on the horizontal axis, organizational context is shared. The variety of leadership models are categorized with these factors in mind.

TABLE 6.1 Jago's Leadership Research Matrix

	Universal	Situational
Trait	Leadership traits, including abilities, personality, physical, and social characteristics	Research that focuses on a set of conditions under which certain leadership traits are effective
Behavior	Leadership styles with a focus on how leaders behave when interacting with followers	Leadership models depend on the situation and define leadership in terms of behaviors

Source: Adapted from Olson, D. (2000). *How do leadership practices affect employee satisfaction?* [Ph.D. dissertation]. University of Minnesota, Minneapolis, MN.

Traits are generally associated with characteristics you are born with, for instance, personality or motivations. Behaviors are more attributed to skills you have learned. A primary focus either on traits or on behaviors is one of the distinguishing characteristics that define different leadership models as is the type of organizational approach—universal or contingent. Theories involving universal approach to leadership state that there is only one way to lead, whereas theories supporting a contingent approach to leadership believe how to lead is contingent upon the unique needs and situations of the organization. In other words, leadership approaches under a contingent model should vary if the situation dictates doing so.

Examples of these different leadership models include the following.

Great Man Theory

Leadership traits theories began with the **Great Man Theory** established in the 19th century by proponents such as historian Thomas Carlyle, who put forth the idea that the world's history is nothing more than a collection of biographies belonging to great men. The Great Man Theory centers on two main assumptions that leaders are born possessing certain traits that enable them to rise and lead and that great leaders can arise when the need for them is great. The Great Man Theory remained the popular and predominant theory for explaining and understanding leadership until the mid-20th century. As the behavioral sciences grew, so did the idea that leadership is more of a science that can be learned and nurtured. Those with opposing views say great leaders are shaped and molded by their times, as the traits necessary to lead are learned and honed.

Transformational Leadership

One of the more recent popular trait theories is **transformational leadership**, which is relevant at all levels of an organization and to all types of situations (Bass, 1996). To be effective, these leaders have a "contextual intelligence" that gives them "an almost uncanny ability to understand the context they live in—and to seize the opportunities their times present" (Mayo & Nohria, 2005). Transformational leadership theory has four key assumptions:

- **Individualized Consideration:** The leader acts as a mentor or coach to employees, and effectively listens to their questions or concerns. The leader makes sure someone does not feel like a "number."
- **Intellectual Stimulation:** The leader stimulates and encourages new ideas and changes to followers.
- **Inspirational Motivation:** The leader is able to create a vision and goal that their followers can believe in.
- **Idealized Influence:** The leader can be a good role model for their followers. This means the leader has high ethical standards, instills pride, and obtains high levels of respect.

The transformational leadership model has been more prevalent in the acute care administration literature and has never not gotten as much traction in the LTC services and supports field.

Fiedler's contingency theory was created in the mid-1960s by Fred Fiedler, a scientist who studied the personality and characteristics of leaders. The model states that there is no one best leadership style. It also holds that group effectiveness depends on an appropriate match between a leader's style (essentially a trait measure) and the demands of the situation (Yukl, 1989).

Behavioral Theories

Behavioral theories focus on leadership behaviors primarily learned over time with experience. These are often referred to as competencies that one must possess in one's field. One early behavioral theory model, y, suggests that behaviors of effective managers and leaders must fit into different categories such as task-oriented, relations-oriented, and participative leadership (Yukl, 2006). The **task-oriented** manager is focused on planning, coordinating, and providing resources rather than doing the same kind of work as their subordinates and is an effective manager when delegating responsibility appropriately. Effective managers display **relations-oriented** behaviors when they are supportive and considerate to subordinates. They initiate efforts to understand subordinates, keep them informed, listen to their ideas, recognize them, and empower them. Effective managers also practice **participative leadership**. Rather than just providing individual supervision, they use group activities to facilitate and encourage subordinates to work together and participate in decision-making (Yukl, 2006, p. 54). Leaders are more effective when they consult with subordinates if they lack essential information or if the subordinates may not share the leader's goals or accept an autocratic decision. The leader should empower a group to decide if the leader and subordinates share the same goals and the group is fully informed and capable of making a quality decision. Because leaders remain responsible for all decisions and their results, it is important that leaders practice participative leadership when they have communicated their vision and goals effectively and provided subordinates with the right tools and support (Yukl, 2006, p. 93).

Path goal theory is a theory based on specifying a leader's style or behavior that best fits the employee and work environment in order to achieve a goal (House & Mitchell, 1974). The theory states that a leader's behavior is contingent to the satisfaction, motivation, and performance of their subordinates (House, 1971).

Other Leadership Models

There are certainly other approaches to leadership bearing mention and consideration by health services executives. One of these is **emotional intelligence** (Goleman, 1995), which is the capacity to be aware of, control, and express one's emotions and to handle interpersonal relationships judiciously and empathetically. There are four key components: self-awareness, self-regulation, relationship management, and social awareness or skills. Emotional intelligence quotient is the level of a person's emotional intelligence, often as represented by a score on a standardized test.

Another model of leadership that fits well with LTC is Greenleaf's concept of **servant leadership** (Spears, 1995), which addresses many of the nuances of LTC. The servant leadership model emphasizes the practices of vision (conceptualization, foresight, building community); change (persuasion, commitment to the growth of people); communication (listening); visible presence (empathy, awareness, healing); and technical (stewardship).

The opportunity to impact the lives of the residents and their family members was richly rewarding. The numerous thank you notes and the expressions of gratitude made the challenges of the profession very manageable. The greatest reward, however, was the opportunity to learn and be mentored through the interaction with residents. The experiences and advice that the residents (and family members) shared with me were the biggest contributors to my professional growth. It truly is a profession that demonstrates the values of Servant Leadership daily.

Ed Kenny, President, LCS Foundation

LEADERSHIP PRACTICE MODELS

Examining leadership practices provides a better link to evaluating effectiveness than do studies of pure traits or behaviors. Two approaches that have gained credibility and support over the past decade are the works of Bass and Avolio (1997) and Kouzes and Posner (2002). These researchers have developed one of the more commonly used and cited instruments for evaluating leadership practices.

The Multifactor Leadership Questionnaire (MLQ) developed by Bass and Avolio (1997) captures the basic elements of transformational leadership. It measures practices that arouse strong follower commitment, including the influence that leaders have on followers' perception of problems, how leaders encourage and support followers, a leader's effectiveness in communicating an appealing vision, how leaders model appropriate behaviors, and how they enforce rules to avoid mistakes. Numerous research studies have validated the MLQ, which is largely focused on the leader practices at the level of personal influence.

Kouzes and Posner (2002) conducted extensive interviews to identify practices related to the best and most fulfilling achievements of managers. They identified five practices that were validated through ongoing surveys of middle and senior managers across the country. Their Leadership Practices Inventory (LPI) assesses (a) challenging the process, (b) inspiring a shared vision, (c) enabling others to act, (d) modeling the way, and (e) encouraging the heart. Challenging the process has leaders searching for opportunities to change the status quo. Inspiring a shared vision is focused on envisioning a future. Enabling others to act is associated with fostering collaboration and building teams. Modeling the way focuses on behavior in pursuit of goals and treatment of people. Encouraging the heart recognizes contributions and celebrates accomplishments. The LPI has a stronger focus on the leader–follower relationship, which can be compared with organizational leadership models and applications concerned with how the organization experiences leadership.

ORGANIZATIONAL LEADERSHIP APPLICATIONS

The **Good to Great** research by Collins (2001) found a unique characteristic in the leaders of organizations who had made a transition from good to excellent performance. These "level 5" leaders had a combination of both professional will and personal humility. Their focus was on the organization's success rather than their own. They took responsibility for the organization's failures but gave credit to others for the successes. The practices of "level 5" leaders were revealed by the embedded characteristics of the organizations they led to transformation. They brought the right people into the organization to help develop and sustain the vision. They kept the organization focused on what it was best at, passionate about, and economically successful in doing. They understood and acted on their current reality while sustaining hope that they would prevail in the end. They created a culture of self-discipline and rigor that enabled them to make key decisions that would accelerate rather than create their momentum. Additionally, there was a follow-up book by Collins and Hansen (2011) *Great by Choice*, which was a retrospective study of successful organizations, including their leadership traits and corporate culture that produced results for the highlighted organizations 10-fold of their peer competitors (dubbing them 10-Xers) that focused on the consistent, disciplined, and thoughtful approach of leaders.

The Baldrige National Quality Program's Criteria for Performance Excellence also provides an excellent model for effective leadership practices in organizations. Three of the categories (leadership, strategic planning, and customer and market focus) form the "leadership triad" of the Baldrige framework. These categories guide how senior leaders set organizational direction and see future opportunities for the organization. The categories are workforce focus, process management, and results from the "results triad." This triad represents the way that the organization's work is accomplished to achieve performance results. The category of measurement, analysis, and knowledge management gives the organization a fact-based, knowledge-driven, continuous improvement foundation for the performance management system. The leadership category assesses how senior leaders lead the organization through vision and values, focus on results, instill workforce communication and engagement, as well as provide effective governance, leadership performance evaluation, and legal and ethical behavior. The program assesses both the effectiveness of the approaches used and the performance results, with emphasis on alignment and integration (NIST, 2018).

SPECIFIC LEADERSHIP APPLICATIONS

In a National Science Foundation study, Potthoff, Grant, Anderson, and Olson (1998) used the framework of the Baldrige National Quality Award Program to customize quality practices to the senior service setting. Olson (2000) used the study to explore how leadership practices impacted the participating nursing homes. The leadership practices were developed using a thorough review of the leadership and quality literature and expert interviews, focus groups, and pilot testing to refine the scale. Using employee satisfaction as the dependent variable, Olson found that three fundamental leadership practices were correlated to higher facility performance (2000). These are as follows:

- **Focused visionary** is the practice of setting a clear future for the organization and is connected to the planning function.

- **Supporting change** is the practice of encouraging growth and innovation at both an organizational and individual level and has a strong influence on the operations of an organization.

- **Effective communication** practices, the creation of a climate of sharing information, had the only direct relationship with employee satisfaction. Being an effective communicator is critical to the success of an administrator.

A visible presence of leaders was important to these organizations, but not empirically significant in the model. The time-tested management by walking around (MBWA) model is considered critically important to build relationships and trust. The need for MBWA was one of the most important messages of the text by Tom Peters and Bob Waterman (Peters & Waterman, 1982), and one could argue that many people still do not practice it nearly enough. It is next to impossible to effectively manage the high touch environment of the health and aging services field without getting out of your office and on the floor on a consistent and regular basis.

A second qualitative study using the Baldridge framework (Olson, Dana, & Ojibway, 2006) focused on effective quality practices of the upper-level American Health Care Association's Quality Award winners resulted in the following themes emerging:

1. Effective LTC managers and leaders develop and align their quality management system with doing the right thing rather than with some extrinsic requirement or incentive.

2. They have a passion for providing superior customer value that takes them well beyond the need to comply with regulations or their own internal standards.

3. They continuously learn and develop effective leadership traits and competencies.

4. They communicate a quality-focused mission and influence positive change.

5. They contribute to a culture of empowerment, innovation, agility, and results.

6. Effective LTC leaders are never satisfied with just good quality.

A study validated the rigor of this quality program using a quantitative method to assess the performance of the upper-level award winners (Castle, Olson, Patel, & Hansen, 2016). Unfortunately, there are not lot of other references or comprehensive evidence to suggest the impact that leadership has in senior care, yet the most notable evidence is that experience and stability of leadership has operational significance (Castle, 2001; Castle, Ferguson, Olson, & Johs-Artisensi, 2015; Castle, Olson, Hyer, Ferguson, & Wolf, 2015).

Triple Bottom Line

At the end of the day, a phrase made popular by Harry Truman, "the buck stops here," is still important for leadership in senior living organizations to accept, because leaders are ultimately judged on the results of the organization. It is essential to remember the triple bottom line: care and service, people (human resources), and money (financial results). Competent leaders need to keep a watchful eye on these three outcome areas.

A variety of factors impact leadership and the triple bottom line, yet there are some universal truths across service lines within the field of LTC services and supports that guide effective leadership practices. They are as follows:

1. Leaders must create and establish culture within the organization that portrays a sense of caring. This includes the need to personally exhibit a compassionate perspective for the needs of others and to serve as a role model for others.

When you walk by, make sure that you acknowledge me. I am a person. Please don't forget that your staff is taking care of me. You must remember that every day they are helping me go the bathroom, bathing me, and assisting me to get ready for the day or for bed. They are angels to me. How do you see them?

Phillip Machmeier, deceased resident and former teacher, talking to new students on what he looks for in an administrator

2. Leaders must build effective relationships with their staff. The high touch, labor-intensive nature of providing LTC services and supports with a predominately nondegreed labor force makes it possible and imperative to build relationships with as many staff as possible. The so-called "flat" organizational structure encourages management to build relationships in the LTC environment (Leader–Member Exchange Theory, Yukl, 2006, chap. 5).

3. Leaders need to role-model and practice what they preach as it relates to a commitment to lifelong learning. This spirit must play out with preparing their management team to be successful and lead. The biggest payoff for a leader is when proper investment is made by the leader with their management team. It also becomes an extremely positive influence for the benefit of the management team. Most management groups may not have a lot of preparatory management training, and too often in senior living organizations, underinvestment in the group is the norm. The next generation of employees and managers expects development and looks for it in their employers, especially their leaders. If you do not provide this type of environment, you will lose the high-performing stars you want to keep.

So building your team must be a number one priority. This includes celebrating differences, including race, gender, age, and other factors that are considered important for a diverse and an inclusive environment that starts with leadership. A leader who includes the team in deliberations and decisions sets a tone of inclusiveness and participation. An example of this would be respecting the expertise of a clinical leader, such as the Director of Nursing or Home Health services, and making sure they are consulted or empowered when it comes to any significant care or service decisions or policy changes. This leadership style would be applicable with any of the specific disciplines of the management team or with the overall group.

CONCLUDING THOUGHTS

A few words of wisdom (or at least some good thoughts to consider) for both current and future leaders in this noble profession are as follows:

- When it comes to hiring for your management team, hire for character, passion, and energy. You can always teach skills.

It is clear in today's healthcare marketplace, supply is not keeping up with the demand for seasoned, skilled competent leadership staff with the work ethic required to provide quality of care and service to our resident population with available resources. Even though this is true, it cannot be used as an excuse to lower one's expectations as to how key personnel must function in performing their daily obligations to the residents and the organization. Therefore, when seeking department heads do not focus solely on experience, educational background, and job knowledge, but through the interview process, determine if the prospective staff members have the personality that blends with their peers and more importantly yourself. You can teach some of the essential management functions. Also look to see if the individual has demonstrated a work ethic that allowed them to accomplish areas of responsibility beyond the norm. One should also look to see how they present themselves; much can be determined by the way a person takes what they have and expresses a positive self-image. Finally, do you believe that you can trust this person and are you willing to invest in them as part of your team during your career?

Larry Slatky, Executive Director, Shaker Place
Rehabilitation and Nursing Center

- A positive spirit and a glass half full outlook is critically important in this noble profession for not only yourself but also your team.

"In my classroom, or when I am with management teams, I usually pose the following question. Given the choice, whom would you rather work with: Winnie the Pooh or Eeyore?" (Olson, 2020). Whom do you think is the predominate answer? Of course, Pooh.

- Know and accept that one of your key roles is to inspire hope and lead through challenging and difficult times.

When things are running smoothly, you should celebrate that time. One recommendation to consider going forward is that during challenging times, for example, major weather event and personal staff issue, these can be an opportunity for authentic leaders to shine in times of adversity.

- Last, but not least, if you have done your job and you have a competent, strong team, you need to empower them and get out of the way!

SUMMARY

Leadership and management competencies are essential for the health services executive. It is important to understand the various models of leadership not only for your own individual awareness and growth but also for your role in helping to develop your management teams. The impact of effective leadership and management is a core driver of performance results so you can achieve the triple bottom line. The health administration and aging services profession has key opportunities to make a difference for their clients or residents, staff, and the broader community and is counting on the next generation of leaders to champion effective leadership practices.

KEY POINTS

The student will be able to do the following:

- Distinguish between leadership and management.
- Understand the development process for emerging leaders.
- Explore different leadership models and senior services applications.
- Analyze the influence of leadership on organizations.
- Highlight critical practices of effective leaders.
- Do not forget the intrinsic, soft skills of people.

LEADERSHIP ROLES

Individuals who serve as health services executives have an incredible opportunity to make a difference combined with a tremendous responsibility to lead an organization entrusted with the care of frail, elder adults. One of the ways to ensure that both the personal and professional maturity is in a good place is to have a keen understanding of the leadership profession.

HIGH-IMPACT PRACTICES

1. Be knowledgeable about the context of leadership within senior care and service.
2. Clearly be able to leverage the leadership and management talents of your team.
3. Ensure that as an individual you have an awareness of your own strengths and limitations.
4. Support the development of your management team on an ongoing basis.

QUESTIONS FOR DISCUSSION

1. How does a health services executive share leadership and management information and resources with their senior management team?
2. What are some of the most important leadership and management responsibilities of a health services executive?
3. What are the challenges that one might face when trying to develop both yourself and your team? How can you overcome these obstacles?

CASE PROBLEMS

1. A skilled nursing facility has been operating as a traditional care facility and is beginning to feel the challenges of lower occupancy due to a shrinking market for these types of services. The management team is not open to change. The health services executives have approximately 3 months to change their

perspective. List at least three things that would be helpful for the team to shift their perspective.

2.   An assisted living community has been experiencing relatively good performance for the past 6 months and is preparing to apply for a quality award. One of the weaknesses of the organization is a lack of alignment between the management team and staff on the key strategies of the business. Does the management team need to address this issue? Why or why not? How would you approach this?

3.   In an adult day center that has an attached child day care setting, a variety of communication issues exist within the organization. These include staff working different areas and shifts, the workforce representing different generations, and customers and their families having a wide range of expectations of service and benefits. What are the leadership practices and responsibilities that need deployment by the manager of this entity? Discuss some possible approaches or communication systems to try or to put in place.

NAB DOMAINS OF PRACTICE

50.17 Lead organizational change initiatives. This task requires the Administrator to demonstrate leadership by carefully assessing the facility needs, strategically developing effective methods to meet these needs, and then communicating the need for change(s) to the individuals affected. All changes should include providing clear and concise purposes related to the change and then to effectively train, validate, and celebrate those who participate in the change.

50.18 Facilitate effective internal and external communication strategies. This task requires the Administrator to develop methods of effective communication, internally and externally. The Administrator must establish a hierarchy of individuals who communicate with each other via an organizational chart. The chart should be available to residents, families, and staff so that it is clear who is responsible and has the authority to provide information. This includes creating clear and concise messages so that all staff are aware of how and what is to be communicated and when the need for assistance in communication is necessary. No employee should ever feel that the total weight of providing information rests on them. Training and strategies should include not only verbal and written communication but also electronic media such as Facebook, blogs, and Twitter.

50.19 Promote professional development of all team members. This task requires the Administrator to purposefully assess team members' training and experience and to facilitate an environment that allows employees opportunities to grow professionally. This would include internal and external opportunities for employees motivated to develop themselves professionally.

Source: Reproduced with permission from the National Association of Long-Term Care Administrator Boards. (2016). *Annotation of tasks performed and knowledge and skills used across lines of service in long term care.* Retrieved from https://www.nabweb.org/filebin/pdf/Annotation_of_Tasks_Performed_Across_LOS_in_LTC.pdf

REFERENCES

Association of University Programs in Health Administration. (2007). *Special announcement.* Arlington, VA: Retrieved from https://www.aupha.org

Bass, B. M. (1996). *A new paradigm of leadership: An inquiry into transformational leadership.* Alexandria, VA: U.S. Army Research Institute for the Behavioral and Social Sciences.

Bass, B. M., & Avolio, B. J. (1997). *Full range leadership development manual for the multifactor leadership questionnaire.* Palo Alto, CA: Consulting Psychologists Press.

Bennis, W. G., & Nanus, B. (1985). *Leaders: The strategies for taking charge.* New York, NY: Harper & Row.

Buckingham, M., & Coffman, C. (1999). *First, break all the rules.* New York, NY: Simon & Schuster.

Castle, N. G. (2001). Administrator turnover and quality of care in nursing homes. *The Gerontologist, 41*(6), 757–767. doi:10.1093/geront/41.6.757

Castle, N. G., Ferguson, J., Olson, D., & Johs-Artisensi, J. (2015). Quality of care and long-term care administrator's education: Does it make a difference? *Health Care Management Review, 40*(1), 35–45. doi:10.1097/HMR.0000000000000007

Castle, N. G., Olson, D., Hyer, K., Ferguson, J., & Wolf, D. (2015). The value study: The importance of professional membership of nursing home administrators. *Journal of Health and Human Services Administration, 37*(4), 538–560.

Castle, N., Olson, D., Patel, U., & Hansen, K. (2016). Do recipients of an association sponsored Quality Award Program experience better quality outcomes than other nursing facilities across the US? *Journal of Applied Gerontology, 37*(11), 1368–1390. doi:10.1177/0733464816665205

Collins, J. (2001). *Good to great.* New York, NY: Harper Business.

Collins, J., & Hansen, M. (2011). *Great by choice: Uncertainty, chaos, and luck: Why some thrive despite them all.* New York, NY: Harper Collins.

Dana, B. (2005). *Developing a quality management system: The foundation for performance excellence in long term care.* Washington, DC: AHCA.

Goleman, D. (1995). *Emotional intelligence.* New York, NY: Bantam Books.

House, R. J. (1971). Path goal theory of leader effectiveness. *Administrative Science Quarterly, 16*(3), 321–339. doi:10.2307/2391905

House, R. J., & Mitchell, T. R. (1974). Path-goal theory of leadership. *Journal of Contemporary Business, 4*(3), 81–97.

Jago, A. G. (1982). Leadership: perspectives in theory and research. *Management Science, 28*(3), 315–337.

Kotter, J. P. (1990). *A force for change: How leadership differs from management.* New York, NY: Free Press.

Kouzes, J. M., & Posner, B. Z. (2002). *The leadership challenge* (3rd ed.). San Francisco, CA: Jossey-Bass.

Mayo, A. J., & Nohria, N. (2005, October). Zeitgeist leadership. *Harvard Business Review 83*(10), 45–60, 156.

National Institute of Standards and Technology. (2018). *Baldrige national health quality program criteria for performance excellence.* Gaithersburg, MD: NIST. Retrieved from https://www.nist.gov/baldrige

Olson, D. (2000). *How do leadership practices affect employee satisfaction?* [Ph.D. dissertation]. University of Minnesota, Minneapolis, MN.

Olson, D. (2020). *Personal lecture materials.* Eau Claire, WI: UW-Eau Claire.

Olson, D., Dana, B., & Ojibway, S. (2005, April). Mapping the road to quality. *Provider* 69–72.

Peters, T., & Waterman, B. (1982). *In search of excellence: Lessons from America's best-run companies.* New York, NY: Harper Collins.

Potthoff, S., Grant, L., Anderson, J., & Olson, D. (1998). *Performance improvement in long-term care organizations.* A National Science Foundation Study, University of Minnesota, Minneapolis, MN.

Spears, L. (Ed.). (1995). *Reflections on leadership: How Robert K. Greenleaf's theory of servant-leadership influenced today's top management thinkers.* New York, NY: Wiley.

Yukl, G. (1989). Managerial leadership: A review of theory and research. *Journal of Management, 15*(2), 251–289. doi:10.1177/014920638901500207

Yukl, G. (2006). *Leadership in organizations* (6th ed.). Upper Saddle River, NJ: Prentice-Hall.

ADDITIONAL RESOURCES

Boyatzis, R. E. (1982). *The competent manager*. New York, NY: Wiley.

Carlyle, T. (1840). The hero as divinity. In *Heroes and hero-worship*. The University of Adelaide Library, South Australia. New York, NY: Wiley.

Castle, N. G., & Fogle, B. (1999). *Skilled nursing facilities led by professional administrators show evidence of higher quality care*. Alexandria, VA: American College of Health Care Administrators.

Clark, K., & Clark, M. (1990). *Measures of leadership*. New York, NY: Leadership Library of America.

Dana, B., & Olson, D. (2007). *Effective leadership in long term care: The need and the opportunity*. Paper commissioned by American College of Health Care Administrators. Retrieved from https://achca.memberclicks.net/assets/docs/ACHCA_Leadership_Need_and _Opportunity_Paper_Dana-Olson.pdf

Fries, K. (2018, February 8). *8 Essential qualities that define great leadership*. Retrieved from https:// www.forbes.com/sites/kimberlyfries/2018/02/08/8-essential-qualities-that-define-great -leadership/

Gilster, S. (2005). *Changing culture, changing care: S.E.R.V.I.C.E. first*. Cincinnati, OH: Cincinnati Book Publishers.

Haimann, T. (1990). *Supervisory management for healthcare organizations*. New York, NY: Brown & Benchmark Publishers.

Jensen, E. (2005). *Teaching with the brain in mind* (2nd ed.). Alexandria, VA: Association for Supervision and Curriculum Development.

Kotter, J. P., & Cohen, D. (2002). *The heart of change*. Boston, MA: Harvard Business School Press.

Ovans, A. (2015, May 5). *How emotional intelligence became a key leadership skill*. Retrieved from https://hbr.org/2015/04/how-emotional-intelligence-became-a-key-leadership-skill

Sample of Current Leadership Assessment Tools

Baldrige Self-Assessment
Emotional Intelligence 2.0
Leadership Practices Inventory
StrengthsFinder
Transformational Leadership Scale

CHAPTER

Strategic Thinking and Innovation: Positioning for the Future

INTRODUCTION

The field of senior care has a history of being reactive rather than proactive largely due to the vast demand of required services by a burgeoning aging population and the involvement of government as a driving force. One of the refreshing changes in the past decade has been that many senior care organizations across the continuum recognize the importance of taking a more healthy, proactive approach to looking to the future for their customers, employees, and overall business.

The Baldrige National Quality Award Program (National Institute of Standards and Technology [NIST], 2018) does a great job of outlining the different elements of strategic planning. One of the first necessary tenets is the distinction between the broader development of strategies and the more deployment-oriented tactics. Clearly, both items are necessary, yet they are fundamentally different. Leadership is more focused on the development of the broader strategies or goals, whereas management is usually involved with the implementation of tactics and operational actions. One needs to consider the relevance of the age-old quote applied to leadership: "Do not get lost in the forest so that you can't see over the trees."

STRATEGIC PLANNING BASICS AND APPROACHES

To understand strategic planning, it is critical to be grounded with solid definitions of the foundational elements. The first essential components are understanding the differences and importance of an organization's mission and vision.

- The "mission" defines the purpose of the organization.
- The "vision" describes the desired future state of the organization.

Mission and vision are considered together because these two ideas are consistent and work together. The mission is the overall long-term goals and beliefs of the facility, and the vision is the plan for tomorrow to keep your mission going. In other words, in order to properly achieve and pursue your mission statement, you should always have visions that align with it. The vision's intent is to satisfy the mission over time. Together, these should answer the three questions:

1. Who are you?
2. What do you value?
3. Where are we going?

The answer to all of these should aim to improve the quality of life of residents, tenants, and clients, ensure staff satisfaction, and constantly work toward quality improvements. As a leader, you need to look at the long-term mission and be able to strategically plan a vision for how to create a constantly improving organization.

"Values" are underlying principles the organization embraces and are what needs to be prioritized to succeed while considering the needs of the different stakeholders. Specifically, for long-term care (LTC), the values of a facility, community, or service should pay attention to or reference the values of the clients, tenants, or residents. Expectations from residents should be well known and addressed with each area of care and service. It is important for ideas and beliefs to be heard by everyone in a facility. Customer values should be given the most attention while still attempting to minimize inefficiencies or waste. In short, values are what are important to the organization and practiced by everyone involved.

A breakdown on how to ensure value in your company that would be helpful to review would be Jim Collins's article "Aligning Actions and Values" (Collins, 2000), which has some great suggestions to consider for your management team. One quote taken from one of his books, *Built to Last: Successful Habits of Visionary Companies*, is: "Core values and sense of purpose is beyond just making money— that guides and inspires people throughout the organization and remains relatively fixed for long periods of time" (Collins & Porras, 1994, p. 48). This is a good practice to follow within your senior living organization.

Next, one of the long-practiced approaches for the beginning stages of the strategic plan development is to take a hard, honest long look at the strengths, weaknesses, opportunities, and threats (SWOT) of your organization. An example of a starting point for a senior care community is illustrated in Exhibit 7.1.

Some questions that a SWOT analysis will additionally generate include the following:

- What is working and can become even better?
- What is not working and needs to be fixed?
- What is not working and must be discontinued?
- What are we not doing and need to start?

EXHIBIT 7.1 Strengths, Weaknesses, Opportunities, and Threats

Internal	Strengths Examples: • Reputation of organization • Service focus of senior services	Weaknesses Examples • Age of LTC product • Regulation challenges
External	Opportunities Examples • Demographics of the United States • Technology advances, e.g., EHR	Threats Examples • Lack of available workforce • Changing government reimbursement

EHR, electronic health record; LTC, long-term care.

These are approaches and questions senior leadership needs to be addressing with both their ownership, board, or respective stakeholders, along with their management team.

Next, what does success look like for everybody's own organizations?

- Goals can be both short term or long term, and best practice would advocate for each goal to have effective tactics and measurable outcomes.
- Critical success factors or CSFs are the essential areas of activity that must be performed well if you are to achieve the mission, objectives, or goals for your business or project. Some examples include the following:
  - Organizational: Consistent staff assignments, prevent the need for hospitalization, more person-centered care.
  - Clinical: Reduce infections and medications.
  - If we were completely successful: All needs would be met in financial performance, resident/family requirements, clinical outcomes, employee measures, and regulatory compliance.

It is important to take the time to evaluate a CSF's relative importance to successful outcomes for the organization and to ensure there are not too many to take on. A clear and aligned focus with associated activities will positively contribute to your chances of success. It is important to note that you should have your ownership group, board, and entire management team on the same page before you even consider addressing this alignment interest with the entirety of staff. There is a concept called the "Hedgehog Concept" in the *Good to Great* literature and on their website (Collins, 2019). This concept is not a goal, strategy, intention, or plan to be the best. Rather, it is an understanding of what you can be the best at and focus on that. The distinction is crucial for your senior leadership team.

Leaders also need to understand the terminology and the relationships among key strategic planning concepts. A few of these are listed here.

- **Strategic:** This is the broader more inclusive view of planning over a period of year(s).
- **Long Range:** This concept is associated with longer term view of the plan (3–5 years).
- **Operational:** This is focused on the annual operationalization or deployment of the plan.
- **Developmental:** For our senior living context, this could include fundraising approaches to support the plan.
- **Budgeting:** This is fiscal context or depiction of the plan, usually associated with the operational plan.
- **Capital:** These are dollars dedicated to major expenses, projects over the period of years.
- **Marketing:** This is the plan associated with the required sales of services. You can also expect a connection between both the community and public relations activities and goals of the organization.

The business of planning impacts the entire organization, and the cycle of planning connects with a broad array of organizational efforts.

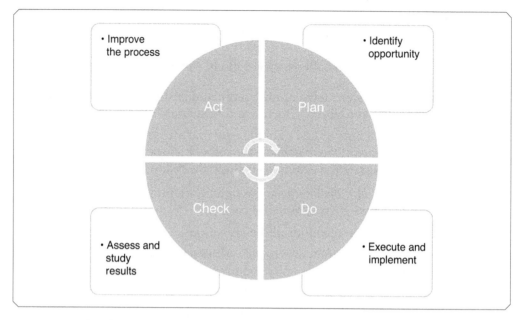

Figure 7.1 Plan, Do, Check, and Act (PDCA) Methodology

A successful planning process also includes other actionable items that further define the approach. These can include the following:

- Objectives, which outline or focus on what you are trying to achieve or accomplish. Here is an example in the healthcare field:
    - Improve the quality of life by establishing support, strengthen the workforce, and improve outcomes
- Action plans, which are detailed plans outlining actions needed to reach one or more of the goals.
- Use data to analyze and solve problems—look at what is necessary and what is extra, be smart on how, where, and when to collect data.
- Know the core knowledge about the area or focus of your plan. This may require an investment in training and development.
- Use a cycle of improvement methodology, such as plan, do, check, and act (PDCA; see Figure 7.1) so that you have a disciplined approach embedded within the plan.

Contingencies are also important to consider as you go down a path of action and achievement, because everything does not always go as expected.

Advice from Stephen Covey, the world-renowned author of *The 7 Habits of Highly Effective People* (2004), educator, and speaker, suggests that you should "Begin with the end in mind," which will help you envision what success looks like. This is habit #2 and means to begin each day, task, or project with a clear vision of your desired direction and destination (Covey, 2004). All of Covey's seven habits are worth paying attention to by any developing leaders in the senior care field.

A few other processes that are linked to effective strategic planning include (but are not limited to) the following well-known systems. The first are the SMART goals (Doran, 1981) that stand for: S—specific; M—measurable; A—Assignable;

R—realistic; and T—time based. These SMART concepts and approaches provide a simple, straightforward guide to help managers be successful in both the development and deployment of their goal areas.

A second concept is total quality management (TQM), which has eight principles (American Society for Quality [ASQ], 2020):

1. **Customer Focused:** The resident, tenant, or client determines the level of quality and service. No matter what a leader or organization does to advance continuous quality improvement, the customers we serve determine if any improvements in care and service standards are meeting their needs.

2. **Total Employee Involvement:** Getting everybody on board with an organization's goals is no small task. Employee engagement depends on trust, empowerment, and a good work culture. Senior care organizations have seen some successes with examples of cross-functional clustered work areas, team scheduling and accountability, and management sessions on units, areas, shifts, or locations.

3. **Process Centered:** A focus on getting better and using a continuous quality improvement approach has helped senior care organizations focus on the whole process. Many organizations are consistently using process improvement tools with either encouragement from association resources, government initiatives, or their own leadership with the end goal of better results.

4. **Integrated System:** In senior care organizations, there may be a variety of functional and service areas or departments that at times focus their efforts on their own silos of responsibility. A good systems approach encourages thinking about process more broadly with the attention and work reaching across these traditionally organized structures. Quality improvement committees or councils often work in parallel to the organizations and allow for a greater consideration of all parts of the process. This is a necessity in senior care delivery to many direct and support functions that need to work together for the end goal of satisfied residents, tenants, or clients.

5. **Strategic and Systematic Approach:** Another part of quality management is to have a good strategic plan in place that reflects the organization's vision, mission, and goals. This process, called strategic management, includes a broader view of the strategic planning process incorporating the organization's quality approach as a foundational underpinning. This fits well for the type of health and aging services organization that strives to get better.

6. **Continual Improvement:** Senior care organizations have historically focused on quality assurance or monitoring but more recently have embraced the concept of continuous quality improvement, which focuses on the cycle of ongoing evaluation and subsequent action.

7. **Fact-Based Decision-Making:** Using data for information is key to the quality improvement for senior care organizations, so they know how they are doing. Senior care organizations have advanced to a level that has a lot of data being captured and subsequently aggregated. This is used for both decision-making and evaluating performance outcomes. In healthcare, this would be referred to as evidence-based decision-making.

8. **Communications:** Senior care organizations require extensive communication due to the sheer number of interactions and people involved in both care and

services. Communication plays a critical role for implementing both changes and day-to-day operations. Successful leaders are very good at communicating using a variety of formats.

As one can see, there is a significant connection with the "big Q" —organizational quality—and strategic planning and management.

Another widely accepted business model is the balanced scorecard approach. Kaplan and Norton (1996) advance four fundamental processes that include translating the vision, communicating and linking, business planning (which includes building a scorecard), and feedback and learning. They propose that these elements are all necessary for a comprehensive management system. It is interesting to note that the recent interest in dashboards throughout the healthcare services industry can be traced to back to this early work.

There are many different aspects that go into developing success and being known as "successful" as an administrator and as a facility. Organizational consistency is a vital aspect of success. Facilities and individuals should always be organized and stay focused. This can help ensure minimal waste of effort and resources and fosters a cohesive outlook among leaders, managers, and staff in the facility or organization. Organizational performance is one of the most important aspects of success. Examples of clinical outcome measures are low infection rates or medication errors, two key metrics for demonstrating quality of care for residents. Although facilities and organizations can be seen as successful, they should always be striving to get better with outcomes concerning finances, resident and family experiences, clinical performance, employee engagement and productivity, and regulatory compliance.

OTHER CONCEPTS IMPORTANT TO SENIOR CARE AND STRATEGIC PLANNING

Variation

Additional concepts that contribute to the outcome of success require leaders to understand and reduce variation as a key to success. A few comments that leaders should be aware of based on this concept include the following:

- Variation in healthcare can be opportunity for improvement.
- Identifying variation improves cost and quality of healthcare.
- Reducing variation requires analytics.
- Being together with a group from the ground up reduces variation.
- Appreciating some variation is both normal and uncontrollable.

To sustain high performance, it is important to understand and reduce variation as much as possible. Variation in healthcare is something that is very closely monitored to help ensure good quality. By identifying the variations in spending, processes, and procedures, it can help show opportunities for improvement in the quality of care and service. Many analytics go into reducing and further looking into variation, and it is important to have a consistent focus on reducing variation. This includes getting staff involved and the promotion of sharing ideas. When variation of a certain area in a community is analyzed, it is important to have the head of that department involved in the process. This can help to get their opinions and experiences involved in the process to reduce the variation and ensures greater buy-in. A caveat to the concept of reducing variation is that it should not inhibit the ability of an organization to meet the person-oriented, flexible needs and wants of their senior care and service customers.

Environmental Scanning

Environmental scanning is a process that systematically surveys and interprets relevant data to identify external opportunities and threats. An organization gathers information about the external world, its competitors, and itself. This process locates and identifies themes and trends with healthcare. For instance, a leader may look at the statewide trends of the Medicaid program. Understanding the climate and direction of healthcare and specific elements of each of the factors can help us to:

- shape ideal approaches and systems,
- be proactive and ready for the future, and
- find the best approach or services.

A good specific policy example could be Medicaid-funded LTC, which is trending toward even more home- and community-based options. National policymakers and state Medicaid leaders across the country are paying greater attention to better management of long-term supports and services. A specific resource example might be the report that describes Medicaid-funded long-term supports and services (Engquist, Johnson, & Johnson, 2010) and gives snapshots ofinnovative initiatives from across the nation offering alternatives for reforming the delivery of Medicaid-funded LTC.

Baby Boomer Demand

One of the obvious trends and changes that impact strategic planning in senior care today and tomorrow are the rapidly aging baby boomers who will produce a significant demand and need for LTC and aging services. Baby boomers bring not only a greater generational population needing care and supports but also different expectations for how they want care provided—they expect to feel in control and expect full trust of caregivers. Their differences from the greatest generation may drive new approaches to strategic planning. Given the wave of new customers expected, organizations are trying to anticipate changes and trends so they can be ready for them rather than react to them. One example of the changing model of the demand of services is illustrated in Figure 7.2.

The goals and objectives set by the organization to accomplish the mission will change as the environment changes. This can easily be seen in today's increasingly competitive healthcare environment. As the environment changes, it will become necessary to determine whether the organization can accomplish its original mission. For example, many healthcare organizations were established to provide a full range of healthcare services. Because of the greater competition, some providers can no longer provide the full range of services and remain financially viable, or find themselves in a position where they cannot expand their line of services soon enough to be viewed as the continuum of choice in their market.

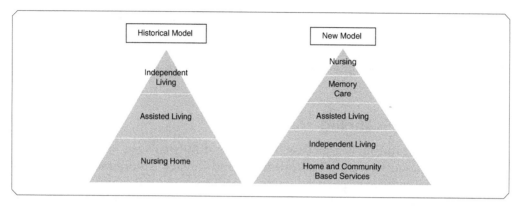

Figure 7.2 Comparing Demand of Services Models

THE ART OF CHANGE

Strategic planning is an intentional process to improve the performance and positively impact results. Change is required to make progress with an organization. Moving from point A to point B requires an intentional direction. The key to positive results for an organization is leadership embracing and influencing the direction and type of change.

A few key principles to keep in mind for a good change process include the following:

- Establish two-way trust and integrity with all coworkers.
- Manage the process of change.
- Create a system for frequent, ongoing communication.
- Develop a thorough training program.
- Have mechanisms for measurement, feedback, and redesign.
- Pay sustained attention.
- Involve coworkers in the plan and design of change.

These are some of the fundamentals of managing a healthy, successful change process that concurrently supports progress toward the goals of the strategic plan.

When fostering a successful culture for change, trust and integrity play big roles for coworkers and fellow employees, which lead to their increased capacity to accept and adopt the change. Generally, trust and integrity link teams of people and motivates workers to contribute their efforts during transitions into a process of change. "They also reduce uncertainty and discomfort that are normally associated with change that can impair individual and group adaptability and will encourage employees to take risks that are associated with the new process" (Coff & Rousseau, 2000; Rousseau, 1995). Furthermore, trust has two-way flow and takes two forms: top-down trust and bottom-up trust. Top-down revolves more around competence and leaders trusting their coworkers to have the proper skill set and intelligence to successfully adapt to the new change. On the other hand, bottom-up trust is based on the workers' perceptions of the manager's or organization's integrity and ability to perform well.

Once trust is established, creating a successful process to foster successful change is contingent on five important factors. To begin with, ongoing communication is essential for coworkers being able to adapt. Frequent, ongoing communication is a key ingredient and powerful facilitator of change. Keeping open communication about the mission and vision driving the change being made will help employees be more comfortable and increase job commitment. Aside from communication, proper training is essential in order to adopt new roles and responsibilities. Managers have the power to implement change supported by training processes to make sure coworkers are prepared when the change is implemented. After change has been implemented, there should also be various channels for feedback to measure its success and adjust when needed to achieve the maximum effectiveness. Consistency also will make sure that the change is sustained and not forgotten. Managers should always follow up with employees, continuously training and asking for feedback so the change becomes ingrained in the organization. The last major rule that managers should follow when creating change is allowing workers to be involved in the planning and design of the new process. They are the hard-working individuals on the floor and in the home, who will have to carry out the change implemented. Involving them in the direct planning is crucial.

EFFECTIVE MODELS OF CHANGE

Planned change management dominates the literature and is based on theories that look at the context of the field, group dynamics that impact the organization, and action research. Action research advocates for an approach for analyzing a situation, identifying possible solutions, and determining the best course of action based on the nature of the situation to drive actions and alternatives toward a solution.

Several models have been advanced to create understanding and provide frameworks to successfully implement planned change or change management. Lewin's three-step model provides a good overall context for how organizational change happens. The model advances a three-step sequence of change: unfreezing, moving, and refreezing. The first stage of the model, unfreezing, involves destabilizing the status quo by creating buy-in for change and ensuring that organizational members appreciate the need for change. The second stage, moving, draws from field theory and group dynamics to first identify what needs to be changed and then develop an implementation strategy that will resonate with the change targets. Once an ideal state has been obtained through the change process, refreezing must occur to stabilize the change or group at a new place. This model is used by Antwi and Kale (2014) to frame a chart to compare and evaluate other frequently used change models (see Table 7.1). The authors drew on Bullock and Batten (1985), Lippitt, Watson, and Westley (1958), and Kotter and Kohen (2002).

The visual depiction of the various change models in Table 7.1, although not all inclusive, gives the senior care leader an understanding of the phases or steps of change. The second model of change shown in the table focuses on the cycle of change described in terms of four phases and comes from Bullock and Batten, and fits the Lewin framework quite well. The third model of change outlined in Table 7.1 is the Heart of Change by Kotter, summarized in the following from the Kotter website (Kotter, 2019):

1. Establishing a sense of urgency
2. Forming a powerful coalition

3. Creating a vision

4. Communicating the vision

5. Empowering others to act on the vision

6. Planning for and creating short-term wins

7. Consolidating improvements and producing still more change

8. Institutionalizing new approaches

This model works well in the field of health and aging services, and the website and text has a large array of additional suggestions and resources to use within any senior care organization.

The final model of change shown in Table 7.1 takes the approach of envisioning the use of a change agent to help the organization navigate the process and was developed by Lippett. This model of change also highlights the cyclical nature of change.

The authors are not advancing a recommendation that there is any best model, yet we share these models for the purposes of providing an awareness of the basic elements of change. Furthermore, any model one chooses to use as a foundation of understanding and guidance probably has additional explanation and resources for the aspiring leader and respective teams.

TABLE 7.1 Change Models Compared Using Lewin's Framework

Lewin	Bullock and Batten	Kotter	Lippitt
Unfreezing	*Phase 1—Exploration:* The organization has to make a decision on the need for change. *Phase 2—Planning:* Understand the problem.	*Step 1:* Establish a sense of urgency. *Step 2:* Create a guiding coalition. *Step 3:* Develop a vision and strategy.	*Phase 1:* Diagnose the problem. *Phase 2:* Assess motivation and capacity for change. *Phase 3:* Assess change agent's motivation and resources.
Moving	*Phase 3—Action:* Changes identified are agreed upon and implemented.	*Step 4:* Communicate the change vision. *Step 5:* Empower employees for broad-based action. *Step 6:* Generate short-term wins.	*Phase 4:* Select a progressive change objective. *Phase 5:* Choose appropriate role of the change agent.
Refreezing	*Phase 4—Integration:* Stabilize and embed change.	*Step 7:* Consolidate gains and produce more change. *Step 8:* Anchor new approaches in the culture.	*Phase 6:* Maintain change. *Phase 7:* Terminate the helping relationship.

Source: Courtesy of Smith School of Business. (2014). Change management in healthcare. Retrieved from https://smith.queensu.ca/centres/monieson/knowledge_articles/files/Change%20Management%20in%20Healthcare%20-%20Lit%20Review%20-%20AP%20FINAL.pdf

The Change Process: Sharing Information With Employees

As part of the change process, the value of the timing—concerning when to share information with employees—cannot be underestimated. This is an art, not a science. The two extremes—sharing too early or too late—best illustrate this judgment of when to share information for the leader. The first extreme is to share information too early, when a plan is not fully developed and has too many unanswered questions or responses. This can create anxiety and resistance before you even have a chance to consider approaches or alternatives. It also makes it difficult to stay creative and even more importantly have a chance to implement a good solution. On the other end of the spectrum, not sharing any information can create voids of communication, which ultimately get filled with misinformation, gossip, and rumors. This can result in distraction and having to devote extra time to address any misinformation. The optimal balance is characterized by sharing enough information as you go through a change process. This helps staff feel comfortable yet not lock you or your management team into a premature approach.

The role of leadership is to encourage an open and honest environment with an understanding that you will need to be a cheerleader during the initial phases of any change and be responsible for sharing regular updates of progress. One should also never underestimate the power of humor and fun. The best leaders in health and aging services are skilled at the art of change in what some people would describe as a relatively change-resistant environment.

IMPORTANCE OF ORGANIZATIONAL ALIGNMENT

Recent research has suggested that when connections are made among organizational direction, strategies, goals, and purpose, it will increase the likelihood of sustained performance within the company. Furthermore, one study has shown that when people understand and are excited about the direction of their organization, the company's earning margins can be twice as likely to be above the median (Nautin, 2014).

When making these connections, a team and individual approach should be taken. Aligning the entire workforce is effective, but being able to get everybody on board at an individual level is hard to do. In terms of creating a vision, to achieve success, five factors are important:

1. Visions must be broad enough to be understood by everyone in the organization.
2. Visions must differentiate your organization from the competition when possible.
3. Visions must also be enduring enough to have sustainability while allowing for some implementation adjustment.
4. Visions must be both lofty and realistic.
5. A vision's message or story should appeal to individuals, teams, customers, the organization, and society (Zohar, 2000).

Lastly, after forming a compelling vision, a strategy must be created that supports a tangible set of organizational goals and desires. Together, the vision and strategy outline where the organization's competitive advantage will be in the senior care environment (Nautin, 2014).

Another stage of alignment goes back to being able to communicate the vision and strategy more broadly across the company and with the right timing. The biggest challenge is when to communicate the transformation is happening. If it is done too early, then coworkers will fail to see the evidence associated with the change that it is important and may work against it. Once again, if the communication comes too late, especially if it leads to turnover, then it can damage employee morale. Picking when to inform all employees of the upcoming change or transformation is crucial.

Your primary responsibility as a leader is strategic visioning and planning that will leave your organization in a better place after you are gone and ensure its viability far into the future.

By enhancing the breadth of programs and services and new innovative models of care, you ensure your organization's ability to respond to rapidly evolving industry dynamics and changing demographics and expectations of current and future residents. You enable your organization to protect and strengthen its abilities to meet market demands through capital improvements and programmatic innovation to deliver care to current and future residents within and outside of the walls of the communities. By actively identifying traditional and non-traditional strategic partnerships and relationships, you will improve and expand the mission of your organization. This may include new delivery systems, new markets, new programs and services, affiliations and partnerships with healthcare providers which respond to dynamic industry trends. There is the old cliché that if you are not changing, you are dying.

Tim Dressman, Vice President of Development,
CHI Living Communities

INNOVATION

When it comes to strategic planning, the role of board, owner, or governing body is to provide the overall direction working with management to more fully develop and implement the plan. It is imperative that the governing body allow the leader and their management team to operate the organization. Innovation and change are often used interchangeably, which is inaccurate.

Change is more about a process or system. Innovation is more associated with a new idea or approach. Change can happen without innovation, yet innovation would require change for anything new to happen. An openness to innovation or an innovative spirit is necessary for senior leadership to keep in mind. Innovation often occurs in strategic planning as people look outside their organization or field for new approaches or ideas. Leadership certainly needs to keep their "periscope up!" as they move forward with a thoughtful strategic planning process. Best practices in the senior care field are usually all around us if we just take a look. Dining is one example of an area that has moved from a very traditional meal approach to a much more flexible, restaurant style option for many residents, tenants, or clients of senior care and service organizations. The built-in external analysis or scanning will result in the creation of potentially innovative idea or approach.

Is new better? It may or may not be the case for your organization. There are several considerations that will help leaders and managers be more successful with this discernment:

- **Risk/Reward:** Evaluate both your appetite and ability to take on a new approach.
- **Evidence-Based Practice:** Carefully review existing information and literature.
- **Process for Evaluation:** Build evaluation into any addition of a new idea or approach.
- **Benchmarking:** Assess both your use and others' experience.
- **Trial Period:** A simple go- or no-go time period is a smart expectation.
- **Celebrate Effort:** This can be for both successes and failures you have learned from.

These are all good practices and certainly honor the need to know that there is value in the business and healthcare market to have an image of being an "innovator."

There are two components to innovative leadership. First is an innovative approach to leadership. This means to bring new thinking and different actions to how you lead, manage, and go about your work. The second component is leadership for innovation. In this component, leaders must learn how to create an organizational climate where others apply innovative thinking to solve problems and develop new products and services.

> One simple way that leaders encourage innovative thinking with their management teams is to have their regular management meetings in a different place or even at a different service-related organization. The change of environment and service approach is often all it takes for some to think differently about how they have always done something.

One of the benefits of innovation in the healthcare market is that standard business thinking is based on deep research, formulas, and logical facts. Deductive reasoning and inductive reasoning are favored tools. Business thinkers are often quick to make decisions, looking for the right answer among the wrong answers. Business thinking is about removing ambiguity and driving results. On the other hand, innovative thinking is not reliant on past experience or known facts. It imagines a desired future state and figures out how to get there. It is intuitive and open to possibility. Rather than identifying right answers or wrong answers, the goal is to find a better way and explore multiple possibilities.

One of the important elements to consider with both change and innovation is continuous discernment or taking a reflective stance to develop oneself, one's organization, and community. This requires leaders to grasp, comprehend, and evaluate clearly ideas, distinguish between what is real and what is not, and continuously link actions to results. Continuous discernment enables one to continuously link the results one is honestly observing to their causes or inspiration allowing adaptive action. In the field of health and aging services, there can be a lot of information to sort through, so this can be a critical skill. Discernment is valuable because it is focused on facts, finds the best from the rest, helps individuals avoid snap decisions and mistakes, encourages asking the right questions, and encourages ownership of any decision. In senior care environments, there is a lot of activity going on with residents, clients, families, staff, business partners, and other stakeholders every day 24/7, and it is easy to get caught up in what needs to be done the next minute, hour, or day. Effective leaders work hard to develop the perspective and skill to stay in the moment when necessary, yet to also have the ability to look ahead or beyond to how things could or may be done differently for better care or service for people. A good example could be progressive leaders partnering with businesses to help empower staff to explore more efficient uses of technology for both saving time and providing better response to the needs of their residents, tenants, or clients.

The importance of celebrating effort and accomplishments is a good way to finish the conversation of strategic planning and change management. It is critically important to celebrate the everyday efforts and successes of your management team and staff and other critical stakeholders of the organization. It takes "juice" to get things done, and avoiding discouragement and staying positive is one of the key ingredients and skills of effective leaders.

SUMMARY

Being a visionary and strategic thinker is an important skill for an effective leader. A senior care organization is never standing still; they are either getting better than or falling behind the competition. It is the role of a leader to make sure that there is a spirit of change in senior care organizations and that staff of communities are engaged and open to exploring different possibilities. An effective leader knows how to create a culture that embraces opportunities for a desired new or refined care or service approach.

KEY POINTS

1. The foundations and key elements of strategic planning need to be understood.
2. Strategy and tactics are important to understand, as well as their key roles toward improving performance.
3. Strategic planning is about setting goals and being consistent.
4. Change is an art yet does have models that help guide efforts.
5. Leaders need to lead planning efforts, embrace change, and encourage everybody
6. Innovation and change are different yet related concepts.
7. The chief goal of innovation is to find a better way and explore multiple possibilities.
8. Leaders must celebrate successes with their team, as well as support the notion that failure is also something we learn and grow from.

LEADERSHIP ROLES

1. Ownership of the planning process rests with leadership.
2. Leaders are responsible for guiding the process with all stakeholders.
3. Leaders need to serve as cheerleaders.

HIGH-IMPACT PRACTICES

1. Always keep the number of significant goals to things you can count on one hand and stay focused with your efforts and your team
2. Visit other healthcare and non–healthcare businesses with your leadership team to help encourage them to think outside the box.
3. Comfort with discomfort requires leaders to know that they have little control over some things and that is okay, recognizing that some of the best organizational insights and growth come during uncomfortable times.

QUESTIONS FOR DISCUSSION

1. Describe the key elements of strategic planning that a new administrator should understand prior to undertaking the strategic planning process.
2. What are some of the models of organizational change and how do you use them to support the improvement of the organizational outcomes?
3. What are some of the major differences between lines of service that should be considered when it comes to strategic planning?

CASE PROBLEMS

1. Many years ago, when I was a young administrator, I was confronted with a building that needed some updating to keep it market relevant. The Board of Directors approved several items, and one of them included some common space and hallway carpeting to be installed over some existing tile floors. I approached this opportunity not expecting much resistance, but then I met Linda. She was a housekeeper who was a long-time employee, was respected by many of her peers, and was very proud of her assigned floors for their cleanliness, exactly what you would want from your staff. The only issue was that she kept her tile floors spotless and was in no way a fan of carpeting the floors. Being an informal leader among her peers, she was creating quite a resistance to this carpeting project. We knew the project would go better if we could win her over. What would you do?
2. The "Good to Great" research literature (Collins, 2001) talks about getting everybody on the same bus. Refer to Figure 7.3 developed by a colleague (McDougall, 2010), with Part A depicting an organization with lots

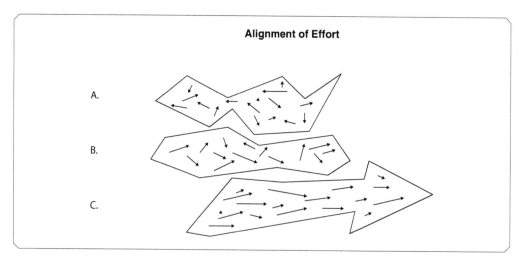

Figure 7.3 Alignment of Effort Diagram

Source: Courtesy of Duncan McDougall.

of activity, Part B an organization that is somewhat aligned, and Part C an organization that has everyone on the same page with values and goals of the organization.

How would you describe organizations you have worked for and what type of organization would you like to lead and why?

You should also list a few things you would do to get your organization to a better place with alignment.

3. Consider a home care agency that has been recently acquired by a senior care community that has skilled nursing, assisted living, and independent living. Home care agencies have a very diverse and geographically spread out workforce that create opportunities and challenges when both developing and deploying a strategic plan. Using a SWOT approach, outline the areas that your senior leadership team should be considering for the annual strategic planning retreat that is planned for 3 months after this transaction has occurred.

NAB DOMAINS OF PRACTICE

50.16 Develop, implement, and evaluate the organization's quality assurance and performance improvement programs.

50.17 Lead organizational change initiatives.

50.18 Facilitate effective internal and external communication strategies.

Source: Reproduced with permission from the National Association of Long-Term Care Administrator Boards. (2016). *Annotation of tasks performed and knowledge and skills used across lines of service in long term care.* Retrieved from https://www.nabweb.org/filebin/pdf/Annotation_of_Tasks_Performed_Across_LOS_in_LTC.pdf

REFERENCES

American Society for Quality. (2020). *What is Total Quality Managment (TQM)?* Retrieved from https://asq.org/quality-resources/total-quality-management

Antwi, M., & Kale, M. (2014). *Change management in healthcare: Literature review.* Kingston, ON, Canada: Monieson Centre for Business Research.

Bullock, R., & Batten, D. (1985). It's just a phase we're going through: A review and synthesis of OD phase analysis. *Group and Organization Management, 10*(4), 383–412. doi:10.1177/105960118501000403

Coff, R., & Rousseau, D. (2000). Sustainable competitive advantage from relational wealth. In *Relational wealth: The advantages of stability in a changing economy* (pp. 27–48). New York, NY: Oxford University Press.

Collins, J. (2000). *Aligning actions and values.* Retrieved from https://www.jimcollins.com/article_topics/articles/aligning-action.html

Collins, J. (2001). *Good to great.* New York, NY: HarperCollins.

Collins, J. (2019). *Good is the enemy of great.* Retrieved from https://www.jimcollins.com/

Collins, J., & Porras, J. (1994). *Built to last: Successful habits of visionary companies.* New York, NY: Harper Business.

Covey, S. R. (2004). *The 7 habits of highly effective people: Restoring the character ethic* (Rev. ed.). New York, NY: Free Press.

Doran, G. T. (1981). There's a S.M.A.R.T. Way to write management's goals and objectives. *Management Review, 70*(11), 35–36.

Engquist, G., Johnson, C., & Johnson, W. C. (2010). *Center for Health Care Strategies Report. Medicaid-funded long-term supports and services: Snapshots of Innovation.* Retrieved from https://www.chcs.org/media/LTSS_Innovations.pdf

Kaplan, R., & Norton, D. (1996). Using the balanced scorecard as a strategic management system. *Harvard Business Review, 74*(1), 75–85.

Kotter. (2019). *8-step process.* Retrieved from https://www.kotterinc.com/8-steps-process-for-leading-change/

Kotter, J. P., & Cohen, D. S. (2002). *The heart of change.* Boston, MA: Harvard Business School Press.

Lippitt, R., Watson, J., & Westley, B. (1958). *The dynamics of planned change.* New York, NY: Harcourt, Brace & Company.

McDougall, D. (2010). *Developed for the use of planning consulting engagements.* Lake Elmo, MN: Pathway Health Services.

National Institute of Standards and Technology. (2018). *Baldrige national health quality program criteria for performance excellence.* Gaithersburg, MD: NIST. Retrieved from https://www.nist.gov/baldrige

Nautin, T. (2014). *The aligned organization.* Retrieved from http://www.mckinsey.com/search?q=The%20aligned%20organization

Rousseau, D. (1995). *Psychological contracts in organizations: understanding written and unwritten agreements.* Thousand Oaks, CA: Sage.

Smith School of Business. (2014). *Change management in healthcare.* Retrieved from https://smith.queensu.ca/centres/monieson/knowledge_articles/files/Change%20Management%20in%20Healthcare%20-%20Lit%20Review%20-%20AP%20FINAL.pdf

Zohar, D. (2010). Thirty years of safety climate research: Reflections and future directions. *Accident Analysis and Prevention, 42*(5), 1517–1522. doi:10.1016/j.aap.2009.12.019

ADDITIONAL RESOURCES

Association Websites

American Association of Quality: https://asq.org

Baldrige Performance Excellence Program: https://www.nist.gov/baldrige

Kotter, Inc.: https://www.kotterinc.com

Good to Great Diagnostic Tool: https://www.jimcollins.com/tools/diagnostic-tool.pdf

Other

Bartling, A. (1997). 25 pitfalls of strategic planning. *Healthcare Executive, 12*(5), 20–23.

Burnes, B. (2004). Kurt Lewin and the planned approach to change: A re-appraisal. *Journal of Management Studies, 41*(6), 977–1002. doi:10.1111/j.1467-6486.2004.00463.x

Healthcare Success. Retrieved from https://www.healthcaresuccess.com/blog/medical-advertising-agency/swot

Lewin, K. (1951). *Field theory in social science; selected theoretical papers.* New York, NY: Harper & Row.

CHAPTER 8

Marketing and Public Relations for Senior Living Organizations

INTRODUCTION

The history of marketing in senior care has been an interesting road traveled. Healthcare, in general, has had less of a marketing emphasis in the past due to the lack of perceived value or need by providers. This could be attributed to healthcare being viewed as less of a business product and more of a traditional employment benefit service that is often government funded. In the 1970s and 1980s, this started to change; however, the focus was less on comprehensive marketing and more on advertising and promotion. Increased competition and consumer choices in the healthcare sector continued to move organizations to the full adoption of marketing efforts by the turn of the 21st century (Berkowitz, 2011). Senior care led the charge in many ways due to its unique differences—serving many private pay consumers and with a growing market of senior housing and assisted living across the country. The home care and skilled nursing services providers brought an understanding of the importance of their referral sources and managing those relationships. Marketing today is an essential component of every service provider and a skill set that all leaders need to have to effectively manage their respective organizations.

Marketing is the process or technique of researching, promoting, selling, and distributing a product or service. In senior care organizations, this function is both an authorized and recognized activity led by management. One of the keys to success is ensuring that marketing is a proactive process with both an internal and external focus. Even though management is driving marketing and public relations efforts, it is also essential that everyone within the organization understands the role they play in the overall marketing efforts of the organization.

To truly understand how to effectively lead and manage marketing efforts, one must understand what makes marketing different in senior care. The following is a list of several factors that influence marketing of services to the aging and disabled populations.

- Choosing services or living arrangements is a very personal decision and service.
- The products and services are very staff intensive to deliver.
- The consumer is generally a very vulnerable population.

- It is important to note that the actual decision-maker may not always be the consumer.

- The costs of service and payer sources can be very complex.

- The role of government has a significant impact on access, cost, and quality.

All these elements have an impact on your marketing efforts and plans and need to be paid attention to to make sure that you are successful with your marketing activities and focus.

Across lines of service, there are also unique aspects that can impact how to effectively market externally to your customers and consumers. A good indicator of how to approach your marketing efforts in senior care given these factors is to understand who the decision-maker is for various settings and services and how that might influence your marketing approach. Here are some of the unique aspects to keep in mind:

- *Home care* decisions will be affected by the level of service the patient might require. For example, if it is a service that is covered by Medicare or insurance, the payer's plan may impact your choices, which is different than a caregiver who is providing services on a private fee basis. The patient, family, and plan are involved in the decision in part dependent on the patient's functional capacity (which is true for almost all decisions).

- *Senior housing* is generally paid for privately, and the future tenant(s) is usually very involved in the decision.

- *Assisted living* decisions usually involve the partner or family much more often in the process.

- *Skilled nursing* placements for shorter stays are more like a home care decision process, whereas skilled nursing placements for longer stays may involve a partner, family, or even designated healthcare proxy in the overall process.

- *Clinics and hospitals* typically work with designated insurance plans that are in network for the patient. In these scenarios, the marketing involvements are broader in most cases and include both the physicians and plans a bit more.

The rationale for outlining these decisions across the broader continuum of services is to help you identify the key stakeholders you are directing your marketing efforts toward. They do vary to some degree with each respective service or setting.

Marketing in skilled nursing is often based on an acute event and has also become much more partnership driven today. Government and health system involvement has required an ever-increasing eye on the quality of the services, which is often a part of the marketing agenda and message. Assisted living is more proactive and often based on anticipated needs by the person and their family.

Mike Schanke, NHA
Administrator and Owner of Oakridge Gardens

RELATIONSHIP TO OTHER FUNCTIONS

Marketing does not operate independently and is best done when fully integrated into the organization's priorities and plans. It is also important to understand how some of the related "marketing" concepts all come together (Thomas, 2010).

- Public relations is a strategic communication process that builds mutually beneficial relationships between organizations and their publics (Public Relations Society of America, 2012). Public relations include press releases, website news, and social media to name a few. Press releases in the senior care community are some of the best ways to reach the general public. Local newspapers are always looking for activities and interest stories, and your residents have a high human interest factor that they are looking for. When you supply them with the context of an event or initiative with a picture or two (with the appropriate releases), you can generally count on them using your organization's stories on a regular basis. Social media serves some of the same purpose yet is much more in the control of the organization or the individuals working for an organization. There are several nuances associated with social media, including crafting clear messages, managing the exchange with a variety of users and stakeholders, and always protecting the privacy of the individuals you both serve and work with.

- Community relations refers to the various methods companies use to establish and maintain a mutually beneficial relationship with the communities in which they operate. This happens both formally and informally with an organization and its community. A couple of examples of formal community relations could be sponsoring a local little league team or hosting a community event in the common space of the senior care organization. An example of an informal relationship may be some of the management team participating and serving on local service organizations, such as the Rotary Club. All these connections make a difference, and more progressive organizations are very intentional and thoughtful about their presence in the fabric of the community.

- Strategic planning is integrally linked to marketing with market assessment and research being one of the foundation elements of a good strategic plan. Knowing your current and future customers drives many of the actions and strategies of the plan to both attract and meet the needs of your target population. Being on target with this assessment drives the occupancy and use of services. Ultimately, the projections of occupancy and use of services drive the revenue stream for the organization and impact the financial health and success in both the short term and long term for any of the lines of service in the senior care market.

Clearly, the leader of the organization must understand how everything fits together and both complements and supplements other functions (Figure 8.1).

FURTHER EXPLORATION OF CONCEPTS IN HEALTHCARE ENVIRONMENT

Marketing is the comprehensive approach and tools that aim to influence consumers' purchasing decisions and are deployed to motivate people to buy services. The

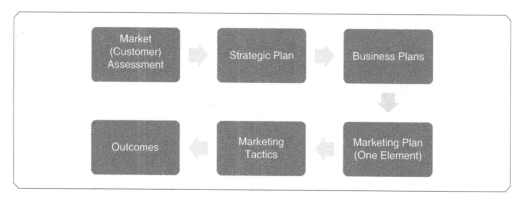

Figure 8.1 Integration of Strategic Planning and Marketing

main goal is to increase sales and revenue of the organization and meet the needs of the community and populations within the geographic area.

Public relations uses communication tools that create positive perceptions and aims to influence consumers' attitudes and perceptions. The main goal is to increase favorable public opinion using press releases, newsletters, brochures, and social media or the Internet.

Selling in the senior care market is best done by building trust, avoiding any associated tactics anchored in anxiety or fear of what's next for the consumer, and maintaining a relationship after the move in or use of services. One of the high-impact practices in the very personal area of marketing and selling to seniors is the use and sharing of positive resident stories.

Research and **benchmarking** are critical steps in the development of a marketing plan. Benchmarking is an intentional review of an organization's strengths and weaknesses. It is also a careful look at the ability of the organization and corresponding quality level of performance. Some of the purposes are to help better satisfy customers' needs and to promote change and encourage improvements in service. One of the ways organizations can do external research is with the use of secret shoppers that pose as patients or a patient's friend or family member to assess the quality of patient experiences in either your own agency or community (Pinnacle, 2019). This approach can also be used to explore how your organization compares with other organizations in your defined service area. A multitude of strategies can be used to get this valuable information, for example, phone calls, walk-through visits, and even patient visits. Knowing how your organization provides services and stacks up to others is critical knowledge to have for the respective leadership team.

Focus groups are another common qualitative research technique done for marketing research. The groups are generally between 6 and 12 individuals, and the focus group is conducted by a moderator. The selection and recruitment of participants is generally determined by the goals of the market research, which determines whether they are existing customers, prospects, or decision-makers. Organizations may contract with an external organization to do these for them or may do them internally. The latter approach requires some additional training for the in-house person. This individual should be someone with whom participants would feel comfortable and safe enough to give their honest feedback.

In the marketing application, an organization must know what its target audience is and how the market is segmented. Generally, one thinks of the primary audience as those over 65 years old who have either an increase in chronic conditions, need help with additional activities of daily living, or require either memory care, assisted living, or other supportive services. Although many times this is true, other key market stakeholders that need to be paid attention to are the adult children, in their 40s and 50s, of individuals needing services who would be providing guidance and support for their parents (Pew Social Trends, 2013). Additionally, the needs and preferences of future customers also need to be factored into the planning for future delivery of services and living arrangements.

> A simple way to understand the needs of stakeholders is to use an example from the senior services field. In many new assisted living buildings, the resources allocated for a nice fitness center are not always directed only at the customer. Sites want to make sure that the daughter or son is satisfied that their loved one will have facilities and equipment available to maintain their flexibility and strength, and they have a perspective of their own about fitness spaces. These perspectives usually are not the same, but both people are involved in the decision-making and must be sold.

MARKETING APPROACHES

When marketing senior services, it is essential to implement an approach that discretely breaks down marketing focused on internal and external strategies. Understanding the differences and devoting resources to both channels can help focus your marketing efforts. Here are important distinctions and key aspects to keep in mind:

- **Internal marketing** involves leveraging and utilizing the key information assets within your organization and aligning your mission and vision with your branding, messaging, and other visible marketing tools. This approach also appreciates the power of the voice of your employees, residents, and families and emphasizes working hard to ensure that their experience and message is positive. Organizations that understand this pay attention to satisfaction surveys and have advisory councils in place. Word of mouth is a powerful form of marketing, and these internal stakeholders are an extension of your marketing team.
- **External marketing** is much more focused on both getting and keeping your name visible in the community. This is accomplished with a variety of marketing tools including electronic media, print media and promotion materials, newsletters, and other formal mechanisms. External marketing is also accomplished with both formal and informal relationships with community groups and other associated healthcare providers, most notably hospitals and clinics.

With both approaches, some commonsense things need to be kept in mind, and a checklist of questions is included at the end of this chapter as an example of one way to ensure that activities are grounded in day-to-day operations (see Box 8.1). Your marketing mix of products will change over time. An organization always needs to be prepared to serve new clients, excels when it has friendly and cooperative staff, and consistently meets customer expectations.

Box 8.1 Internal and External Marketing Questions

Internal—Supporting What You Say You Are

How clear, visible, and welcoming is your signage (outside and inside)?

Are the grounds well kept? Is the building in good repair? Is your entrance presentable?

What is your staff retention and turnover? How is staff morale? Do staff understand their role in marketing?

Do you do employee and resident/family satisfaction surveys? Do you pay attention to them?

Do you have regular communication with family members?

Is the medical director effective and stable? Is the medical director someone that will serve as a spokesperson when asked?

Do you have an advisory council in place? Do members serve as ambassadors for your organization?

External

What are you doing with digital media (radio, TV, Internet, website)?

How are using print media (newspapers, brochures, flyers, bulletins)?

Are you doing a community newsletter (decide what you want to say)?

What would the community say about the facility today?

How good is your hospital/hospice/home health relationship?

Do you have a transportation program? Does it advertise your organization?

How is your media relationship? Do you talk with them when they need expertise or a story?

Are you involved in community sponsorships?

Are you and your leadership team involved with community groups?

Source: Adapted from marketing lecture with Jim Diegnan, Consultant, Eau Claire, Wisconsin.

"Who wants to go to a nursing home?" is the wrong question. The better question is—"If you need services, what do you want your care and support services to be like?" What are the things a prospective customer will value?

MARKETING AND BRANDING CONCEPTS IN SENIOR CARE

In senior services, customers are fortunate that there is a diverse set of services, including independent senior housing, home- and community-based services, assisted living care, and skilled care services (both short and long term). This variety also brings a set of challenges from a senior care marketing perspective. A good rule of thumb that can help you establish your efforts is to first understand the set of services your organization provides. By knowing your services fully, you can highlight a specific product through a niche marketing approach within the broader market strategy. This can be a very effective approach when competing for customers who are also debating what sets of services are right for them (Lindsay, 2007).

Senior Care and the 4Ps

The continuum of senior services is also impacted by the traditional marketing mix, also known as the 4Ps—place, product, price, and promotion, but with subtle yet important twists. For instance, in senior care, place carries such great importance that it should be mentioned before product. The following describes unique aspects in the senior care field that impact marketing and branding.

- **Place** in senior services makes location most important, whether it is a rural or urban setting. The proximity to family, closest kin, or friends can be a significant impact on the choice of location or services, and this impacts how marketing needs to be approached

- **Product** is largely based on what makes your services unique and of quality to customers including services that offer the least restrictive environment and encourage the greatest freedom and quality of life, both of which are major factors that can distinguish your product.

- **Price** has a more significant impact on the services that are not covered in full and that have the least amount of government or insurance involvement in the reimbursement for services. Marketing strategies must take into account the types of services that are not generally covered by the payer or government.

- **Promotion** is important to keep in the forefront, but it must be understood that customer needs cannot always be proactively targeted. The purchase and use of many care services are often decided because of a changing health condition or crisis for the prospective customer.

Another related concept that is important in the senior care space is the idea of product mix. Some of the fundamental decisions organizations need to make are who is their target customer, how are they going to attract them, and in what numbers (or percentages). A good example of this is: What is the percentage mix of a skilled nursing facility targeting private pay or Medicaid eligible individuals? This could also be true for any of the lines of service including Medicare recipients as well. **Branding** is creating a unique name and image for a product in the consumers' mind, mainly through advertising campaigns with a consistent theme. Branding aims to establish a significant and differentiated presence in the market that attracts and retains customers (Nelson, 2015). Branding takes into consideration a variety of factors, including a company's image, consistency of service, perceived and earned trust, and the core beliefs of the organization, often expressed in its mission, vision, and value statements (Thayer, 2003). An extension of branding is a concept called "top-of-mind awareness" (TOMA), which refers to a brand (or product) being first in customers' minds when thinking of a particular industry or category. At the market level, TOMA is more often defined as the "most remembered" brand or organization names. The significance of this concept is understated in the senior care and support arena, which are services that are generally decided upon in a short amount of time and often based on what organization first comes to mind. Having top-of-mind brand awareness in your community can give your organization a "leg up" on competitors in the senior care sector.

Conveying the Message

All these marketing concepts are aimed at relationship building with a wide variety of stakeholders. Principles of education are an understated powerful force for marketing. Leaders with good teaching skills are very good at conveying and sharing the message. Providing educational seminars around topics that are front and center for future customers can be very powerful marketing tools. They are less intimidating and build an organizational awareness for when they do need services. Strong communication with customers, media, and the public is imperative to achieve an effective marketing program.

SALES IN SENIOR CARE AND SERVICES

Sales is not always the first thing one thinks about when marketing senior care services, but it is a necessary business skill in senior care. For many of the products and services offered in the senior care field, especially those based on a private pay market, understanding sales concepts is critically important. Assisted living and senior housing are two market areas that have a large influence on the sales maturity of the senior care field. The development of sales careers, such as sales counselors and representatives, in this field has been driven by senior housing and assisted living.

Argentum (2019), a national association that represents assisting living providers, has developed a specific sales counselor certificate program. This program focuses on industry knowledge, marketing strategy, and a consultative sales process. This program is offered to people that are either new or have been in the field and was launched in 2016. This "new" program is an example of the increased recognition of the important role sales has in the senior care market, especially in the largely private pay markets of assisted living and independent housing options.

"Marketing in senior living requires the skill set needed in marketing for any other industry but with an increased level of sensitivity and empathy for the residents and their families. At every level, senior living marketing efforts should be the embodiment of 'listening to the customers,' understanding their concerns and needs, and, just as important, their aspirations for an improved quality of life. Successful providers market not only what's different about their communities and programs, but also speak to the positives of senior living concepts. We are marketing to families and teams of loved ones, sometimes in emotionally charged moments, and at the same time to individuals whose dignity and choice must be honored. The executive director and marketing leaders need to be 'joined at the hip'—aligned

on goals and responding to needs of the customer and their family. Education specific to senior living goes a long way toward successfully meeting these complex and sometimes competing goals."

James Balda, President and CEO, Argentum

These sales people, and in smaller settings the administrator or manager, have the responsibility to highlight and "sell" the benefits and features of the services being offered to prospective customers. The length of the sales cycle in senior care generally is viewed as short (less than 2 weeks) for an immediate health crisis with skilled care and home care, and then increasing based on descending need for care and services. For instance, adult day care may be closer to under a month; assisted living is generally projected to be around 45 days followed by more independent senior housing at closer to 3 months or more (depending on if it is a rental, cooperative, or investment arrangement; Anderson, 2014). The responsibilities of managing the relationship with the prospective customer are a process and begin with the first point of contact or referral until the actual move-in or use of service by the resident, client, or tenant.

CUSTOMER PERCEPTION OF SERVICES

Any administrator or leader of a senior care organization or service would be also well served by putting themselves in the shoes of the customer. One of the best ways to do this is by evaluating and researching what are the things they would be looking for. There are several resources and opinions on some of the shopping tips that customers will be using or paying attention to and include the following few examples:

- How is the hygiene and grooming for residents? Evaluate hair, teeth, and even fingernails of residents entrusted to their care. The rationale is that if hair, teeth, and nails are good, everything else is probably running smoothly, because they are often the final care duties.
- What is the perspective of the resident on the food served? Look at the food and see if the plates are empty or near empty, which means people probably enjoyed the meal.
- What are the attitudes of residents, staff, and visitors? Are there lots of smiles? Getting the sense of individual's happiness is a good indicator of a good or positive culture.
- What is the average length of employment for staff? Ask about the employee retention rate, because other quality measures are highly correlated to the stability of staff.

An example of a great resource that every management team should read is *The New Nursing Homes: A 20-Minute Way to Find Great Long-Term Care* (Rand, Popejoy, & Zwygart-Stauffacher, 2002). This book was written to serve as a resource for finding great facilities that feel like home, treat your loved one like family, and provide quality, personalized care. There are other guides available that would be very helpful to have for the management and marketing teams (Gresham, 2018; Schoch, 2019; Wisconsin Department of Health Services, 2018).

MARKETING PLANS

Marketing plans are an essential element of an overall business plan. During the initial assessment phase of the strategic planning process when an organization may be using a SWOT (strengths, weaknesses, opportunities, and threats) analysis, questions about your market position and marketing presence will often be uncovered by the team. A good marketing plan needs to complement and support your organizational goals, especially those related to use of services. The marketing plan also needs to be adequately funded with time and money, practical with specific activities, and have both methods and measures to determine success. Marketing plans serve as an annual road map for staff and leadership.

Marketing Plan Approaches and Tools

There are several approaches and tools that inform marketing plans, providing important feedback as well as communicating and disseminating information to stakeholders. Tools that serve as forms of feedback include surveys, focus groups, personal interviews and observation of care, service areas, and new systems. Information can be communicated in a few different ways, and some examples include tours, a website, newsletters, and brochures. The dissemination of information happens informally with word of mouth, formally with prepared media or news items, and more formally such as when media want a direct comment from a senior care leader regarding a specific activity, issue, or initiative. Administrators are well served by having a policy in place to designate who speaks to the public and manages any press contacts.

Marketing plans within the senior care and service field have undergone a shift in recent years. Once, there had been plans with a greater emphasis in giveaways or other special gift packages as tools to attract customers. In the current landscape, there is a greater emphasis on relationship building among key stakeholders, and organizations are using technology and other outlets to connect with their consumers. Obviously, technology has had a significant impact on marketing with the move from the Yellow Pages to websites with video and virtual tours (Henderson, 2017), and this is likely to continue to shape how promotions are crafted to highlight product and services especially in a competitive marketplace. The impact of marketing activities through technology is also increasingly being tracked with more sophisticated measures. One of the benefits of this increased public relations pressure and measurement capability is that more of the right things are probably being done to educate and inform both today's and tomorrow's consumers.

Marketing and Leadership

As far as the field of marketing has come in senior care, there remain a few common mistakes that leaders make with this important activity.

- The lack of focus on the development and implementation of specific marketing strategies happens to be one of the fundamental problems that exists in the marketing field, and quite often, this occurs due to the lack of designated responsibility.

  Solution: Make sure your organization has an annual marketing plan that is aligned with the organization's goals and has both staff and resources assigned to the plan's tactics.

- The lack of accuracy or research on the target audience or potential customers can be a problem that can cause a poor allocation or use of resources producing little results.

  Solution: Make sure your organization pays attention to the changing marketplace and has regular customer focus groups with both current and prospective clients.

- Another issue is the lack of initiative or consistent marketing effort, which can be seen in organizations that are distracted with an external challenge. Another type of organization that may have a challenge with a consistent marketing effort is one that is experiencing a high level of occupancy and/or use of services. They do not feel the need to keep the energy directed toward a marketing plan, and ultimately, they end up with a lag in volume.

  Solution: As part of your healthcare organization's business plan, include regular marketing activity and outcomes metrics to be reported at regular time intervals.

- A final challenge often faced by senior care services is the lack of a marketing background or skill of the personnel involved in the planning and delivery of the marketing efforts of the organization.

  Solution: Commit to regular marketing training and updates for key personnel engaged in resident, tenant, or client outreach for your senior care organization.

All these issues can be addressed by an organization with the right attention and resources, and the key is to not get too far behind before pinpointing the problem.

One of the other emerging marketing awareness needs is the use of social media. This new channel of marketing and public relations requires navigating social media platforms, developing strategies and content, and targeting audience engagement, all needing to be done correctly and consistently. Leaders would be wise to do their homework and understand the potential opportunities presented with social media, which is only expected to increase as a publicly used resource. Organizations also need to use care to respect the privacy of their residents, families, and employees with any social media approaches.

Marketing Roles and Responsibilities

The responsibility of marketing ultimately rests with the CEO or administrator of a service or setting. The effective administrator or director delegates responsibility to another person or position within the organization. In a larger setting or service, this might be the marketing or public relations director. In a skilled nursing or assisted living facility, this responsibility may be associated with social service or admissions staff. In home care, it probably rests with the agency director or referral manager. In these organizations, making sure everybody understands their role in marketing is one of the best messages to send to your staff. Clarifying who does what and holding people accountable for marketing is a key requirement of leaders in this field.

The administrative role is multifaceted when it comes to marketing. First, the senior service leader has a responsibility to be a presence in the community and ensure that a large network of community and healthcare individuals and organizations have an awareness of the scope of services and setting for their organization. Second, there is a coordinating role within the organization to ensure that all the related marketing and public relations functions are carried out on a consistent basis. Third, the leader serves as a spokesperson for the organization with the media and the public. Last, executives must make sure the right amount of resources and support are in place to carry out each of the marketing activities necessary for the organization to be successful. This may seem daunting for one individual, yet with the right team in place, the responsibilities can be accomplished with reasonable effort and focus.

SUMMARY

Marketing is a skill set required of health services executives today. It is necessary for leaders to develop and deploy a marketing strategy that works for the organization. One of the essential ingredients is an understanding of all the key elements of a comprehensive marketing approach within a unique set of settings and services focused on the changing needs of an aging client or customer. The impact of effective marketing on the overall health and reach of the organization cannot be underestimated.

KEY POINTS

1. Healthcare marketing in the senior care field is different with some specific nuances based on both the type of services and the very personal nature of services.

2. The marketing function is important to pay attention to, and understanding how it relates to other management areas is helpful.

3. All the elements that make up an overall marketing plan and activities are important to understand.

4. Key roles are taken on by staff and residents, both inside and outside the facility or service.

LEADERSHIP ROLES

Health services executives serve as the key leader for marketing. The leader serves as a champion, coach, and cheerleader for the organization when it comes to marketing. Effective leaders know how to allocate marketing responsibilities, effectively delegate tasks, and hold people accountable for these critical activities. Being on top of your game when it comes to marketing is about making sure there is a consistent and on-target set of activities happening all the time to raise awareness and ultimately use of the care and services of the organization.

HIGH-IMPACT PRACTICES

1. Do focus groups with your target market to make sure the organization has the right message and focus for your audience.

2. Engage the entire organization in the role of marketing and promoting your care and services to everybody.

3. Always keep looking outside the organization and the field for fresh new marketing ideas to consider every year.

QUESTIONS FOR DISCUSSION

1. How are marketing concepts in senior care and services emphasized differently than at other businesses?

2. What marketing information or data can be most practical in your healthcare setting or service?

3. What different types of marketing strategies can be used when comparing long-term care (LTC) and acute care?

4. What are the elements of marketing that appear easier or more natural to you?

CASE PROBLEMS

1. Skilled nursing facilities sometimes referred to as "nursing homes" have a problem with a negative public perception. As an administrator, what are some of the areas you would focus on when it comes to developing a brand for your organization? How would you use this information to develop or support the brand of the organization?

2. An assisted living facility has been struggling a bit with occupancy, and the owner has come to visit the site that you as the director oversee. The owner wants to know the key metrics you are paying attention to. List three of the most important measures that your community tracks that have a significant impact on referrals and occupancy.

3. A home care agency with a great brand and reputation wants to expand to another geographic urban market within the same state. Put together a communications plan and marketing strategy for the opening and first few months of operation, including identifying the key stakeholders and prioritizing the activities you are willing to spend money on.

NAB DOMAIN OF PRACTICE

50.14 Develop, implement, and monitor comprehensive sales, marketing, and public relations strategies.

This task requires the Administrator to develop an effective marketing strategy designed to help the consumer, resident or responsible party, and staff to know about the features, benefits, and amenities of the community/organization. The community/organization should have clear policies, standards, and protocols to build consumer confidence.

Source: Reproduced with permission from the National Association of Long-Term Care Administrator Boards. (2016). *Annotation of tasks performed and knowledge and skills used across lines of service in long term care.* Retrieved from https://www.nabweb.org/filebin/pdf/Annotation_of_Tasks_Performed_Across_LOS_in_LTC.pdf

REFERENCES

Anderson, J. (2014, May 7). *The length of our sales cycle.* Retrieved from http://partners.aplace formom.com/2014/05/07/moves-sales-cycle-length/

Argentum. (2019). *Industry training that supports rapid onboarding.* Retrieved from https://www .argentum.org/sales-counselor-certificate/

Berkowitz, N. E. (2011). *Essentials of Healthcare Marketing, 1*(1), 1–442.

Gresham, T. (2018, July/August). 10 amenities adult children seek in senior communities. *Senior Living Executive, Argentum,* 32–36. Retrieved from https://www.argentum.org/magazine -articles/10-amenities-adult-children-seek-in-a-senior-living-community/

Henderson, G. (2017, November 29). Content marketing in 2018: Trends and tools for success. *Forbes.* Retrieved from https://www.forbes.com/sites/forbesagencycouncil/2017/11/27/ content-marketing-in-2018-trends-and-tools-for-success/

Lindsay, M. (2007). Today's Niche Marketing is all about narrow, not small. *AdAge.* Retrieved from https://adage.com

Nelson, M. (2015). *Behind the rebrand: Improving senior living occupancy and image.* Retrieved from https://seniorhousingnews.com/2015/10/27/behind-the-rebrand-improving-senior -living-occupancy-and-image/

Pew Social Trends. (2013, January 30). *The sandwich generation.* Retrieved from https://www .pewsocialtrends.org/2013/01/30/the-sandwich-generation/

Pinnacle. (2019). *Mystery shopper.* Retrieved from http://pinnacleqi.com/products/mystery _shopper/

Public Relations Society of America. (2012). *A modern definition of public relations.* Retrieved from http://prdefinition.prsa.org/index.php/2012/03/01/new-definition-of-public-relations/

Rand, M., Popejoy, L., & Zwygart-Stauffacher, M. (2000, December 19). *The new nursing homes: A 20-minute way to find great long-term care.* Minneapolis, MN: Fairview Press.

Schoch D. (2019). Finding a nursing home: Don't wait until you need one to do the research. *AARP.* Retrieved from https://www.aarp.org/caregiving/basics/info-2019/finding-a -nursing-home.html

Thayer, L. (2003, September/October). Mission-driven branding. *AAHSA Best Practices, 2*(5), 6–10.

Thomas, R. K. (2010). *Marketing health services.* Chicago, IL: Health Administration Press.

Wisconsin Department of Health Services. (2018, January 23). *Consumer guide to health care: Finding and choosing a nursing home.* Retrieved from https://www.dhs.wisconsin.gov/ guide/nursing-home.htm

ADDITIONAL RESOURCES

Healthcare Marketing Association: http://healthcaremarketingassociation.com/

Home Care Association of America: https://my.hcaoa.org/hcaoa-store

Moore, J. (2001). *Assisted living strategies for changing markets.* Fort Worth, TX: Westridge Publishing.

Robbins, K. (2016, December 21). Key marketing strategies for long term care facilities. *Health System Management.* Retrieved from health-system-management.advanceweb.com/key -marketing-strategies-for-long-term-care-facilities/

Senior Care Marketing and Sales Summit: https://www.seniorcaremarketingsummit.com/

The Society for Health Care Strategy & Market Development: http://www.shsmd.org/

Critical Thinking and Operational Practice for the Health Services Leader: Pulling It Together

INTRODUCTION

It is important for the health services executive to have critical thinking skills that they use on a consistent and regular basis. Critical thinking is the ability to think reflectively and independently in order to make sound decisions. By focusing on the root cause of issues, critical thinking helps you avoid future operational problems that can result from your actions.

To put in more simply, having critical thinking skills allows you to take a step back and see the forest through the trees. In the spectrum of senior services, the day-to-day challenges can consume the attention and energy of leaders so that it is difficult to strategically approach issues for the individual, management team, and the organization. Effective leaders understand the need for thoughtful reflection and systems to navigate operational issues and make solid decisions.

MODELS FOR APPLICATION

The adoption and use of a problem-solving model by the organization is a step that must not be overlooked in the senior service field and that is heavily dependent on a variety of individuals including caregivers and support team members. Team members do better when they learn to expect a consistent approach from their leaders.

Plan, Do, Check, and Act

One of the most commonly used models is the simple Deming cycle, the plan, do, check, and act (PDCA) approach (as introduced in Chapter 7, Strategic Thinking and Innovation: Positioning for the Future). This approach is broken down into the four steps summarized in the following:

1. *Plan:* Plan the change or improvement.
2. *Do:* Conduct a pilot test of the change.

3. *Check*: Gather data about the pilot change to ensure the change was successful.

4. *Act*: Implement the change on a broader scale. Continue to monitor the change and iterate as necessary by repeating the cycle (Deming, 1986; Tague, 1995).

This model is well accepted across a variety of disciplines and was later modified by Deming to be referred to as plan, do, study, and act or PDSA. Another variation that has been advanced is FOCUS–PDSA with the FOCUS standing for:

Find a process to improve.

Organize an effort to work on the improvement.

Clarify knowledge of the process.

Understand process variation.

Select a strategy for the improvement.

This was developed by the Hospital Corporation of America, and after the FO-CUS steps are done, the PDCA cycle is used to test implementation of the chosen strategy.

The DECIDE Model

There are also several other approaches and models, including five-, six-, and seven-step models (and even 14 if you include Minnesota Hamilton's problem-solving model, University of Minnesota, 2019) with more in common than different. An example of a six-step problem-solving approach is the DECIDE model, which has the following components:

1. D = define the problem,
2. E = establish the criteria,
3. C = consider all the alternatives,
4. I = identify the best alternative,
5. D = develop and implement a plan of action, and
6. E = evaluate and monitor the solution and feedback when necessary.

The DECIDE model is another example of a resource for managers when attempting to use a thoughtful process for decision-making (Guo, 2008).

Problem Identification

All these approaches require good problem identification, so energy and effort are being directed in the right place. Finding the specific cause of an issue or problem is a major step, and often root cause analysis is used to get at the core of the issue or problem. Getting to the root cause of a problem is an extremely important critical skill to learn and requires an intentional inquiry. Here are a couple of techniques that are commonly used in the healthcare and the senior care field.

- **The Five Whys** is a simple problem-solving technique that helps to get to the root of a problem quickly. This strategy involves looking at any problem and drilling down by continually asking "Why?" or "What caused this problem?"

- Another common technique is using a **fishbone diagram**, which uses cause-and-effect brainstorming to identify possible causes of a problem by sorting ideas into useful areas or categories. A fishbone diagram is a visual way to look at cause and effect. The problem or effect is displayed at the head or mouth of the fish with contributing causes listed on the smaller "bones" under various cause categories. A fishbone diagram is helpful in identifying possible causes for a problem that might not otherwise be considered by directing the team to look at the categories and think of alternative causes (Center for Medicare, 2019).

Other common elements of root cause analyses are the development of a variety of approaches, the implementation of a solution, and a measurement process for "circling back" to make sure an implementation is working or to determine if the approach needs adjustment or refinement. In order to ensure solutions are found, problem identification of the main problem is paramount.

An important concept that new emerging leaders need to understand is that every one of their decisions has both expected and potentially unexpected causes and effects. When a decision is made in one area, e.g., staffing, it will have an impact on another area, e.g., customer satisfaction, and they need to pay attention to these effects when leading or managing their senior care business. Every decision has a cost associated with it.

David Wolf, PhD, MSJ, MSOL, Fellow ACHCA,
CNHA, CALA, CAS
Professor, Bellarmine University

PEOPLE AND TEAMS

Sound operational practices also depend on another element that is critically important to success, which is the effective use of teams. A seasoned senior services administrator knows how to engage others in moving toward a solution, which requires establishing a team with diverse perspectives and skills. One should also consider team composition, because you will want to make sure that some members have knowledge of the processes and systems involved in the problem being addressed. It is also a good practice to make sure that a team works as a task force focused on a specific project and does not turn into an ongoing committee. Management and staff grow weary of too many committees being put in place, and in time-limited projects, task forces are a much better approach. The department head, management team, or second lieutenants of an organization are often used for problem-solving or consultation when teams are formed.

Key considerations for engaging teams include:

■ How does an issue or challenge relate to the mission, vision, and values of the organization? Paying attention to these pillars of the organization keeps them alive and in the forefront of people's attention.

■ How does your overall strategic planning connect and tie together with your problem-solving processes? You should expect that your plan is paid attention to and will be fluid.

■ What are various roles of team members and staff? Clarity of roles helps individuals be even more effective with their contributions in this or any process.

These are all critical elements for leaders to understand and master as part of their overall leadership of the community, site or services being delivered for the residents, and tenants or clients they serve every day. A leader of a senior care organization has the responsibility to be cognizant of the overall operation and its goals.

Communication With Staff and Teams

Valuing the many voices of an organization, including customers, family, staff, and the broader community, is hard work, yet it is a mindset that permeates the culture of the organization. Communication with key stakeholders sets the tone that you care and respect others' ideas and opinions. Communication involves a commitment of attention and time to both listening and responding to others through a variety of mediums, including personal conversations, meetings, written commentary, and others. Often, leaders complain they need to communicate a message two or three times, which can be frustrating, yet the bottom line is that individuals require repetition to help make sure everyone has heard the information.

One can also categorize communication as internal or external, which is a productive way of thinking about this effort. The sheer volume of people and interactions in this service field makes it imperative to establish a routine and a sustainable communication strategy.

There are a variety of mechanisms and skills that require deployment for effectively managing improvement. Senior care leaders must be good at managing effective meetings, whether they are the regular on-site management meeting or an off-site retreat. In today's world, they also need to be proficient in using technology when necessary for remote or teleconference meetings. There are also other information or news sharing tools, such as a regular newsletter, daily/weekly/shift announcements or updates, and the use of social media.

Leaders who are good communicators through all sharing tools have much more success in bringing the entire organization along and onboard with implementing changes and solutions.

During consultative visits with senior care organizations over the years, I have seen a variety of levels of commitment to ensuring good communication. This can be evidenced by the varying approaches to employee communications or newsletters. Some organizational leaders do this in a very limited fashion by posting updates by the time clock as compared to other organizational leaders who have a much more intentional strategy of targeting each individual employee with a printed regular newsletter update or a well-considered text update system.

*Douglas Olson, PhD, Professor, UW-Eau Claire
and Senior Advisor, Pathway Health Services*

EXECUTION

Getting from point A to point B is mandatory. No matter if an organization is changing for better or worse, it is still changing. A leader, in order to be effective, must be proactive and deploy solutions consistently in order to continuously improve an organization. A great resource to study from and guide you from point to point is *The 4 Disciplines of Execution* (McChesney, Huling, & Covey, 2012). The four disciplines or steps include the following:

- Identify the goals described as wildly important.
- Figure out how you are going to measure success, especially using lead measures.
- Assign clear accountability for any initiative or responsibility.
- Keep score and report how things are going on a regular basis.

These are four clear guideposts that help you overcome the day-to-day healthcare activities that keep leaders and their respective teams from implementing and executing programs that drive real change.

Accountability and Alignment

Accountability is a concept that can be both liberating or defeating depending on the situation. It is a very hard concept for new, emerging leaders to practice when they do not leverage the strengths and skills of their team, because they personally feel the weight of all the actions of an organization. Delegating responsibility goes hand in hand with empowerment, and there must be consistent practices and support for this to work. There is nothing more frustrating than a micromanaging leader who swoops in and pulls the rug out from under someone given responsibility to lead a change or process agreed to by an assigned team. Management staff and other informal leaders must allow their employees time to fulfill responsibilities and make decisions. By empowering team members, you create a culture of accountability that can help your organization move forward toward its goals. This can also contribute to greater alignment within the organization. The importance of everybody being on the same page really helps an organization and its respective leaders leverage and harness all the collective energy of all staff. Together accountability and alignment play an important role when monitoring performance of the organization.

Measuring Performance

What you measure matters. Monitoring and evaluating performance improvement throughout the organization allows leaders to assess their strategic outlook including their goals, objectives, and actions toward achieving desired results. A strategic outlook is encouraged of leaders, because it informs an organization's ongoing operational assessment. An operational assessment is the regular monitoring of the standard business outcomes that are reported on a consistent basis. In the field of senior care, these generally revolve around customer or resident services, human resources, and financial outcomes. In Table 9.1, there are some example lead and lag measures used to assess outcomes in each area. When monitoring outcomes, it is important to spend time figuring out what is either important or urgent to focus your time and energy on in the month or quarter ahead.

A trend for monitoring the measures and outcomes of an organization are dashboards. Dashboards are an information management tool that visually tracks, analyzes, and displays key performance indicators, metrics, and key data points to monitor the health of a business, department, or specific process.

Senior care and service leaders that are not driving their business decisions using data are going to falter or fail. The field has started to more fully embrace using the available aggregate data they have readily at their disposal to make decisions on a timely basis rather than wait until the end of the week or month. The use of dashboards and mobile applications has further made data available in a usable, visual format, and information today is literally at your fingertips.

Jim Hoey, President, Prime Care Technologies

Quality Management

In the 1970s and 1980s, the industry began to see the need for an efficient and organized approach to respond to the growth in complexity of financing and regulatory systems. Financial results were emphasized as changes in Medicaid reimbursement, and Certificate of Need laws limited competition and gave focus to efficiency through larger homes and acquisitions. Publicly traded multifacility providers grew rapidly through acquisitions. The short-term bottom line focus, absence of standards, lack of consequences for poor performance, and the lack of competition resulted in some poor quality and the promulgation of standards through laws and

TABLE 9.1 Lead and Lag Example Measures

Area	Example Lead Measure	Example Lag Measure
Resident services	Call light response time	Customer satisfaction
Human resources	Weekly follow-up visits with a new employee	Turnover or retention
Financial outcomes	Daily occupancy level	Net operating margin

regulations. The ability to manage well and maintain an organized approach to delivering care and services was the new trademark of a successful organization and administration. This time in the industry was often referred to as the "business era." The culture of management was prevalent in many organizations, and the corporate chains began to invest time and resources in systems that enhanced efficiency and control.

Events beginning in the 1990s and extending to today signaled the need for a change in the approach to leadership. Changes in elder consumer preferences, growing quality and service expectations, human resource limitations, challenging finances, and an increasingly competitive marketplace have raised the bar for the profession of health and aging services administration. The margin for error in maintaining optimal operations has become slimmer, and boards and owners of healthcare organizations demand effective management. Furthermore, change in the field is constant, and leadership is now required to continuously look for ways to maintain or bolster organizational creativity and innovation while at the same time making sure that the basics of clinical care and other essential practices are achieved. Trends today include continued nursing home transformation, rightsizing (e.g., skilled nursing facilities decreasing their number of beds by often conversion to single rooms) and expanding the array of community- and facility-based service options available to baby boomers and their parents. Proficiency in both management and leadership is required for organizations to survive and thrive.

Unfortunately, senior care administrators often view quality as the management of satisfactory levels of clinical and service outcomes and regulatory compliance. In his book, *Juran on Leadership for Quality*, Joseph Juran (1989) uses big Q and little q to describe the difference in perspectives on quality. Little q thinking is narrowly focused on specific outcomes or tasks such as clinical measures and survey deficiencies. Big Q requires broader thinking to develop systems that align all functions of the organization to contribute to performance excellence and customer satisfaction. Visionary thinking does not replace the need for knowledge of geriatric principles and practices, or the knowledge of what constitutes excellent care and services, or the ability to discern reality from expectations. Rather, visionary thinking connects the best care and service standards to the resident's or client's expectations, productivity to satisfied employees, and person-centered culture change to the rigor of managing effective processes and systems.

The more recent public policy–directed quality models for this diverse set of senior care services across the continuum have evolved with government partnership. The following captures a few of the key thrusts for each of these separate areas that require attention:

- Skilled care facilities are required to have a quality assurance and performance improvement (QAPI) program in place, which the Centers for Medicare & Medicaid Services and many others have invested time and attention to. A rich set of resources are available to help guide this effort.

- Assisted living providers have largely focused on advancing standards that are self-reported and that have an element of quality improvement within their various areas of focus. This is an evolving area with a variety of states taking different positions on their level of involvement.

- Home care agencies that are Medicare certified are required to collect and report Outcome and Assessment Information Set (OASIS) data. This information is used for multiple purposes including calculating several types of quality reports, which are provided to home health agencies to help guide QAPI efforts.

The moral of the story is that if public funds are accessed, there is a direct correlation with some set of quality oversight and a push toward greater transparency by organizations, such as the five-star program advanced by the CMS.

OTHER QUALITY MODELS

The basics of quality include an understanding of the various levels of focus of quality management models. These are often broken down by the following descriptions:

- Quality assurance that is the focus on monitoring quality metrics.
- Quality improvement that encompasses the cycle of improvement.
- Total quality management that encompasses the broader view of quality, including quality assurance and improvement, and the importance of engagement of all stakeholders in the process.

For the new leader understanding that when it comes to quality, it is critical to have a systems perspective. Anytime a person tries to reduce things to one dimension they are more likely to miss something. It is also important to know how to use data, including the right data, for understanding a problem or situation and advance improvement. Continuous quality improvement depends on both of these factors to help the organization get better at what they do for the residents, tenants, and clients they serve every day.

Cathy Bergland, Vice President of Christian Culture and Leadership Development, Presbyterian Homes & Services

Some of the approaches in the senior care field today include the following established models.

The Baldrige Program

The Baldrige Program is the nation's public–private partnership dedicated to performance excellence. The Baldrige Program states the following goals:

- Raises awareness about the importance of performance excellence in driving the U.S. and global economy.
- Provides organizational assessment tools and criteria. The organization has a wide variety of products available on their website.
- Educates leaders in businesses, schools, healthcare organizations, and government and nonprofit agencies about the practices of best-in-class organizations.

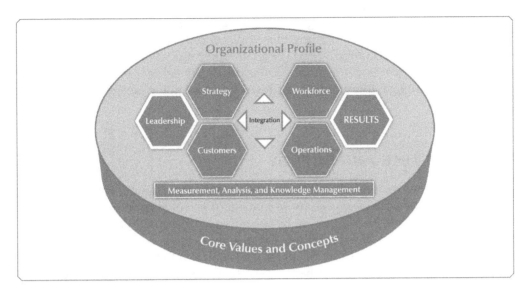

Figure 9.1 Baldrige Model

Source: Baldrige Performance Excellence Program. (2019). *2019-2020 Baldrige Excellence Framework: Proven leadership and management practice for high performance (health care).* Gaithersburg, MD: U.S. Department of Commerce, National Institute of Standards and Technology. Retrieved from https://www.nist.gov/baldrige/publications/baldrige-excellence-framework/health-care

- Recognizes national role models and honors them with the only Presidential Award for performance excellence.

This model is used as a foundation for the American Health Care Association's Quality Award program and is also a tremendous resource for individuals and organizations (Figure 9.1). There are several other quality award programs sponsored by consulting groups, providers, vendors, and associations with varying approaches that are connected with effective performance improvement.

Six Sigma and Lean

A couple of other established models of operational improvement include Six Sigma and Lean. Six Sigma is a method that provides organization tools to improve the capability of their business processes. The goal of Six Sigma is an increase in performance and a decrease in process variation. It helps to reduce defects and improve profits, increase employee morale, and provide better quality of products or services. Six Sigma uses a methodology to define, measure, analyze, improve, and control. Lean management's core idea is to maximize customer value while minimizing waste. Waste, or *muda* in Japanese, is defined as the performance of unnecessary work as a result of errors, poor organization, or communication. The eight lean mudas can be remembered using the acronym DOWNTIME and include (a) defects, (b) overproduction, (c) waiting, (d) nonutilized talent, (e) transportation, (f) inventory, (g) motion, and (h) extra processing.

Simply put, lean means creating more value for customers with fewer resources. There is also a new model combining these two concepts known as Lean Six Sigma (American Society of Quality, 2019). There are other models that could be considered, such as ISO, yet surveying the landscape of the senior services field, these appear to be the most commonly considered paradigms for improving quality in our industry.

MANAGING TIME AND ENERGY

Time management relates to quality management on a personal level. An effective quality leader also understands how to manage themselves and their time. There are a few key tenets to keep in mind. Be proactive by planning what you are going to do and do what you plan on doing. You also need to be aware of the need for a flexible approach and the ability to adjust. The concept of slack time, which means having some open time in your schedule, is also a good one to keep in mind in this very people-oriented service business. Slack time allows the innovative leader to take care of the time-consuming, execution-oriented tasks that result from changes that might slow down projects.

Another central theme is understanding how you are spending your time. The concept of the Four Quadrants of Time Management by Covey (1989) is a good one to both grasp and consider. The central message is to be proactive and spend as much time as possible on the activities that really matter (the top two boxes in Exhibit 9.1).

An effective leader knows that there are certain activities that will happen that are outside of their control, such as a storm or other crisis, which you will need to manage and which will take your time. There are other things that happen and take time that you will have more influence over, such as interruptions or busy work (bottom two boxes in Exhibit 9.1). Although it needs to be understood that these less

EXHIBIT 9.1 Four Quadrants of Time Management

IMPORTANT AND URGENT MATTERS	IMPORTANT ALTHOUGH NOT IMMEDIATE
Emergencies/Employee Crisis. Examples: health department survey or shortage in staff caused by weather or other crisis	Planning for Improvements. Examples: donor relationship development or implimentation of an employee retention program
NOT IMPORTANT BUT ROUTINELY HAPPEN IN SENIOR CARE ORGANIZATIONS	NOT ESSENTIAL OR IMMEDIATE
Distractions/Interruptions. Examples: employee socialization, routine, scheduled meetings	Busy work/Time Wasting. Examples: Internet surfing, completing duplicative resident forms, certain calls, texts or emails

Source: Reproduced with permission from Covey, S. R. (1989). *The 7 habits of highly effective people: Restoring the character ethic.* New York, NY: Simon & Schuster.

important activities are part of your daily administrative life, they should be either avoided or limited as much as possible, because there are only so many hours in a day. One good current example in today's environment is how effectively a person manages their personal mobile device. Ultimately, the time an effective leader is protecting is for the critical activities spent on planning, thinking, and reflection on the big rocks that need to be in the forefront of their organizations. Examples of these include time spent on the development of an employee program with a longer term impact on the stability of your workforce or paying attention to changing senior staff's interests and how that impacts the demand for your current care and service portfolio.

One wants to manage Q1, focus efforts in Q2, avoid Q3 situations, and limit Q4 activities. One of the goals for an individual is to secure some time for planning, thinking, and reflection on the big rocks that are in the forefront of your organizations, such as changing senior interests and how that impacts your current care and service portfolio.

Managing your work–life balance should not be underestimated, because this profession can be both rewarding and taxing. Your professional career is not a sprint and requires endurance with family and wellness being reservoirs of extra energy and support.

TECHNOLOGY

Technology is a critical tool for operational practices and one that requires a thoughtful integrative way of thinking when it comes to electronic systems. A few areas to note when analyzing hardware or software needs at a senior care organization include the following:

- Decision-making steps: Systems selection is generally done with a request for proposal process, which should include a well thought-out implementation plan.

- Redundancy is an area that advancing electronic health records is helping to solve as "systems" are better able to communicate important information.

- An Internet/cable provider system is becoming the standard expectation of consumers and employees today. The ability to be able to access the Internet for any number of uses is critical to the satisfaction of your residents, clients, and tenants. Employees are also dependent on access to both do their job and manage their time.

- Hardware, network, and software advances are hard to keep up with and is one of the key issues that CEOs and leaders report that they are uncomfortable with as an ongoing decision and need.

- Cybersecurity is also a current topic of discussion and concern with lots of training and resources being dedicated to the root causes of many breaches (i.e., the human factor). This is also a responsibility for leaders to protect resident and employee information and ensure a secure electronic system that follows Health Insurance Portability and Accountability Act standards.

There are also lots of other technology factors that are a significant influence in senior care settings, including the following:

- Electronic medical records are required for every resident, tenant, or client. They advance the effectiveness of care and service, and ensure the appropriate level of care and service need, which often drives reimbursement.

- Financial systems that are part of the overall system are also systems either built, customized, or purchased for the important accounting functions related to operations, such as accounts receivable and billing, accounts payable, and general ledger and payroll.

- One of the key advances many people and organizations are wanting to see even better integration between is the care and services, and the financial data systems. The expectation is that there will continue to be progress made in this arena, as many companies and business partners work to fill that gap.

- Staff these days could not function without an email or in-house phone or communication system. Technology is breaking new ground in the senior care setting to serve as a support system for employees and to make their jobs more efficient and less dependent on more traditional forms of passing information along between shifts, departments, and functional areas.

- Call systems and medical alert systems have been significant technology advances for people wanting to be safe in the least restricting setting. One of the great strides made in the senior care field allows aging individuals to live in the least restrictive setting with the aid of technology that can monitor any changes or potential problematic issues or events.

- Wandering prevention has also seen great strides in both cost and effectiveness and allows those with advancing stages of dementia to be safe and unrestrained.

- Fire safety and security are generally found in local and life safety codes and followed by providers of service; technology has served to increase the response time for any such incidents.

- Maintenance and environmental services have been a major benefactor of technology advances. New technologies allow for better workflow and the preventive maintenance scheduling of equipment and systems, which is a current standard of practice. Many vendors are integrating this service as part of their portfolio of services, for example, TELS from Direct Supply. There are also numerous applications for the effective operation of transportation and the management of vehicles.

The years ahead have great potential for the effective development and use of technology that assists and enhances the care and delivery of senior care services. A few examples include the following:

- Life enrichment and memory preservation technologies are making steady progress with new approaches being advanced with groups like the Alzheimer's Association.

- Health informatics and predictive analytics continue to progress with some potential applications of data that influence and optimize decision-making for both individual and organizations.

- Assistive devices and durable medical equipment have seen lots of advances and progress over the past decade, including the ability to share data and information electronically with the resident or client medical record.

■ Robotics is a future area with the potential to help support both the customer and staff by providing supportive resources or tools in postacute care and rehabilitation service areas.

Technology will continue to be a growing, evolving asset for leaders and organizations. By using the right information informed by technology, the right way, at the right time, you can successfully add value to your senior care organization. Because technology is ever-changing, it would be a word to the wise for emerging leaders and all leaders to be positioned to stay abreast and current with new technological solutions for the services they provide. Leaders will be able to gauge the appropriate amount of money and time to allocate to the use of the latest technology from a return on investment standpoint.

SUMMARY

Leaders need to be both thoughtful and intentional in their deliberations and actions. Furthermore, the true test of a successful administrator in senior care services depends on their ability to get things done. The importance of having a grounded, systematic way of thinking is a critical skill set for individuals involved in directing and managing senior care organizations.

KEY POINTS

1. Senior care and service leaders need to be aware of problem-solving approaches.
2. Execution is a critical skill for senior care and service executives and is the critical link to getting things done.
3. A variety of quality models exist and can serve as resources for organizational leadership.
4. Effectively focusing time and attention in the right places is necessary on both a personal and professional level for operational excellence
5. Technology is an important component that helps support the effective delivery of care and services.

LEADERSHIP ROLES

1. Leaders need to drive the operational practices of an organization.
2. They must have a high level of awareness of the variety of problem-solving models available and be committed to using a consistent approach within the organization.
3. Leaders need to engage their team in the process to ensure buy-in.
4. Accountability is linked to keeping score and is an expectation that people want.
5. Technology decisions are required to optimize customer service, staff time, and the best use of all resources.

HIGH-IMPACT PRACTICES

1. Share models of problem-solving with management staff and have a discussion with them to consider what would be the best approach to use within your organization.

2. Talk to staff to better understand their perception of how they perceive the ability of the organization to get things done.

3. At professional conferences, seek out vendors that are advancing new technology solutions for the delivery of care and services.

QUESTIONS FOR DISCUSSION

1. In this high-touch, labor-intensive field, what are the key factors related to that characteristic that must be considered when making decisions?

2. What would you describe as the key leadership practices that you need to develop to effectively get things done within a senior care organization?

3. Do the different models of problem-solving and quality management apply the same or differently across all settings of senior care and service?

4. How will you ensure that you are up to date with technology in your career?

CASE PROBLEMS

1. A challenging issue in the skilled care environment is staffing, which is a consistent problem for this field across all lines of services. You work as a facility administrator for a regional provider of postacute rehabilitation that is experiencing a significant retention problem with nearly half of the staff hired leaving within 90 days. What are the steps you would take to investigate the issue? How would you involve staff and advance any changes?

2. Many assisted living leaders use a self-assessment approach of the services they provide and plan to monitor and promote an environment that provides exceptional care and service for residents. What are some of the different ways you think they do this for their organizations? How do you think they use this information with future customers? What are some creative ways that they could involve external or independent stakeholders in this quality process? Identify the stakeholders including the expertise or resource they would bring to the table and their respective role.

3. Home- and community-based services could gain from a better technological approach to monitoring care delivery and health of their customers in home- and community-based settings. Investigate some of the more promising technology opportunities for this sector of care and services. What criteria would you use to determine which new technologies to invest in? Lastly, consider any steps required for the implementation of any new technology enhancement for both clients and staff.

NAB DOMAINS OF PRACTICE

50.07 Identify, foster, and maintain positive relationships with key stakeholders.

This task requires the Administrator to determine who key stakeholders are and develop a working relationship/understanding with each of them. This task includes creating an atmosphere of trust and understanding. This should be tempered with providing necessary information to work jointly on projects and systems that benefit the organization. At no time should the impression be given that any key stakeholder is asked to assist in leading the facility/organization.

50.09 Solicit information from appropriate stakeholders for use in decision-making.

This task requires the Administrator to set up protocols/standards of practice to use all available input from trusted resources to make effective, fair, and timely decisions. The Administrator must have the ability to weigh the situation/circumstance and the time used to make decisions. While the Administrator is accountable for the decisions they will make, it is important for the Administrator to know that sometimes a good decision is better than the best decision when time or the lives of others is a factor.

50.13 Implement, monitor, and evaluate information management and technology systems to support service providers operations.

This task requires the Administrator to meet all federal, state, and community requirements for information management of health records, financial information, and Health Insurance Portability and Accountability Act. Safeguards to employee, patient, resident, and client information must be in writing and show evidence of training/competency of all employees. In addition, the administrator must ensure that there is a process in place to protect access to information, to secure and track passwords, and to back up and protect all data in the community servers. Attention must also be given to ensure that all technologies are designed to save employees time and allow more time for patient/resident/client care.

50.16 Develop, implement, and evaluate the organization's QAPI programs.

This task requires the Administrator to develop an effective QAPI program. This includes following CMS guidelines related to QAPI and establishing specific procedures, policies, and systems to perform an effective QAPI program. This also includes ensuring the program is designed to meet the ever-changing needs of the facility/organization.

Source: Reproduced with permission from the National Association of Long-Term Care Administrator Boards. (2016). *Annotation of tasks performed and knowledge and skills used across lines of service in long term care.* Retrieved from https://www.nabweb.org/filebin/pdf/Annotation_of_Tasks_Performed_Across_LOS_in_LTC.pdf

REFERENCES

American Society of Quality. (2019). *What do you want to do?* Retrieved from https://asq.org

Baldrige Performance Excellence Program. (2019). *2019-2020 Baldrige Excellence Framework: Proven leadership and management practice for high performance (health care).* Gaithersburg, MD: U.S. Department of Commerce, National Institute of Standards and Technology. Retrieved from https://www.nist.gov/baldrige/publications/baldrige-excellence -framework/health-care

Covey, S. R. (1989). *The seven habits of highly effective people: Restoring the character ethic.* New York, NY: Simon & Schuster.

Deming, W. E. (1986). *Out of the crisis.* Cambridge, MA: Massachusetts Institute of Technology, Center for Advanced Engineering Study.

FOCUS-PDCA Model, The Hospital Corporation of America. UCLA Health System A3/A4. Retrieved from https://www.uclahealth.org/nursing/workfiles/Education%20Courses/ RR-SMH-MagnetResources/CombiningModels-EBPModel%2CFOCUS -PDCA%2CA3-A4%20%281%29.pdf

Guo, K. L. (2008). DECIDE: A decision-making model for more effective decision making by health care managers. *Health Care Management, 27*(2), 118–127. doi:10.1097/01. HCM.0000285046.27290.90

Juran, J. M. (1989). *Juran on leadership for quality: An executive handbook.* New York, NY: Free Press.

McChesney, C., Huling, J., & Covey, S. (2012). *The 4 disciplines of execution: Achieving your wildly important goals.* New York, NY: Free Press.

Tague, N. R. (2005). Plan–do–study–act cycle. In *The quality toolbox* (2nd ed., pp. 390–392). Milwaukee, WI: ASQ Quality Press. (Original work published 1995)

U.S. Centers for Medicare & Medicaid. (2019). Retrieved from https://www.cms.gov/ Medicare/QAPI/downloads

University of Minnesotas. (2019). *About the MHA founder.* Minneapolis, MN: University of Minnesota. Retrieved from https://www.sph.umn.edu/academics/degrees-programs/ mha/master-healthcare-administration/mhafounder/

ADDITIONAL RESOURCES

ACHCA Quality Award: https://www.ahcancal.org/quality_improvement/quality_award/

Aging 2.0: https://www.aging2.com

Argentum Standards for Senior Living: https://www.argentum.org/wp-content/ uploads/2017/01/Argentum-Standards.pdf

Baldrige: https://www.nist.gov/baldrige/self-assessing/baldrige-sector/health-care

CMS resources: https://www.cms.gov/Medicare/Provider-Enrollment-and-Certification/ SurveyCertificationGenInfo/LTC-CMP-Reinvestment.html; https://www.cms.gov/ Medicare/Quality-Initiatives-Patient-Assessment-Instruments/HomeHealthQualityInits/ index.html

Comagine Quality Awards (formerly Health Insight): https://healthinsight.org/quality-awards

HIPAA: https://www.hhs.gov/hipaa/for-professionals/security/laws-regulations/index.html

The Joint Commission: https://www.jointcommission.org/accreditation/long_term_care.aspx

National Council for Aging Care: https://www.aging.com/7-ways-technology-has-improved -senior-care/

CHAPTER 10

People: Human Resources and Relationships

INTRODUCTION

In this chapter, we take a deeper dive into the nuances of effectively establishing and building a workplace culture that fosters professional and personal growth, engagement, fulfillment, and favorable outcomes for the organization and for those served by it. This does not happen by spontaneous generation. It takes a leader who:

- consistently demonstrates vision, empathy and compassion, discernment, integrity, transparency, and stamina;
- recognizes the potential each person brings to the table and is willing to invest not only in developing the person's skills but in them as a person;
- can successfully nurture the multidirectional relationships on which top-performing provider organizations rely to advance their mission.

WHO SUCCEEDS?

The Qualified

Competence in performing a particular skill or task should not be confused with either **proficiency** or **mastery**. The people we serve, who may already feel compromised or vulnerable, understandably want some reason for trusting their caregiving team and its leaders. Accordingly, various levels of "credentialing" have evolved among the health professions, in general, and for administrative leaders across the postacute care continuum, in particular.

Credentialing protects the public's interest by establishing professional standards of practice on which people can rely in selecting a service provider. In healthcare, the most common jurisdiction for enforcing those standards are state boards of licensure, although some local governments might impose additional requirements.

In order to receive a professional credential in the healthcare field—whether an academic degree, certificate of completion, or government-issued license—it is standard practice to require at least some demonstration of a person's fundamental command of the information relevant to the discipline. An academic program awards someone who successfully completes a prescribed course of study such as associate's, bachelor's, master's, or doctoral degree. Also, a person who already holds an academic degree and wants to learn more about a particular subject, such as gerontology or accounting, but do so without acquiring another degree, might earn a certificate from an academic program that offers such an option.

The terms **certificate** and **certification** are sometimes either used interchangeably or confused for one another. However, they are *not* the same thing. **Certification** is typically awarded by a nongovernmental organization, generally a professional membership society that represents the interests of that profession, to someone who demonstrates advanced proficiency in their discipline (e.g., Professional Certification in Nursing Home Administration or Assisted Living Administration by the American College of Health Care Administrators).

Health professionals who must acquire a state-issued license to practice are typically expected to also engage in continuing education activities in order to renew their license periodically (commonly every 1–2 years). This is intended to ensure that health practitioners keep current with the latest developments in their field.

Nursing Home Administrator

Effective in 1971, the federal government mandated that each state create a board of licensure for nursing home administrators (Social Security Act). An unintended consequence of the relatively short timeline for complying with that mandate was the emergence of rules and standards that varied—sometimes considerably—across the states. The National Association of Long-Term Care Administrators (NAB), to which each state licensing board belongs, has developed standards for approving continuing education, accrediting academic programs in long-term care administration, and other regulatory guidelines to enhance its members' ability to effectively meet their public protection charge.

Assisted Living/Residential Care Administrator

There is not yet a comparable, national set of state-administered licensing standards for someone leading an organization that provides assisted living or residential care. Some states have begun moving in that direction, the earliest of which were Idaho in 1993 (Idaho Administrative Rules, 2019) and Virginia in 2008 (Virginia Code, 2019). The Argentum (formerly known as the Assisted Living Federation of America), the national association representing the interests of organizations that operate assisted living communities, introduced in 2017 a professional certification program. According to its website, earning the Certified Director of Assisted Living (CDAL) credential "demonstrates attainment of consistent, relevant, measurable and industry-recognized standards of practice in the assisted living executive director role" (Argentum, 2019).

Home- and Community-Based Services Administrator

Although considered by many as the fastest-growing segment of the postacute care continuum, professional standards for home- and community-based services (HCBS) leaders have been slower to emerge than for those leading organizations providing either nursing care or assisted living and residential care. Accompanying the anticipated growth in the number of people that this service line affects will be a rise in public scrutiny, including expectations for professional competence, accountability, and transparency.

The Rewarded and Fulfilled

Everyone has a unique set of motivations for working. The reasons people work vary widely, but all people receive some combination of rewards from their work, ranging from monetary support for basic sustenance and quality of life to a sense of accomplishment and contribution to others (Heathfield, 2019). A career in any postacute care setting is definitely not for the faint-hearted or for someone who seeks the comfort of routine and predictability!

Some people are drawn to the postacute care setting by their love of the work itself; others work for personal and professional fulfillment. People who like to feel they are contributing to something larger than themselves or have an overarching vision for what they can create typically thrive in this field. Others simply love what they do or the clients they serve—and the life stories that are abundantly shared. Some like the interaction or camaraderie formed with residents and coworkers. Some workers like change, challenge, and diverse problems to solve.

However, almost *everyone* works for money. Whatever it is called—compensation, salary, remuneration, bonuses, or benefits—it pays the bills. Money provides food, shelter, clothing, healthcare, education, leisure activities, and retirement. Unless one inherits enough to be considered independently wealthy, working is, at least in some part, about earning a living.

Competitive wages and benefits are foundational building blocks for recruiting and retaining committed staff members. Researchers at global human resources consulting firm Watson Wyatt Worldwide have found that to attract the best employees, an organization should expect to pay more than its average-paying counterparts in the marketplace (Pfau & Kay, 2001). Money provides basic motivation.

Most people also want more from work than money. In a study of workers and managers sponsored by the American Psychological Association, managers predicted that the most important motivational aspect of work for people they employed would be money. Instead, it turned out that personal time and attention from the supervisor was cited by workers as most rewarding and motivational for them at work (American Pyschological Association, 2014).

Another study that involved more than 200,000 employees in more than 500 organizations explored a number of different management topics, such as culture, recognition, growth opportunities, and motivation (Drzymalski, Gladstone, Troyani, & Niu, 2014). A question the survey asked was, "What motivates you to excel and go the extra mile at your organization?" Employees could choose from 10 answers. Interestingly, money—often assumed to be the major motivator—was seventh on the list:

1. Camaraderie, peer motivation   (20%)
2. Intrinsic desire to a good job   (17%)
3. Feeling encouraged and recognized   (13%)
4. Having a real impact   (10%)
5. Growing professionally   (8%)
6. Meeting client/customer needs   (8%)
7. Money and benefits   (7%)
8. Positive supervisor/senior management   (4%)
9. Believe in the company/product   (4%)
10. Others   (9%)

The Reliable and the Dependable

Movie celebrity and comedian Woody Allen is credited with saying, "Eighty percent of success is showing up" (QuoteInvestigator, 2013). There are very few workplaces for which this adage has more meaning than postacute care organizations. Particularly in clinical roles, not only are clients counting on everyone who is scheduled to work to arrive—on time—but so are the clients' families and coworkers.

Attendance

Of course, attendance has at least two key characteristics: presence and engagement. It is possible to arrive, clock-in, and report to an assigned work location but to be less than fully engaged and productive.

Some of the most commonly occurring distractions that can erode a person's engagement level include the following:

- **Illness:** If someone can simply not financially afford to miss work, it may be the only viable choice to report for duty and do the best they can—realizing it may put both clients and coworkers at risk, as well as potentially increase the employee's own risk of either injury or worsening the illness.

- **Exhaustion:** It is not uncommon for staff members, particularly in lower-wage positions, to either work extra shifts or have outside employment to earn more money. This can also occur with older staff members due to age or disability, not driven by income, and can be addressed by re-evaluating job duties to minimize its impact on attendance.

- **Transportation:** Whether it is a personal vehicle or public transit, if the means for getting to work fail for some reason and there are limited backup options, this can present an attendance barrier.

- **External Pressures:** These range from a sick child or family member to harassment by a collection agency regarding past-due bills and from domestic strife to issues that require a personal appearance over which they have little control (maintaining public benefits eligibility or a court hearing).

- **Slippery Onboarding:** If the person feels either unwelcome or excluded, or worse, hazed by more established coworkers, is it worth coming back? It is quite a paradox that longer-tenured staff members would treat new arrivals as anything less than the cavalry or EMS coming to their rescue, and forget that they, too, were ever new to the organization. This is *the* most actionable contributing factor for leadership to address, and it both deserves and requires a shared commitment throughout the organization.

According to the U.S. Bureau of Labor Statistics, the 2019 absence rate for full-time employees in America was typically about 2.8% (2020). Among all healthcare workers, that figure is slightly higher (3.4%), and among senior living staff, it is even higher (over 10%). On any given day, a postacute care provider organization with 100 employees could expect to have 10 staff members missing! If a disproportionate share of those have direct care roles, it can negatively impact both care outcomes and morale.

Punctuality

Punctuality is showing up when one is expected to arrive, ready to perform the duties of the position. The prevalence of steadily declining punctuality among American workers is not unique to postacute care. More than one of four employees admit to being tardy at least once a month, and 16% are late once a week, or more (Smith, 2013). In our settings, however, this creates more than a mere inconvenience or delay. Depending on how late the staff member arrives—and whether they called to report the anticipated late arrival—job duties may get reassigned and need to be changed again when the late-arriving staff member arrives, disrupting the day for clients and coworkers, alike.

There is not enough room in the appendices of this book to include a list of the excuses offered by associates when they were "running a little behind." A survey conducted in 2012 by Harris Interactive asked more than 2,600 employers to share some of the most memorable and outlandish excuses they have heard from employees who were arriving late (Smith, 2013). They range from blaming an angry spouse (who froze the car keys in a glass of water) or unexpected acts of nature (a bear attacking the car or having to stop to help deliver a stranger's baby) to self-generated mishaps (driving to one's previous employer's location or leaving the house wearing the shoes of one's spouse).

"Employees panic," says Rosemary Haefner, vice president of human resources at CareerBuilder. "Instead of just telling the employer the real reason they were late, they go for the big story, and unfortunately, it raises red flags and hurts them in the long run." Employers realize that from time to time, things that are out of an employees' control are going to happen and they will be late, she says. "But it escalates to a problem when the behavior becomes repetitive, causing employers to take disciplinary action." In fact, more than one third of hiring managers reported they had to fire someone for being late (Smith, 2013).

IMPORTANCE OF EFFECTIVE SUPERVISION

Leading a team of people effectively involves four critical elements—planning, organizing, directing, and monitoring. Inspiring others to work together toward a set of common goals calls for cultivating a *culture* of communication.

Planning

"Plan what you do, and do what you plan," advises Dr. Robert Slaton, Kentucky's former Commissioner of Health (Jackson & Slaton, 1993). Best-selling author Stephen Covey recommends, "Begin with the end in mind" in his widely acclaimed *The 7 Habits of Highly Successful People* (1989). Whether it is for current operations—budget, staff scheduling, dining menus, preventive maintenance, or floor care – or for envisioning a strategic direction for the future, planning is essential to success and a hallmark of effective leadership.

Planning should be an ongoing process, allowing for adjustments to be made when either internal or external influences or circumstances change. It is a journey, not an event with a starting and ending date. For instance, when an area's unemployment rates decline, recruiting and retaining employees may become tougher because the organization is increasingly competing against businesses in multiple sectors, not just with postacute care employers.

Effective planning engages as many different stakeholders—people with a vested interest in the outcome—as possible. Depending on the issue, a stakeholder might come from the ranks of clients and their families, team members and their families, volunteers, clinical contractors and suppliers, community and civic leaders, or even regulators. Including a variety of perspectives helps build a more thorough plan, as well as enhancing the probability of success by inviting shared "buy-in" and ownership of the plan.

Organizing

According to Merriam-Webster's Dictionary (2019), organizing is "to arrange by systematic planning and unified effort." Metaphorically, it is not only selecting the members of a work team, it is also getting everyone on the team rowing in the same direction and at the same rhythm in order to optimize performance and reach the desired destination or goal. Business author and Stanford University professor Jim Collins, in his book *Good to Great* (2001), suggests that the most effective leaders continuously ask, "First who, then what?"

You are a bus driver. … You have to decide where you are going, how you're going to get there and who is going with you. Most people assume that great bus drivers (read: business leaders) immediately start the journey by announcing to the people on the bus where they're going – by setting a new direction or by articulating a fresh corporate vision. In fact, leaders of companies that go from good to great start not with "where" but with "who." They start by getting the right people on the bus, the wrong people off the bus, and the right people in the right seats. (Collins, 2001, p. 44)

Recruiting, screening, hiring, training, and developing talent are fundamental functions of managing human resources. However, here are some additional suggestions for effectively *organizing* effort among team members.

- **Champion:** Every project should have a lead person, a champion, who coordinates all team members in order to ensure that the project progresses smoothly, on time and within budget, and meets or exceeds relevant professional and regulatory standards. An effective champion demands (and gets) excellence from the team and helps team members in their personal development and motivation.
- **Task Assignments:** Competent distribution of responsibilities among team members boosts each one's overall efficiency, reduces the risk of duplication or working at cross purposes, and fosters group ownership in the organization's success. Also, if there is a question about a project or procedure, there is a greater probability of finding the person with the best answer.
- **Cross-Training:** Equipping people with the knowledge and skills to perform assignments outside of the realm of their normal position adds flexibility and bench strength for the operation, as well as widening their career paths.

What matters most, at the end of the day, is that each team member leaves feeling connected to the organization's mission and that their efforts contributed in a meaningful way to advancing that mission. Designing—and flexibly and appropriately adjusting—how responsibilities are assigned, shared, measured, and rewarded is an essential factor in leadership success.

Directing

An effective leader not only oversees employee performance but also instructs, guides, and inspires—*coaches*—the growth and development of each member of the work team in order to most effectively and efficiently achieve desired goals and objectives. Planning and organizing are merely interesting exercises without an organization's leadership providing solid direction. Direction typically has the following characteristics (Juneja, 2019):

1. **Pervasive Function:** Required at all levels of organization, from work team leader to CEO.

2. **Continuous Activity:** Ongoing activity throughout the life of an organization; a journey, not an event.

3. **Human Factor:** People have diverse needs, life experiences, skills, expectations, and perceptions; channeling those in ways that positively influence advancing the organization's mission takes skilled direction.

4. **Creative Activity:** Converting plans into performance is only rarely successful in a "paint-by-numbers" environment; leveraging people's creativity can foster the feeling of ownership and improve the prospects for success.

5. **Delegate Function:** One can delegate authority, but not responsibility. A leader can deputize someone to complete a particular task or project—to make binding decisions about resource allocation, procedures, or other business matters. However, that "delegate" is an extension of—a surrogate for—the leader who made the assignment. In traditional management and leadership environments, the delegating leader always retains *responsibility*. However, more contemporary organizations find that "self-directed teams" can often replace this approach and produce better, more lasting results.

Self-Directed Work Teams

Self-directed teams in the workplace were first demonstrated as effective and popularized in the manufacturing sector over a half-century ago. It does not mean trading law and order with chaos and anarchy. Instead of the traditional supervisor and subordinate model that prevailed during the Industrial Age, people accept greater levels of planning, organizing, directing, and monitoring in their work as a team, from personnel scheduling to purchasing and from workflow to performance metrics.

Numerous highly successful companies have applied this approach for decades. However, service organizations, in general, and health and human services providers, in particular, have been slow to embrace the abundance of evidence supporting the many benefits that can result from adopting this model. In many ways, the healthcare field has remained firmly entrenched in the belief that a single manager is better at making decisions than the 10 people who report to that manager. The underlying premise of self-directed work teams is that the 10 people most affected by a decision will be better at making it.

It is becoming increasingly clear that in order for a senior living organization to thrive, a contemporary health services executive must find ways to create and nurture the development of teams without traditional managers. Self-directed teams produce results because this approach fosters a culture of mutual respect, capitalizes on people's creativity and desire to belong to a winning team, and invites ownership in the success of the organization. Ownership has been shown to be one of the most powerful motivators in a variety of business settings (Blakeman, 2014).

Many companies have benefited for decades from giving people back their brains. These companies grow faster, are more productive and more profitable, have lower turnover, and have increased longevity. As more and more owners and investors see the numbers, they will demand that their companies move in this direction. It is simple, but it is rarely easy. A century of "bosses" have taught people they are not quite as smart and motivated as managers. You have to reverse that notion, and it will take time for people to trust you really are doing it. Here is one path for moving forward (Blakeman, 2014):

1. Form a team around an *objective* (i.e., 4–12 people).
2. Have them *first* clearly define the desired *result*.
3. Then have them define the *process(es)* needed to get that result.
4. Then, *they* set *metrics* for steps in the process.
5. *Pay them based on the result* desired (quality, quantity, speed, etc.).
6. Finally, *they decide* what happens if the metrics are not met and how to move team members along if they are not contributing appropriately.
7. Leadership *approves*.
8. Run it.

Safeguarding the Organization's Future

Today, people want a job that does more than pay the bills; they want work that allows them to be fully human, make decisions, and own their stuff. As more companies leave their Industrial Age management structures behind and invite people to decide, they are more likely to retain the great people they have. Embracing the concept of self-managed teams is one great way to give people back their brains.

If you treat people like they have brains, they will use them!

Robert E. Maten, Store Manager
S.S. Kresge, Inc.

Monitoring

It is important to review conducted work and determine what went well and the mistakes that occurred in the process. Try to get to the core of identified mistakes. It is possible—even likely—that behind an error there was some good intention or logic. There was just some kind of impediment on the way toward success. Collective reflection and analysis will make any team more unified and powerful for higher achievements going forward.

Monitoring is an important feature of a quality assurance and performance improvement (QAPI) program. QAPI has roots in the work of W. Edwards Deming, who recommended that business processes be placed in a continuous feedback loop to identify and change the parts of the process that need improvement (Arveson, 1998). He labeled the four key steps in this model: plan, do, check, and act, now commonly referred to as the "PDCA cycle."

In addition to the morale-building benefit of an effective monitoring process, ideas for measurable performance improvement should surface. Maintaining a culture that encourages people to share their ideas—and have confidence that they will at least be considered, if not actually tried—is essential. Without such an environment, there is an inherent risk of people developing fear of either failure or worse yet, reprisal.

Motivation

Reward and recognition expert, Bob Nelson, suggests that employees want to be valued for a job well done by those they hold in high esteem (Box 10.1). He adds that people want to be treated as if they are "adult human beings who think, make sound decisions, try to do the right thing, and don't need a caretaker watching over their shoulders" (Nelson, 1999).

BOX 10.1 Key Workplace Motivators

- **Control or Influence:**
  - Ability to have an impact on decisions
  - S.M.A.R.T. goals (Specific, Measurable, Achievable, Realistic, and Time-bound)
  - Job enrichment
  - Recognition for achievement

- **Insider Membership:**
  - Smooth on-boarding and effective orientation
  - Receiving timely information and communication
  - Understanding leadership's approach to decision-making
  - Opportunities for participating in team and organization-wide meetings
  - Visual documentation and posting of work progress and accomplishments

- **Growth and Development:**
  - Education and training (including cross-training)
  - Career pathways and mentoring

(continued)

BOX 10.1 Key Workplace Motivators (*continued*)

- Team participation
- Succession planning
- Recognition for growth

- **From Leadership:**
  - Understand leadership's vision for the future
  - Alignment with the mission and values of the organization
  - Respect
  - Consistently fair and equal treatment
  - Transparency and sincerity

Source: Adapted from Heathfield, S. (2019, January 4). *What people want from work: Motivation*. Balance Careers. Retrieved from https://www .thebalancecareers.com/what-people-want-from-work-motivation-1919051

People who feel consistently rewarded and find their work fulfilling tend to stay with the organization longer, and they are typically more productive because of their familiarity with the duties of the job and with the needs and preferences of the clients. An effective leader learns the needs and rewards that are the most meaningful to *each staff member* and develops a strategy and tactics to provide them (Heathfield, 2019).

Connectivity and "the Knack"

A "knack" is simply the art of doing things with ease. Virginia Bell and David Troxel, creators of the widely acclaimed "Best Friends™ Approach to Dementia Care" (2016), applied this concept as a central element in their formula for success in serving persons with Alzheimer's disease and related disorders. It is also relevant to achieving optimal outcomes across the entire postacute care continuum, and not merely for how staff members can more effectively serve clients. It applies equally well to the relationships among coworkers. More than an *aptitude,* the "KNACK" reflects an *attitude* and set of skills that entail the following:

- **Knowledge:** Understanding of the client's disease and the experience of that person; applying common sense; setting realistic expectations; and planning ahead
- **Nurturing:** Making care relevant to each person; empathy; maintaining caregiving integrity; maintaining optimism; using humor and spontaneity; remaining nonjudgmental; and valuing the moment
- **Approach:** Effectively communicating on the client's cognitive level; respecting the basic rights of people; employing finesse appropriately; exercising patience and flexibility; remaining focused; and exuding confidence
- **Community:** Facilitating inclusion and fostering a sense of belonging; and leveraging the client's life story for cueing
- **Kinship:** Including family and friends in the care program and taking care of oneself

Communication

A recurring theme throughout this book is the importance of effective communication. Stakeholders want—and deserve—to know what is going on. The days of keeping people on various levels of "need-to-know" status are rapidly being replaced by expectations for transparency. Some have suspicions reinforced by reminders in the daily news about corporate leaders' misguided attempts at insider trading and acting as though the rules (sometimes laws) simply do not apply to them. Others simply want to contribute to improving the organization's performance—and could do so *better* if they were fully aware of the full picture. Instead, opportunities to fully leverage stakeholder engagement to improve operations are often missed due to ineffective communication by an organization's leaders.

TRUST AND CONFIDENCE

Trust is generally earned, not declared. Sometimes you get the benefit of the doubt, and people's trust is considered yours to lose. Regardless, once it is harmed or erodes, it is definitely much harder to win back. Most people want to follow a leader who is trustworthy and in whom they have confidence to apply rules fairly and consistently. Here are some tips about maintaining a culture of trust:

1. **Honesty:** Your word is your bond; exercise honesty when giving any sort of promise.

2. **Manage Expectations:** Goals can be both aspirational and realistic—they are not mutually exclusive. However, make every effort to keep people apprised of the organization's progress, acknowledging and celebrating successes as well as soliciting input for overcoming obstacles.

3. **Transparency:** Follow up on promises to demonstrate that you meant what you said. Do not conceal or cover up information that fails to support the planned direction.

4. **Anticipation:** Do not wait for someone to ask where things stand; proactively and regularly initiate communication about issues that matter to people about the organization's performance and prospects.

5. **Acknowledgment:** You can never thank someone too much. In order to have its intended effect, it must be perceived by the recipient (and any witnesses, if expressed publicly) as sincere. Gratitude "by-the-numbers" often feels awkward and may even have the unintended consequence of losing the trust and confidence of the very people you are trying to lead!

6. **Perception = The *Only* Reality That Matters:** Communicating in ways that the receivers of the information can understand is essential. Choices about words, phrases, and information vehicles (memo, email, in-person meeting, phone call, etc.) can influence how well the message meets your goal. Start with the intended audience's profile in order to frame what is said, how it is conveyed, and most importantly, how to measure how accurately it is received.

Both competence and character are absolutely critical and in about equal doses! We need individuals in senior living leadership who have deep convictions about serving others, doing so with humility, who embrace empowering others.

Rick Stiffney, PhD,
Owner, Integrated Leadership
and Consultancy, LLC

Visibility and Accessibility

A key element of transparency is availability, making it possible for stakeholders to reach you in a multitude of ways. Drain the moat around your office castle, if people think there is one, and invest time in meandering through the operation so they do not have to work up the courage to come see you. This can be a little more challenging in some home and community based organizations because of its decentralized nature—but where there is a will, there is a way!

Beyond making yourself visible and accessible, it is important to exude confidence without conveying arrogance and to foster optimism without coming across as having your head in the clouds. Finding something positive to say—even in the midst of a seemingly disastrous day—can make the difference between rallying the team and confirming any hopelessness that might be dwelling among its members.

Because most postacute care settings operate on a 24/7/365 basis, part of the showup is regularly outside of traditional business day hours, such as weekends and holidays, evening and night shifts. If people only see their leaders at one of those times because there is a crisis, then it would be natural to expect some bad news when one shows up.

Equal Treatment and Fairness

The regulatory compliance issues wrapped around treating people who are similarly situated both equally and fairly. Achieving and maintaining compliance is certainly important. However, equally or more important is the morale among stakeholders when this is not happening routinely. It is discouraging to staff members to see either favoritism or discrimination, as well as the staff turnover typically associated with either. It is defeating to residents and their families, too, who rely on a competent, stable staff for their comfort and confidence.

One way to cultivate a culture of equal treatment and fairness is to periodically review disciplinary actions that have had the names redacted to see if there is even a hint of a pattern to address with some intervention. QAPI works splendidly in several segments of the operation, not just in *clinical* matters. When there is such a discovery, group problem-solving around it reflects leadership's commitment to championing (not just complying with) equal treatment and fairness.

Confidentiality

The most threatening and potentially harmful phrase spoken in most organizations (generally softly or in a whisper) is "Don't tell anyone you heard it from me, but…"

It does not merely apply to gossip; it can often also apply to facts about a person's personal circumstances that they would prefer *not* to have widely known or discussed. It might be work related or not. The key determinant is who rightfully owns it and ethically should control its dissemination.

An old saying, "Discretion is the better part of valor," holds true today. It is not only more noble to protect someone's confidentiality, but it is a leadership imperative. Your reputation as a trustworthy leader deserving of people's loyalty ties closely to how well you are perceived as someone who respects every person's confidentiality.

Sincerity, Interest, and Compassion

Demonstrating your sincere interest in the well-being of others and showing your genuine interest in their lives—away from the workplace as well as while working—is an indispensable method for connecting with people. People generally sense when someone is sincere, so simply going through the motions or just saying the right words is rarely enough. Demonstrating real concern for the welfare of others takes committing time to do it proactively and practice to do it well.

No senior care community rises above the caliber, compassion, and commitment of its managers, administrator, and director of nursing. The nursing assistants and the clinical staff are the bricks and mortar of quality. Long-term care managers are the engineers and architects of quality in long-term care.

As people managers, they face a formidable challenge. Long-term care, more than other service professions, operates on a relational platform. To begin with, old age often brings physical disability and creates social and psychological challenges. Long-term care creates communities where frail and older people are brought together to spend the last years of their lives in a place, not always built, to promote dignity and privacy.

The social origin and setting of the staff who serve the elders can differ vastly in culture, education, age, and experience. We expect the managers to create a community from these diverse elements. Their background and training may not always adequately prepare them for the task. In addition, overbearing regulations and the predatory ways of lawyers make their task more difficult. Their training, professional requirements, and incentives lean heavily on compliance and avoiding liability rather than compassion and kindness.

The need for leaders who demonstrate compassion to their caregivers typically has not been addressed by education or quality programs. We need to work to infuse a greater emphasis on the need for compassionate leadership.

V. Tellis-Nayak, PhD, Mary Tellis-Nayak, RN, MSN, MPh
Consultants in Postacute Care, Chicago, Illinois

Advocacy: Safe Place

Creating an environment that feels safe to those who weave in and out of it is closely related to the concepts trust, confidence, equal treatment, fairness, confidentiality, sincerity, interest, and compassion. Safety and security are among the most commonly cited reasons for people to move from their homes to a congregate living setting (Liepelt, 2015) and highly rated as concerns for those who remain at home with contracted supports and services (National Institute on Aging [NIA], 2019). Finding a balance between encouraging self-determination and applying cautionary measures to prevent accidents resulting in injury is an ongoing challenge. However, documenting why certain interventions or equipment are in place (or *not*) is beneficial for both compliance and QAPI purposes. Communicating about them regularly—particularly *why* they are in place—with care recipients, their families, and staff is important.

There are, of course, plenty of safety issues pertaining to staff and visitors, as well. They range from potential physical plant hazards, such as a cracked sidewalk or a wet floor to less controllable risks, such as weather events. What is less intuitive, however, is the rising risk of workplace violence caused by an intruder or "active aggressor."

Finally, their place of employment is, for some staff members, the safest setting in their lives. Some live amid a constant threat of domestic violence, facing financial challenges with landlords or collection agencies, living in unsafe neighborhoods or healthy food deserts, depending on unreliable transportation, and much more. Advocating for and providing a safe and secure oasis in their lives can result in a tremendous return on investment in human capital.

LOYALTY

Loyalty has its foundation in an organization's leader paying close attention to building and fostering a culture of mutual trust, confidence and optimism, sincerity and transparency, equal treatment and fairness, and compassion and advocacy. Loyalty can offset many kinds of operational misfires and can serve as a catalyst for quicker and more effective solutions to problems that might surface.

Much like "love," loyalty is hard to describe because it is experienced so differently by people. The common denominator about which many agree, however, is the underlying premise that every person has intrinsic value. The truly "loyalty-worthy" organizations are those that respect the dignity of all who work for and are served by them.

Inclusion

Importance of Participation and Ownership

People tend to work harder toward making a plan that they helped develop succeed. A plan created by people who are directly affected by the outcome tends to produce better results. Inclusivity is more than sharing an action plan with a wide audience; it is asking first, "who has the most to gain or lose, and what can they contribute to solving this problem?"

Teamwork Principles and Practices

There is no "magic recipe" when it comes to organizing people into teams and producing the desired results. However, some defining characteristics of effective work teams that have withstood the test of time include (Levi, 2016; Mosser & Bugun, 2013):

- sharing a common goal and responsibility for achieving it,
- having the authority for taking action to achieve the goal,
- embracing accountability to the organization,
- developing strong relationships,
- positively leveraging interdependency among team members,
- incorporating effective group processes, and
- fostering team members' participation, satisfaction, learning, and growth.

High-performing work teams typically require both good leadership and followership—and for each member to recognize when it is best to engage in either. Followership involves understanding and performing roles needed for achieving the goal, such as a baseball team with players assigned to different positions (Chatwani, 2017).

Planning and Problem-Solving Together

Our contemporary culture seems to increasingly place value on speed and convenience, sometimes at the expense of thorough and thoughtful planning. Healthcare consultant Dennis McIntee holds that reducing the potential for distracting behaviors is often important so that people concentrate on the problem to be solved rather than one another (2018). There is an element of science—gathering and analyzing relevant data. There is also a companion element of art—focusing the group's attention on applying critical thinking skills to developing plausible solutions. The shared ownership of a group-authored recommendation enhances the probability of its success.

Advantages of Workforce Diversity

One way to show respect is to embrace the value of diversity as a strength-building characteristic of an organization. When considered in the context of "loyalty," diversity can perhaps more accurately be described as "inclusiveness" and "well-roundedness." Often limited to discussions about the blend of races, genders and identity, religions, and national origins, the notion of inclusiveness also has implications for shared governance, employee empowerment, balance of perspectives, and depth of engagement. It involves inviting everyone who has "skin in the game" to participate in productive ways to advance the mission of the organization—and *meaning* it.

POLICIES AND PROCEDURES

Developing policies, procedures, and leadership practices that address the topics covered in this chapter—and consistently applying them—earns trust, respect, and loyalty from staff, care recipients, and their advocates. The next wave of culture change in senior living involves relationship-centered care, fostering and nurturing the multifaceted web of relationships among the stakeholders of an elder care community. Adapting them to the various settings across the postacute care continuum of service lines may present challenges, but the foundation to success is honoring people's inherent value and dignity.

SUMMARY

The leader sets the tone for employee relationships in the organization. The human resources of a senior care and service organization is one of its biggest assets. The number of human interactions and relationships is a unique element of these types of organizations. A good leader has an understanding of their role and impact, and knows that their approach and actions contribute to the work culture. An appreciation of all of the different factors and practices will serve leaders well as they lead by example and model what they expect of their management team and others in the organization.

KEY POINTS

1. An health services executive (HSE™)-caliber leader builds a workplace culture that fosters professional and personal growth, engagement, fulfillment, and favorable outcomes for the organization and for those served by it by:

    a. demonstrating vision, empathy and compassion, discernment, integrity, transparency, and stamina;

    b. investing in developing people's skills and knowledge, professionally and personally; and

    c. nurturing multidirectional relationships that produce results.

2. HSE™-level leaders who succeed are

    a. qualified—with relevant preparation and credentials to lead the organization;

    b. rewarded and fulfilled—motivated and fed by this line of service;

    c. reliable and dependable—lead by example, are available and approachable, and are trustworthy and transparent.

3. Effective leadership entails planning, organizing, directing, monitoring, motivating, and communicating.

4. Establishing trust and building confidence demand a commitment to visibility and accessibility, and advocacy.

5. Loyalty is earned through consistently exercising sound executive judgment, treating people fairly and equally, preserving confidentiality, and demonstrating sincere and compassionate interest.

6. High-performing work teams rely on building strong relationships, clearly stating goals and expectations, embracing inclusion and diversity, and a blend of leadership and followership.

LEADERSHIP ROLES

Effectively establishing and building a workplace culture that fosters professional and personal growth, engagement, fulfillment, and favorable outcomes for the organization and for those served by it does not happen on its own; it very rarely develops swiftly; and it is hard work that demands continuous effort by the health services executive.

HIGH-IMPACT PRACTICES

1. **Reliability and Dependability:** It is not uncommon to hold a party honoring a team member who is either retiring or departing for some other reason. How about throwing an event periodically to celebrate the arrival of new employees—the people who will be there tomorrow? Residents, their families, and other staff members want to meet them. If it is a not-for-profit organization, invite board members; if not, invite the owners. Reinforce each new arrival's decision to accept the job offer, and let them go home feeling emotionally attached to their new environment.

2. **Sincerity, Interest, and Compassion:** Here are a few practical methods for achieving them:

   a. **Handwritten Notes:** In an era increasingly dominated by e-communication (emails, texting, and social media), the efficacy of sending someone a handwritten note remains unsurpassed. It takes negligibly more time and maybe some modest expense (if mailed). However, sending a note in your own handwriting—essentially confirming it is really from *you* and not someone you asked to do it for you—sends a strong message about your interest in the relationship with the person to whom you are writing. Aside from being viewed by older cohorts as a sign of respect and good manners (no matter how primitive your handwriting might have become), a handwritten note is uniquely owned by its recipient; not cut-and-paste-able or forward-able in an email. Try it when someone least expects it—catching them off-guard with an acknowledgment about something that there was no awareness about you noticing.

   b. **Names:** Very few things are more important to someone than their name. So make people's names a priority as a way to show your interest in who they are (not just what they do). There are many time-honored techniques for achieving this, but all involve practice and time. *Tip:* Always call a resident/patient/client/participant by their last name initially, waiting for their offer to use a more familiar term, such as a first name. *Bonus points:* Study and learn the names of significant others, such as spouse, children and grandchildren, or important nonrelatives (pastor, neighbor, etc.).

   c. **Calendar Celebrations:** Almost as unique as each person's name are certain dates of importance: birthday, date of hire, wedding anniversary, family member's graduation or wedding, and so forth. Select a category and research it for all members in a group (clients, staff, etc.) or mix them up and have at least one item for every person who receives services from or works for your organization, and enter a reminder in your e-calendar as a cue. (Enter as a recurring item any celebrations that are annual.) Each day, you will likely have at least one person you will want to seek out to surprise.

3. **Culture of QAPI:** Celebrate with great fanfare a project team that seemed to follow all the prescribed steps to find a new solution—but either came up short or the new solution did not produce better results. People are generally risk averse, and their work history may not have included a progressive environment that encouraged self-directed work teams or innovation. In order to achieve widespread confidence that *trying* is important and valued, people need to believe that risk-taking is part of creative problem-solving. Working in an atmosphere that encourages empowerment and expects engagement may be a whole new experience. They may want to believe it is true, but they might need some visible signs that it is "okay to come in the water!"

4. **Reward Valor With Value:** Providing some non-cash incentives or rewards to a work team is generally appreciated by its members—if they are things that are truly valued by the recipient. *Example*: A reserved parking place is not a meaningful sign of gratitude for someone who utilizes public transportation for getting to work; it may actually do more harm than good by exposing unfamiliarity with that team member's circumstances or needs. It is also important to nurture the binding spirit that makes a team feel part of something purposeful and worthwhile. Providing a work team with all necessary tools—such as a comfortable working space, equipment, supplies and supportive, friendly environment—tends to build a trusting relationship and improve brand awareness. There is no better representative of the organization than an engaged and loyal staff.

QUESTIONS FOR DISCUSSION

1. What are key motivators for people to excel in their job roles?
2. What makes treating people both fairly and equally important?
3. How do diversity and inclusion strengthen an organization's prospects for success?
4. Why is it beneficial for an HSE™ leader to pursue visibility and accessibility?
5. Discuss leadership and followership, and the relationship between them.
6. Describe some of the advantages of self-directed work teams? What obstacles might slow down their introduction in a health or human services organization?

CASE PROBLEMS

1. **On the Road Again:** A home health agency serving a three-county, rural area in the South, was experiencing financial pressures related to the rapidly rising price of gasoline. The reimbursement system was not set up to respond swiftly to such abrupt market changes. Although the agency would likely

receive payments sufficient to address the added operational costs, the lag time was expected to approach 18 months. In the meantime, its cash flow had turned negative. The agency formed three work teams that were similar in membership—clinical and nonclinical staff members, clients and family members, and a representative from the agency's primary lender—and initiated a competition for addressing the challenge. **Result:** A combination of cost savings, efficiency, and growth strategies emerged. Everyone working for the agency shared in the healthier bottom line that resulted, customer satisfaction rose, and the organization's bank renewed the line of credit with a higher limit and more favorable interest rate.

Questions:

a.   To what degree do you think the composition of the work teams contributed to the successful outcomes?

b.   What other stakeholder(s) would you add to this approach and why?

2.   **Mayflower Manor:** This assisted living community in a suburban, residential neighborhood, found itself competing for personnel with businesses outside its line of service. It formed the "R-Team" (R = recruitment), with a representative from each department. A series of short video testimonials was launched on social media, predominantly Twitter, Instagram, and Facebook sharing why they loved their work, that it was more of a *calling* than a job. They invited people who were looking for more than a paycheck from their employment to visit Mayflower Manor and "go for a test drive with the R-Team, and find out for yourself how you might qualify to enter the most fulfilling career imaginable and that you never thought of before!" **Result:** Within 3 weeks, applications exceeded vacancies, and Mayflower Manor wound up with a waiting list for new hires.

Questions:

a.   Can Mayflower Manor also expect employee turnover to decline? Why or why not?

b.   What approach would you likely take to enhance the probability that the newest staff additions stay?

3.   **Better Day Adult Day Center:** A collective outreach ministry of an urban, multidenominational faith community organization, this center experienced a transportation challenge due to an unexpectedly powerful snowstorm. The call went out through the participating churches to their respective members that help was needed to transport participants to their homes safely, but the response was not sufficient to complete the task by normal closing time. A few staff members stayed at the center with the remaining participants until very late in the evening, engaging in activities, preparing and serving dinner, and essentially extending the program schedule to fit the new reality. The director sent a handwritten note to the spouse and/or family of each staff member who stayed, thanking them for their sacrifice and for their support in such a challenging situation. Enclosed was a gift card for a home-delivered pizza. **Result:** One of the note recipients mentioned it at church; the pastor called a local TV station reporter who was a member of the congregation, and the story made the noon and evening news. Seven new participants were attributed to families having viewed the story. (Note: The cost of the pizzas

and stamps on the notes totaled just over $30.00; producing and purchasing an advertisement of the same length as the *free* news segment *would have cost $8,000!*)

Questions:

a. What about receiving a personal acknowledgment for doing something that seemed so obviously needed impressed the reverend enough to share the story with the congregant who worked at the television station?

b. In what other way(s) could the director have shown appreciation that would have been valued by those who stayed?

NAB DOMAINS OF PRACTICE

10 CUSTOMER CARE, SUPPORTS, AND SERVICES
10.19 Ensure the provision of a customer service culture that leads to a quality experience for care recipients.

20 HUMAN RESOURCES
20.07 Establish the planning, development, implementation, monitoring, and evaluation of employee satisfaction and organizational culture.
20.12 Promote a positive work environment (using techniques such as conflict resolution, diversity training, and staff recognition programs).
20.15 Establish a culture that encourages employees to embrace care recipients' rights.

40 ENVIRONMENT
40.10 Establish, maintain, and monitor an environment that promotes choice, comfort, and dignity for care recipients.

50 MANAGEMENT AND LEADERSHIP
50.04 Develop, communicate, and champion the service provider's mission, vision, and values to stakeholders.
50.06 Promote and monitor satisfaction of the care recipients and their support network.
50.07 Identify, foster, and maintain positive relationships with key stakeholders.
50.09 Solicit information from appropriate stakeholders for use in decision-making.
50.17 Lead organizational change initiatives.
50.18 Facilitate effective internal and external communication strategies.

A summary of the related knowledge, skills, and core expectations across service lines—and unique features of each service line is available at www.nabweb.org/filebin/pdf/Annotation_of_Tasks_Performed_Across_LOS_in_LTC.pdf

Source: Reproduced with permission from the National Association of Long-Term Care Administrator Boards. (2016). *Annotation of tasks performed and knowledge and skills used across lines of service in long term care.* Retrieved from https://www.nabweb.org/filebin/pdf/Annotation_of_Tasks_Performed_Across_LOS_in_LTC.pdf

REFERENCES

American Pyschological Association. (2014). *Employee recognition survey*. Retrieved from
    http://www.apaexcellence.org/assets/general/employee-recognition-survey-results.pdf
Argentum. (2019). *Certified Director of Assisted Living Program*. Retrieved from https://www
    .argentum.org/assisted-living-executive-director-certification-program/
Arveson, P. (1998). *The Deming cycle*. Retrieved from https://www.balancedscorecard.org/BSC
    -Basics/Articles-Videos/The-Deming-Cycle
Bell, V., & Troxell, D. (2016). *The best friends approach to dementia care* (2nd ed.). Baltimore, MD:
    Health Professions Press.
Blakeman, C. (2014, November 25). *Why self-managed teams are the future of business*. Retrieved
    from https://www.inc.com/chuck-blakeman/why-self-managed-teams-are-the-future-of
    -business.html
Chatwani, N. (2017). *Distributed leadership: The dynamics of balancing leadership with followership*.
    Cham, Switzerland: Springer International Publishing AG.
Collins, J. (2001). *Good to great: Why some companies make the leap and others don't*. New York, NY:
    HarperCollins Publishers.
Covey, S. (1989). *The 7 habits of highly effective people: Powerful lessons in personal change*. New York,
    NY: Simon & Schuster.
Drzymalski, J., Gladstone, E., Troyani, L., & Niu, D. (2014). *The seven key trends impacting today's
    workplace: Results from the 2014 TINYpulse employee engagement organizational culture report*.
    Retrieved from https://www.tinypulse.com/2014-employee-engagement-organizational
    -culture-report
Heathfield, S. (2019, January 4). *What people want from work: Motivation*. Balance Careers.
    Retrieved from https://www.thebalancecareers.com/what-people-want-from-work
    -motivation-1919051
Idaho Administrative Rules. (2019). *Rules of the Board of Examiners of Residential Care
    Administrators (IDAPA 24 Title 19 Chapter 01)*. Retrieved from https://adminrules.idaho
    .gov/rules/2000/24/1901.pdf
Jackson, C., & Slaton, R. (1993). *From green persimmons to cranky parrots: Practice management
    axioms to live by*. San Francisco, CA: W.H. Freeman & Co.
Juneja, P. (2019). *Directing function of management*. Management Study Guide. Retrieved from
    https://www.managementstudyguide.com/role_of_supervisor.htm
Levi, D. (2016). *Group dynamics for teams* (5th ed.). Thousand Oaks, CA: Sage.
Liepelt, K. (2015, November 12). *Top reasons for moving to a senior living community*. Senior
    Housing News. Retrieved from https://seniorhousingnews.com/2015/11/12/top
    -reasons-for-moving-to-a-senior-living-community/
McIntee, D. (2018). *Drama free teams in healthcare: Less stress, more trust, better outcomes for everyone*.
    Jersey City, NJ: Endevis.
Merriam-Webster Dictionary. (2019). *Organize*. Retrieved from https://www.merriam-webster
    .com/dictionary/organize
Mosser, G., & Bugun, J. (2013). *Understanding teamwork in health care*. New York, NY: McGraw-
    Hill Education.
National Institute on Aging. (2019). *Aging in place: Growing older at home*. Retrieved from
    https://www.nia.nih.gov/health/aging-place-growing-older-home
Nelson, R. (1999, February 1). *The ten ironies of motivation*. Workforce. Retrieved from
    https://www.workforce.com/news/the-ten-ironies-of-motivation
Pfau, B., & Kay, I. (2001). *The human capital edge: 21 people management practices your company must
    implement (or avoid) to maximize shareholder value*. Hightstown, NJ: McGraw-Hill.
QuoteInvestigator.com. (2013). *Showing up*. Retrieved from https://quoteinvestigator
    .com/2013/06/10/showing-up/
Smith, J. (2013, February 8). *The most ridiculous excuses from tardy employees*. Forbes. Retrieved
    from https://www.forbes.com/sites/jacquelynsmith/2013/02/08/the-most-ridiculous
    -excuses-from-tardy-employees/
Social Security Act 1903(a)(29), 42 USC 1396(a)(29) and 1396(g), CFR parts 431.700 -7.15. Federal
    Mandate for State Licensure Boards of Nursing Home Administrators.

U.S. Bureau of Labor Statistics. (2020). *Absences from work of employed full-time wage and salary workers by occupation and industry*. Retrieved from https://www.bls.gov/cps/cpsaat47.htm

Virginia Code § 54.1-2400 and Chapter 31 of Title 54.1 Regulations: 18VAC95-30-10 et seq. (2019).

ADDITIONAL RESOURCES

Employee Engagement

Grant, M., & Notter, J. (2019). *The non-obvious guide to employee engagement for millennials, boomers and everyone else*. Oakton, VA: IdeaPress.

Shepherd, M. (2002). *The art of the handwritten note: A guide to reclaiming civilized communication*. New York, NY: Broadway Books.

Teams and Leadership

Rath, T., & Conchie, B. (2009). *Strengths based leadership*. New York, NY: Gallup Press.

Shaw, R. (2017). *Extreme teams: Why Pixar, Netflix, AirBnB and other cutting edge companies succeed where most fail*. New York, NY: Amacom Books (Harper-Collins).

Stevens, R. (2019). *Emotional intelligence in business: EQ – The essential ingredient to survive and thrive as a modern workplace leader*. ISBN: 9781393746188.

CHAPTER 11

Customer Service: How Are We Different?

INTRODUCTION

Describing what is unique about customer service in the senior living setting requires examining how it contrasts with not only acute care but other health and human services along the postacute care continuum. There is not "one glove that fits all sizes" in senior living. Instead, we find some notable variations on the core functions of effective customer service, shaped by the different needs, wants, demands, and expectations of those who might benefit from the organization's services.

For our purpose here, "customer service" differs from public relations or marketing. A high-performing provider organization establishes policies and procedures that enable it to receive real-time feedback from those whom it serves on every aspect of the operation that touched them—positively or negatively—as an essential element of its quality assurance and performance improvement (QAPI) program. Consistently applying that feedback in ways that nimbly and effectively strengthen customer satisfaction is a hallmark of an organization led by a skilled health services executive.

THE SERVICE SETTING MATTERS

Someone seeking acute care typically experiences an injury event, such as a laceration, fracture, stroke, or heart attack, or requires a highly skilled medical intervention or diagnostic procedure, such as surgery or an MRI. Unless the person lives in an area that has more than one hospital, there is only rarely much customer choice involved in the decision about where to seek care. Proximity often serves as a key determinant of the response speed and convenience and typically influences the customer's confidence in and familiarity with the provider organization. The person's physician—the primary care doctor, specialist, or both—also commonly plays a key role in advising them about where to have acute care services performed.

Because the average length of stay in a hospital currently falls short of 1 week, a customer's exposure to the organization is generally limited to the most visible services, such as medical and nursing care, therapies, dining services, chaplaincy, or social services (Organisation for Economic Coordination and Development

[OECD], 2019; Statista, 2019). Without staying longer, it may be difficult to observe and assess support services, such as pharmacy, clinical laboratory, housekeeping, laundry, or maintenance, and even tougher to evaluate "backstage" elements, such as safety and security, medical records and information technology, human resources, purchasing and central supply, administration, and the billing office. All of these also contribute to the customer's experience, of course.

With the exception of short-term, postacute care for rehabilitation, chronic conditions—sometimes multiple, concurrent comorbidities—tend to drive utilization of senior living lines of service.

Some also refer to this as "transitional care," and choosing a provider and venue more closely resembles the process for selecting an acute care provider because it is also "need driven." This places a premium on meeting the need for continuing restorative therapies as a follow-up to the hospitalization. The primary goal is to regain functional independence—regardless of place.

However, when *chronic* conditions—physical, mental, or both—advance to a point that limits or reduces a person's ability to routinely perform their own activities of daily living (ADLs), then the focus turns to acquiring appropriate supports and services that enhance safety, security, and comfort. Examples of chronic conditions that can motivate someone to consider such a lifestyle adjustment range from arthritis and emphysema to dementia. For many people, the set of possible combinations of contributing factors looks more like a Rubik's Cube—three dimensional—than a jigsaw puzzle.

> *The "stay in my home" phenomenon shows little inclination to diminish over the next 50 years. Aggressively explore how your organization's mission, services, values and brand can be extended to them in their context. This begins with listening and adapting technology—it doesn't start with your organization's brick and mortar assets.*
>
> *Rick M. Stiffney, PhD*
> *Owner, Integrated Leadership and Consultancy, LLC*

Who Is the "Customer"?

A complicating factor is that the "end user" of senior living service lines commonly relies on other people for assistance or advice in exploring options, selecting a provider, and evaluating service quality. This might be a family member, medical or social services professional, clergy, friend or neighbor, or a mix of two or more of them. A variety of labels have emerged to describe our core customer, the care recipient, but the dividing lines are sometimes a little blurry. Table 11.1 shows some of the most commonly used terms and the senior living service line with which each is most likely associated.

SERVICE GOAL: CARE VERSUS CURE

The overriding emphasis of senior living is postacute *care*, as compared with a health system's primary objective of *curing* a disease or repairing an injury. This

TABLE 11.1 Customer Titles by Senior Living Service Line

Service Recipient	Description	Acute Hospital	TCU or IRF	SNF	RC/AL	Congregate or Independent Living	Home Health	Hospice	Adult Day
Patient	From the traditional medical model; implied expectation of healing or recovery from injury, illness, or procedure	☑	☑	✓			✓	✓	
Resident	Social/hospitality model term equating service venue to person's place of residence			☑	☑	☑			
Tenant	Holds a renter's (nonowner) interest				✓	☑			
Client	Benefits by utilizing HCBS						☑	☑	✓
Participant	Engaged in offered programs								☑
Customer	From retail and commerce; purchaser or end user				✓				
Representative									
Guardian	Court-appointed custodian	☑	☑	☑			✓	✓	✓
Power of Attorney	Legally recognized agent	☑	☑	☑	☑	✓	☑	☑	☑
Healthcare surrogate	Person-appointed substitute for healthcare decisions	☑	☑	☑	✓	✓	✓	✓	✓
Responsible party	Emergency contact and/or financial guarantor	☑	☑	☑	✓	✓	☑	☑	☑

Key

☑	Primary use
✓	Secondary use (or special subset of the service line; less frequent)

HCBS, home- and community-based service; IRF, inpatient rehabilitation facility; RC/AL, residential care/assisted living; SNF, skilled nursing facility; TCU, transitional care unit.

is a key distinction to recognize in framing an organization's customer service model. Of course, they are not mutually exclusive. There are many instances when postacute care involves rehabilitation or curative treatment of wounds or illnesses. However, customer service metrics in senior living tend to focus more on a person's senses of comfort, dignity, life satisfaction, value, and self-worth.

Over the past half-century, the relationship between a senior living service provider and service recipient has evolved from one based on a medical model to more of a social or hospitality paradigm. Characteristics of a medical model typically include a power differential between the provider—healthcare professional or health system—and the patient. There is a cultural expectation on both sides of the equation that the professional has rank or advantage—is in charge—due to having greater knowledge, skills, and resources for effectively addressing the patient's medical needs. Because of the immediacy of that need, people have historically been willing to accept a modest loss of self-determination in order to benefit from the guidance and services of the provider.

In the arena of hospitality (chiefly hotels and restaurants), customer preferences and satisfaction more commonly drive the list of services offered, the fashion in which those services are delivered, and even the prices charged. Sure, people may have a desire for lodging when traveling or to eat a meal away from home, but the decision about which "provider" to select is decidedly different than the one related to seeking help in the wake of a critical, acute medical episode. There are more choices of establishments competing for one's business. They seem most interested in delivering a customer's anticipated experience.

Not surprisingly, consumers and their advocates have applauded senior living's gradual departure from the medical model that shaped nursing home care for so long (National Consumer Voice for Quality Long Term Care, 2017. The past two decades have seen a steady erosion of the traditional power differential between service provider and recipient. The emergence of "person-centered care" is a prime example of the continuing shift in senior living toward a hospitality model construct. For this reason, the innovative service approaches incorporating this philosophy are often collectively referred to as part of a "culture change" movement, changing the organizational norms to reflect a more customer-centric attitude and operating perspective.

Much of the discussion nationally about culture change in senior living relates to replacing the traditional medical model in nursing homes. However, the long-term care continuum has now broadened to include home- and community-based service (HCBS) lines. It is noteworthy that one of its key components, hospice and palliative care services, actually introduced many of the very same concepts from the start. According to the National Hospice and Palliative Care Organization (NHPCO), hospice care strives to nurture a person's emotional, mental, and spiritual needs on terms expressed as important *by the person*, not necessarily as dictated by the provider (2019). It serves a wonderful example of placing a premium on the service recipient's perspective.

The migration of senior living providers in this direction is more than an altruistic epiphany—it has been shown to be good for business. Multiple senior living innovation leaders report that there is a strong business case that favors moving in this direction. Yet, according to a Commonwealth Fund study, just over one half of skilled nursing care providers either have adopted or are in the process of adopting such approaches to their operations (Doty, Koren, & Sturla, 2008).

CONSUMER EXPECTATIONS

Today's senior living service recipients are mostly either from the birth cohort that former NBC news anchor, Tom Brokaw, dubbed the Greatest Generation in his 1998 book by the same title (born between 1901 and 1927) or from the Silent Generation (born between 1928 and 1945). One key characteristic that is common to both is respect for authority, which may be why a medical model of service delivery has survived for as long as it has in postacute care. However, that attitude is radically different among Baby Boomers (born between 1946 and 1964). Many anticipate that Boomers will have much higher consumer expectations than their predecessors, having first observed service levels and approaches accepted by their parents and feeling underwhelmed. With 10,000 Boomers turning 65 years old every day for the next several years, this is a demographic phenomenon that will surely make a mark on how senior living customer service is defined, delivered, and evaluated.

Furthermore, we live in an era of increasing access to relevant information concerning postacute services. People not only have more available choices, but they know more about them than ever before due to the advent of the Internet and the explosion of its use. The number of people who have experienced some aspects of postacute care and support services for a family member, friend, or neighbor also continues to grow. Add to these factors the current trend of an overall cultural shift toward seeking instant gratification from shopping online and having products shipped to one's door to hailing a driver who appears on demand to transport one to a desired destination (Muther, 2013). The sum is higher consumer expectations for commerce, in general, which has significant implications for the senior living field.

Are those expectations really unreasonable or difficult to achieve? Let us examine some of the most frequently expressed ones: safety and security, quality treatment, and comfort. The challenge for senior living providers has become finding effective ways to learn from service recipients (and their advocates) how addressing each of these can best satisfy them as consumers.

Expectation 1: Safety and Security

Safety and security is at or near the top of any list of concerns prompting the desire to seek senior living services of any kind. It simply reflects the power of Abraham Maslow's classic social theory describing people's "hierarchy of needs," providing first for one's most basic needs for survival. This can mean providing a range—or combination—of protections, from installing monitoring devices and alert systems in one's private residence to locating in a neighborhood with a low-crime rate, accessible healthcare and supportive service options, and transportation. It can also mean living in a setting free of any fear of reprisal from caregivers. Safety and security most certainly includes living among those who treat all with dignity and respect.

Expectation 2: Quality Treatment

Quality treatment has at least three components in the eyes of those served: staffing, relationships, and communication. Consumers typically want to receive care from personnel who are:

- **Competent:** Well prepared, with appropriate knowledge and proficient skills, and effective in performing their roles

- **Respectful:** Courteous, polite, and considerate
- **Friendly:** Welcoming and approachable, warm, and pleasant
- **Available:** Accessible and responsive

Nurturing the relationships among all the related stakeholders is essential to ensuring quality treatment in senior living. A service recipient's relationships with their family, friends or neighbors, other service recipients and their families, the service provider's staff members, and volunteers all contribute to supporting their sense of value and self-worth, comfort, and life satisfaction. Many of the same stakeholders have interwoven relationships with one another, too. Together that matrix of relationships forms a microcommunity that nourishes its members on many levels, whether physically under one roof or not.

Good communication is another important tool for meeting or exceeding a level of quality treatment that consumers seem to value. They tend to expect from us communication that is:

- **Timely:** Proactively initiated by the provider, either in anticipation of a possible problem or issue or as shortly after as possible
- **Transparent:** Complete and accurate information
- **Understandable:** Expressed in terms that are meaningful and informative, not filled with technical verbiage that requires further explanation

Finally, quality treatment includes preserving privacy and confidentiality. The physical layout of the caregiving environment must provide appropriate privacy for the customer, and staff training should emphasize the importance of consistently following procedures that protect individual privacy. The goal is to develop and maintain an organizational culture that enables every customer to reasonably expect that information about their condition, treatment, or prospects are not shared (without express permission) with anyone who is not directly involved with their care, how it is paid for, or who works for a government agency with regulatory oversight authority.

Expectation 3: Comfort

What constitutes "comfort" relies heavily on personal preferences, taste, and/or experience. Basic human comforts typically include shelter (protection from the elements in a clean, temperate, and safe environment), nutrition and water (enough of both to sustain life), and community (social engagement opportunities that minimize the risk of isolation, loneliness, or boredom). Building on this foundation, customer service can be enhanced in a variety of ways to increase the probability of customer satisfaction.

Dining offers perhaps the most fruitful opportunities for enhancing customer service in senior living—people eat every day, they have well-developed preferences, and they come better equipped to evaluate whether they like the meals served than to assess just about any other aspect of an operation. The evaluative criteria that customers generally apply include the following:

- **Taste:** According to the Mayo Clinic, one's senses of taste and smell tend to erode with normal aging, so two of the biggest challenges are satisfying a customer's expectations for sweetness and for saltiness. Having developed dining habits and preferences over a lifetime makes changing expectations even tougher to accomplish. This challenge amplifies when their physician prescribes a special diet that restricts sugar or salt intake for health reasons (Takahashi, 2019).

- **Temperature:** Hot food arrives hot (but not hot enough to risk injury), and cold food arrives cold (especially ice cream).

- **Presentation:** Appealing appearance and arrangement of the food.

- **Texture:** Cooked so that chewing and swallowing are easily accomplished; avoid overcooking meat (making it dry or tough) or serving bread products with thick or hard crusts. Normal consistency; avoid overcooking vegetables (possibly losing body, taste, and nutritional value). A resident with swallowing disorders presents significant challenges here because of their physiologic limitations and corresponding special diet orders (mechanical soft or pureed diet, thickened liquids, etc.).

- **Nutrition:** The U.S. Department of Agriculture (USDA) has developed recommended daily allowances (RDAs) for seniors, a set of guidelines for older consumers about how much of a wide variety of nutrients—vitamins, minerals, fiber, protein, fats, and carbohydrates—to ingest daily for maintaining good health. They are slightly different than RDAs for adults (Frazier, 2019; USDA, 2019).

- **Portion:** Balancing RDAs with a patient's diminished capacity or hunger urge can also present challenges. Furthermore, an elder who grew up during or soon after the Great Depression likely harbors strong feelings about avoiding unnecessary waste. In more highly regulated venues (inpatient rehabilitation facility and skilled nursing facility [SNF]), the tension between compliance with federal standards and satisfying resident preferences generally favors the former.

Consumer Perspective: Performance Rating

Surveying customers—care recipients and their advocates—has many benefits for ascertaining how well an organization is meeting or exceeding its constituency's service expectations. Whether the instrument is developed in-house or administered by an external firm, simply asking people about their customer experience can effectively guide an organization's planning and direction going forward. The key dimensions of such an effort are as follows:

- **Anonymity:** People generally want to have their opinions heard and considered, but many might hesitate to "rock the boat" and risk any form of reprisal as an unintended consequence. Participation rates improve dramatically when a satisfaction survey's input protects one's identity, and a higher participation rate improves the validity and value of the results (Berkowitz, 2016).

- **Frequency:** Depending on the length of stay, senior living providers who request feedback from customers do so during the service period, upon discharge, or both. Although popular, annually performing this process can make it difficult to meaningfully compare sequential results because of turnover among the clients. With a pledge of anonymity, it is hard to know whether impressions changed among the same people. Leading firms in the field of designing and analyzing resident and family satisfaction questionnaires commonly advocate for conducting such inquiries no less frequently than semiannually (NRC, 2019).

- **Length/Depth:** If the instrument is too long, fewer people may complete it. This consideration tends to be more art than science. Priorities set based on survey results from an instrument that was only partially completed by those who participated may be misguided.

■ **Ease of Participation:** Paper questionnaires that must be completed by hand and turned in or mailed are steadily getting replaced by electronic portals— websites or mobile device applications. Regardless of pathway, offering confidential assistance to any resident who has an impairment or other barrier that limits their ability to participate can successfully bolster the participation rate.

■ **Understandable:** Language matters…not only whether it is English, Spanish, or some other language of greatest proficiency, but word choices and complexity. A question that is focused on one issue or concern, easily understood and unlikely to be misinterpreted, is best. Reframe any question that prompts a resident to ask, "What does that mean?"

■ **Reporting:** Sharing the information once it has been gathered is essential for building confidence in the process itself. Failing to do so can hurt participation in future surveys because people might perceive it as a waste of their time and effort rather than a true opportunity to contribute to performance improvement. Communicate with participants, staff, and other appropriate stakeholders:

  ■ **Results:** What was learned?

  ■ **Action Steps:** What will be done about what was learned?

  ■ **Progress:** Periodic updates on the effectiveness of those action steps.

■ **The Ultimate Question:** Coined by MyInnerview, Inc. before it became part of National Research Corporation (NRC), the singly most useful gauge on the provider's customer dashboard is known as the **ultimate question**, "How likely are you to recommend this provider to someone you know who is searching for the same services?" This surpasses in importance any of the other, more specific operational questions posed; it serves as a simple barometer and composite metric that indicates overall customer satisfaction.

Seeking to understand the customer experience—through their eyes and other senses—parallels taking vital signs for clinical assessment, monitoring, and care planning. It is fundamental. Further developing what we are already doing well and enhancing what we are told would be most valued by improving are both consistent with our mission and help the enterprise thrive.

*James L. Farley, MHA, FACHCA
Cofounder and CEO, Nursing Care Management
of America, and Past President, American
College of Health Care Administrators*

Perpetual Training

Expecting staff members to rely exclusively on their own life experiences to shape how they go about delivering great customer service simply leaves too much to chance. Most of us have both fond and not-so-favorable memories of encounters with retail sales personnel, healthcare professionals, or restaurant wait staff. In most commercial exchanges, a staff member's friendly disposition, attentive engagement, profession-al appearance, and good personal hygiene all contribute to our forming a positive impression as customers. However, the unique features of senior living make it imperative to go further by formulating the organization's customer service goals, strategies, and approaches—then communicate with each individual how they fit in the picture. Creating and fostering a **culture** of person-centered, expectation-exceeding customer service requires ongoing training with consistent messaging, clear directions about techniques to employ, and practice, practice, practice.

POLICIES AND PROCEDURES

Although developing and consistently applying human resources policies and procedures is vital to a senior living organization's success, what distinguishes the contemporary health services executive among peers is the extent to which they constantly exercise imagination to identify opportunities to enhance the organization's customer service. Demonstrating core values—not just memorizing them and reciting them—in fresh ways helps embed them in the mind-set of everyone on the team.

SUMMARY

Leaders are drawn to this profession for a variety of reasons, but certainly one of the most critical is that they want to make a difference in the lives of seniors. This value is important to model at all levels of the organization. A leader has to also be aware of the customer's perspective and encourage consideration of that perception on a regular basis. A positive living experience for residents, tenants, and clients, in spite of sometimes difficult circumstances, is paramount to the success of an organization. Being part of this with customers is also one of the ways that many highly respected leaders draw energy and hope to what they do.

KEY POINTS

1. "Customer service" differs from public relations or marketing; it entails meeting or **exceeding** each customer's self-defined expectations.

2. "Customer" in senior living has various labels that are somewhat dependent on the service line: patient, resident, tenant, client, participant, and customer are some of the most common.

3. The customer's representative can also be associated in several ways, including guardian, power of attorney, healthcare surrogate, and responsible party.

4. People with an urgent medical need seek acute care services to treat an injury and diagnose an illness or both, with a goal of "**cure**." In contrast, chronic conditions—sometimes multiple comorbidities—push people in the direction of seeking postacute services, whether for short-term rehabilitation or long-term services and supports, where the greater emphasis may be on "**care**" of and for the person.

5. Senior living is moving from a medical, institution-centric model of service toward a more person-centered, social model of service, with increasing emphasis on recipient-defined expectations.

6. Consumer awareness and access to relevant information about available options for postacute services continue to improve.

7. Senior living consumers and their advocates expect providers to ensure safety and security, quality treatment, and comfort.

8. Through their own life experiences, consumers are best equipped to evaluate and express their satisfaction with dining services; this area offers some of the best opportunities for meeting and exceeding their expectations.

9. The best way to know what customers want is to ask them and to keep asking them how satisfied they are and what they would like to see improve.

10. Continual customer service training is valuable for *everyone* in a senior living organization.

LEADERSHIP ROLES

The health services executive leads by example in many areas of the operation, but few others offer as many opportunities for visibly setting a positive example as customer service. When employees (and customers) observe the organization's leader going to great lengths to demonstrate their commitment to its stated mission and values, confidence builds and engagement rises. The leader also strives to recognize and celebrate instances—big or small—when staff members throughout the organization deliver on the promise to meet or exceed customer expectations.

HIGH-IMPACT PRACTICES

1. **Invest in Simple Pleasures That Go Beyond the Minimum**

   a. **Towels, Wash Cloths, and Linens:** Fluffy, soft, and absorbent towels and wash cloths provide more than high functionality—they convey luxury and hospitality. High-quality sheets evoke a similar response, including an option for seasonal preferences, such as flannel sheets during winter. While considerably more to purchase than those in standard use, this approach can elevate a customer's impression of how special the organization truly considers their comfort and satisfaction.

   b. **Range of Mattresses and Pillows:** Tailoring the firmness of both mattresses and pillows to accommodate individual preferences not only enhances comfort but demonstrates to the customer the organization's commitment to person-centered care.

   c. **Easy Outdoor Access:** Vitamin D deficiency is a common and sometimes serious risk for older adults, regardless of living arrangement (McCarroll, O'Halloran, Healy, Kenny, & Laird, 2019). Vitamin D is not only critical to bone and muscle health but helps regulate cell growth, fight infection, and carry messages through the nervous system. Regular sun exposure provides enough vitamin D for most people, and having opportunities to spend time outdoors is superior to relying heavily on vitamin D supplements. Whether a balcony, walking path, or garden at a congregate living community or house's patio, porch, driveway, or neighborhood sidewalk—making the outdoors readily accessible both is customer centric and supports wellness (Wegerer, 2015).

2. **Title Matters:** Healthcare and human services have deep roots coming from the medical model, which carries a tradition of hierarchy matched only by banking, higher education, and government. In a progressive, truly person-centered environment, the title of each person should tell the customer that person's purpose instead of focusing on just responsibilities. It is equally important to avoid going so far down this path as to get too cute that the positive impact erodes. Here are some favorite examples—high-impact practices—to inspire such thinking.

Traditional Title	High-Impact Practice	Rationale
Activities director	Life enrichment coordinator	Do we want residents who stay *busy* (with activities) or who *live enriched lives*?
Receptionist	Director of first impressions	Typically the face of the organization, figuratively (phone) and literally (greeting visitors).
Housekeeper	Sparkle supervisor	Built-in high expectation of *more* than just *clean*!

3. **Resident Dining Committee:** Formalizing the process for acquiring useful input from residents by forming a committee or council of interested consumers of the food served can pay big dividends. In addition to providing useful retrospective reviews, such a group can also suggest additions to the menu and even serve as a focus group for trying out new items or recipes. This also has the advantage of providing an element of continuity by developing some institutional memory within the group, thereby avoiding unnecessarily repeating discussions about the same topics.

4. **Random Checkup Calls:** The first reaction of a resident/client's advocate—family member or other—when an unexpected call comes from the administrator of the senior living provider where their loved one resides is likely to be something like, "Oh my, what's wrong?" Imagine the sense of relief and affirmation about the decision to select that provider when the administrator replies, "I'm just calling to see how you feel we're doing…what's going well and what, if anything, is not?" In addition to gaining potentially useful information for the organization's customer service QAPI process, the call can trigger a wave of favorable public relations and marketing "testimonial" comments by the call recipient—free!

QUESTIONS FOR DISCUSSION

1. What are the chief characteristics of senior living that make designing and effectively executing strong customer service unique?

2. Who are the most effective ambassadors for a senior living organization and why?

3. Describe the top four skills on which you would likely focus in designing a customer service training program for a provider of

   a. home healthcare services;

    b.   residential memory care (SNF or residential care/assisted living [RC/AL]); and

    c.   short-term, postacute rehab (SNF).

4.   Is a person-centered care approach in senior living:

    a.   a minimum standard or extraordinary customer service? Why?

    b.   achievable in each postacute care service line? Why or why not?

    c.   more or less expensive than provider-centric models? Explain.

CASE PROBLEMS

1.   **Home Health:** *My Old Kentucky Home Angels* (MOKHA) had provided in-home health and wellness services throughout Central Kentucky for nearly three decades when it decided to expand the scope of its service menu to include nonmedical, in-home personal care. The customer referral network it had built for its core business included primarily hospital discharge planners, nursing home social workers, and several specialty physician practices (neurology, orthopedics, cardiology, pulmonology, and urology). The leadership team held as one of the MOKHA's most coveted hallmarks of success the high levels of customer satisfaction it consistently received from those it had served directly, as well as from their families. Because the service line that was about to launch would not qualify for Medicare or Medicaid payment, there was concern about how applicable testimonials or endorsements from its traditional referral sources or clients might be to an all private-pay constituency. It convened focus groups comprised of the area's private practice geriatric case managers, parish/faith nurses, and staff from the Area Agency on Aging. The lead recommendation came in the form of an affirmation: Competent, professional, consistent and reliable, person-centered service will find support among families of those who need the service. In other words, apply the same operating philosophy and customer service that grew the existing business to the new one, even with a narrower pay source, without fear that there is insufficient demand or interest.

   Questions:

    a.   What other stakeholder groups might be important to include in the organization's analysis of this business opportunity?

    b.   How would you approach assessing the community's workforce capacity for launching such a service?

2.   **Residential Care/Assisted Living Administrators:** Downtown Towers, an urban, 10-floor apartment building for middle-income seniors, was opened in the mid-1970s. About two thirds of its apartments were a "studio" design—one bed/living room with a galley kitchenette, full bath, and large closet. As customer expectations shifted over the subsequent four decades, the relatively low cost of living in the small apartments steadily lost ground to consumers' desire for more space and the community's census declined. Reducing the building's capacity by combining studio apartments was

certainly an option, but perhaps cost-prohibitive given the limited revenue potential. Working with current residents and their families, as well as some families of deceased residents, leadership ascertained what services and/or amenities might most likely succeed in attracting potential residents to the location. The leading candidates were congregate dining and service co-ordination. Supported by a federal Community Development Block Grant, with assistance from elected officials, Downtown Towers repurposed space in its lower level to install a commercial kitchen and dining room. It initially served lunch daily and eventually added supper 6 days a week. It also collaborated with a local university's academic program in social work to design and implement a service coordinator position, staffed by faculty-supervised students who took up residence in the building as partial compensation. The net outcome of the two most emphasized service gaps was that Downtown Towers—for roughly one fourth the cost of reducing its capacity through apartment consolidation—returned to full census and with a waiting list, by listening to its customers.

Questions:

a. Once the dining service opened, what next steps would you likely take to establish methods for resident feedback and input about the program?

b. What operational benefits would you anticipate realizing from the in-residence presence of the faculty-supervised social work students serving as service coordinators?

3. **Skilled Nursing Facility:** Oak Knoll Health and Rehabilitation Center, a 120-bed, dually certified SNF had three wings, each with distinct lines of service:

- short-term, postacute rehabilitation, specializing in treating persons who had suffered a stroke or fracture;

- memory care for medically complex and cognitively impaired people; and

- long-term care for those with multiple, disabling chronic conditions severe enough to qualify them for skilled nursing care.

With such a diverse customer profile, seeking input from the residents and/or their advocates presented a significant challenge. The first group had an average length of stay of less than 2 weeks, so their exposure to the service capabilities of Oak Knoll's staff was somewhat limited and their motive for coming was highly focused on improving enough to leave as soon as feasible. The second group did not have the mental capacity—judgment, memory, or both—to provide meaningful evaluation of the services they received, and most of their advocates only witnessed those services in person, intermittently. The third group was in the best position to participate and had acquired the most information through observing daily life there but commonly expressed anxiety about wanting to avoid the label "troublemaker" or about "rocking the boat."

Based on a recommendation submitted anonymously via the "suggestion box" located near the staff break room, leadership decided to try developing a customer service training experience that relied on taking the entire staff (not all at once, of course) to their choice of a well-known, local amusement park or restaurant. Each participating employee was asked to answer three questions as a *customer*:

- What was the most positive part of your experience?
- What was the most negative part of your experience?
- What *one* thing can Oak Knoll learn about customer service from your experience?

The program not only had over 90% participation but cost less than the organization's previous two resident/family satisfaction surveys and two employee engagement surveys combined. We are often our own toughest critic—the resulting list of recommendations became the foundation for Oak Knoll's training program concerning customer service. Sometimes, nontraditional stakeholders can provide very helpful input—if we ask.

Questions:

a. Should management inform the venues to be visited about the underlying purpose of the group outings? Why or why not?

b. What would be your approach to communicating the results of the project?

4. **All Senior Living Service Lines:** A large Midwestern continuing care retirement community (CCRC) received numerous comments from family members of recently deceased residents that it felt awkward to them to continue visiting the residents, staff, volunteers, and other residents' families with whom relationships had formed. Working with a small number of them, the CCRC formed an "Alumni Association" patterned after the model frequently used in the field of education for keeping graduates engaged. Word spread rapidly, and interest in participation took off. Within 2 years of its inception, the new ancillary organization was responsible for adding to the organization's volunteer roster, launching a peer-to-peer orientation program for the families of newly arriving residents, and enhancing the success of the annual giving campaign. All they were previously lacking was a "plug-in" portal.

Questions:

a. Describe at least three motivations for a family member of a deceased resident to participate in such a program?

b. What other operational benefits might likely develop as a result of the program?

NAB DOMAINS OF PRACTICE

10 CUSTOMER CARE, SUPPORTS, AND SERVICES

10.02 Ensure plans of care are evidence based, established, implemented, updated, and monitored based on care recipient preferences and assessed needs.

10.03 Ensure the planning, development, implementation/execution, monitoring, and evaluation of admission/move-in process, including pre-admission/pre-move-in information, to promote a quality experience for care recipient.

10.04 Ensure the planning, development, implementation/execution, monitoring, and evaluation of discharge/move-out process to promote a quality experience for care recipient.

10.05 Ensure the planning, development, implementation/execution, monitoring, and evaluation of programs to meet care recipients' psychosocial needs and preferences.

10.06 Ensure the planning, development, implementation/execution, monitoring, and evaluation of care recipients' activities/recreation to meet social needs and preferences.

10.09 Ensure the planning, development, implementation/execution, monitoring, and evaluation of a rehabilitation program to maximize optimal level of functioning and independence for care recipients.

10.11 Ensure the planning, development, implementation/execution, monitoring, and evaluation of policies and procedures for responses to care recipient-specific incidents, accidents, and/or emergencies.

10.12 Ensure the planning, development, implementation/execution, monitoring, and evaluation of housekeeping and laundry services for care recipients.

10.15 Ensure the planning, development, implementation/execution, monitoring, and evaluation of dining experience that meets the needs and preferences of care recipients.

10.16 Ensure care recipients' rights and individuality within all aspects of care.

10.17 Integrate support service network's perspectives to maximize care recipients' quality of life and care.

10.18 Ensure transportation options are available for care recipients.

10.19 Ensure the provision of a customer service culture that leads to a quality experience for care recipients.

20 HUMAN RESOURCES

20.03 Establish the planning, development, implementation, monitoring, and evaluation of employee training and development programs.

20.07 Establish the planning, development, implementation, monitoring, and evaluation of employee satisfaction and organizational culture.

20.15 Establish a culture that encourages employees to embrace care recipients' rights.

40 ENVIRONMENT

40.02 Ensure the planning, development, implementation, monitoring, and evaluation of a safe and secure environment.

40.08 Establish, maintain, and monitor a physical environment that provides clean, safe, and secure home-like surroundings for care recipients, staff, and visitors.

40.09 Identify opportunities to enhance the physical environment to meet changing market demands.

40.10 Establish, maintain, and monitor an environment that promotes choice, comfort, and dignity for care recipients.

40.11 Assess care recipients' environment for safety, security, and accessibility and make recommendations for referral or modification.

50 MANAGEMENT AND LEADERSHIP

50.02 Promote ethical practice throughout the organization.

50.06 Promote and monitor satisfaction of the care recipients and their support network.

50.07 Identify, foster, and maintain positive relationships with key stakeholders.

50.09 Solicit information from appropriate stakeholder for use in decision-making.

50.15 Ensure that written agreements between the care recipient and the service provider protect the rights and responsibilities of both parties.

A summary of the related knowledge, skills, and core expectations across service lines—and unique features of each service line is available at www .nabweb.org/filebin/pdf/Annotation_of_Tasks_Performed_Across_LOS _in_LTC.pdf

Source: Reproduced with permission from the National Association of Long-Term Care Administrator Boards. (2016). *Annotation of tasks performed and knowledge and skills used across lines of service in long term care.* Retrieved from https://www.nabweb.org/filebin/pdf/ Annotation_of_Tasks_Performed_Across_LOS_in_LTC.pdf

REFERENCES

Berkowitz, B. (2016, January 31). The patient experience and patient satisfaction: Measurement of a complex dynamic. *Online Journal of Issues in Nursing, 21,* Manuscript 1. Retrieved from http://ojin.nursingworld.org/MainMenuCategories/ANAMarketplace/ ANAPeriodicals/OJIN/TableofContents/Vol-21-2016/No1-Jan-2016/The-Patient -Experience-and-Patient-Satisfaction.html

Brokaw, T. (1998). *The greatest generation.* New York, NY: Random House.

Doty, M., Koren, M., & Sturla, E. (2008, May 1). *Culture change in nursing homes: How far have we come? Findings from the Commonwealth Fund 2007 National Survey of Nursing Homes.* Retrieved from https://www.commonwealthfund.org/publications/fund-reports/2008/ may/culture-change-nursing-homes-how-far-have-we-come-findings

Frazier, K. (2019). *USDA recommended daily allowance nutrition guidelines.* Livestrong.com. Retrieved from https://www.livestrong.com/article/276675-usda-rda-nutrition-list-guidelines/

McCarroll, K., O'Halloran, A., Healy, M., Kenny, R., & Laird, E. (2019). Vitamin D deficiency is associated with an increased likelihood of incident depression in community-dwelling older adults. *Journal of Post-Acute and Long-Term Care Medicine, 20*(5), 517–523. doi:10.1016 /j.jamda.2018.10.006

Muther, C. (2013, February 1). *The growing culture of impatience makes us crave more and more instant gratification.* Boston Globe. Retrieved from https://www.boston.com/ uncategorized/noprimarytagmatch/2013/02/01/the-growing-culture-of-impatience -makes-us-crave-more-and-more-instant-gratification

National Consumer Voice for Quality Long-Term Care. (2017). *Fact sheet: Culture change in nursing homes.* Retrieved from https://theconsumervoice.org/uploads/files/issues/ culture-change-in-nursing-homes-fact-sheet-final_(1).pdf

National Hospice and Palliative Care Organization. (2019). *History of hospice.* Retrieved from
https://www.nhpco.org/hospice-care-overview/history-of-hospice/

National Research Corporation. (2019). Retrieved from https://nrchealth.com/ (NRC Acquired
My Innerview in 2009).

Organisation for Economic Coordination and Development. (2019). *Length of hospital stays.*
Retrieved from https://www.oecd-ilibrary.org/social-issues-migration-health/length-of
-hospital-stay/indicator/english_8dda6b7a-en

Statista. (2019). *Average length of stay in U.S. community hospitals since 1993.* Retrieved from
https://www.statista.com/statistics/183916/average-length-of-stay-in-us-community
-hospitals-since-1993/

Takahashi, P. (2019, August 7). *Is loss of taste and smell normal with aging?* Mayo Foundation for
Medical Education and Research. Retrieved from https://www.mayoclinic.org/healthy
-lifestyle/healthy-aging/expert-answers/loss-of-taste-and-smell/faq-20058455

US Department of Agriculture. (2019). *Nutrition for older individuals.* Retrieved from https://
www.nal.usda.gov/fnic/older-individuals

Wegerer, J. (2015, May 1). *Seniors and vitamin D deficiency.* APlaceforHome.com. Retrieved from
https://www.aplaceformom.com/blog/3-19-14-seniors-vitamin-d-deficiency/

ADDITIONAL RESOURCES

Person-Centered Care and Customer Service

Anderson, R. (2014). *Long term care customer service participant resource guide: Evidenced-based
training for skilled nursing homes, assisted living facilities and anyone working with the elderly*
(2nd ed.). Honolulu, HI: Prima Lux Publishing. (Also: Instructor's Guide.)

Family Caregiver Alliance. (n.d.). *National consumer voice for quality long-term care (formerly
the National Citizens' Coalition for Nursing Home Reform).* Retrieved from https://www
.caregiver.org/national-consumer-voice-quality-long-term-care-formerly-nccnhr-0

Lee, F. (2004). *If Disney ran your hospital: 9½ things you would do differently.* Bozeman, MT: Second
River Healthcare Press.

Marshall, C. (2009). *Satisfied customers seldom sue: A guide to exceptional customer service in long-
term care.* Middleton, MA: HCPro.

Maslow, A. H. (1954). *Motivation and personality.* New York, NY: Harper & Brothers.

Papa, K. S., & Marshall, C. (2016). *Customer service in assisted living: Strategies for building
successful partnerships.* Middleton, MA: HCPro.

Measuring Customer Satisfaction: Senior Living

Agency for Health Care Research and Quality, Consumer Assessment of Healthcare Providers
and Systems (CAHPS): https://www.ahrq.gov/cahps/surveys-guidance/nh/index.html

National Research Corporation: https://nrchealth.com (NRC Acquired MyInnerview in 2009)

Press-Gainey: https://www.pressganey.com

Personal Development: Investing in Yourself

INTRODUCTION

Widely acclaimed business author, Dr. Steven Covey, observed in his book *The 7 Habits of Highly Effective People (1989b)* that "we must never become too busy sawing to take time to sharpen the saw." Just as quality assurance and performance improvement (QAPI), total quality management and continuous quality improvement (CQI) processes are critical to the successful operation of a postacute care organization, they apply to the person in the health services executive's (HSE™) mirror. Some of our field's greatest attractions include its multifaceted, constantly changing nature and its demand for leadership's adaptability, critical thinking skills, and commitment to excellence.

HSE™ **leadership** is not an event; it is an expedition. Every journey begins with selecting a destination and preparing a route, planning and acquiring needed provisions, and getting started. This chapter addresses the preparation expected of those about to enter the profession across the spectrum of postacute care service lines, approaches for securing a leadership position, the benefits of engagement in the profession beyond one's employer, and the importance of maintaining a strong commitment to lifelong learning.

CAREER ENTRY

Nursing Home

A nursing home administrator (NHA or LNHA) is licensed as a health professional in every state and Washington, DC, due to a federal mandate that was included in amendments made in 1967 to the Social Security Act. Every state was expected to establish a method for licensing the administrators following foundational guidelines provided by the U.S. Department of Health and Human Services (DHHS, formerly known as the Health Care Finance Administration or HCFA). Those guidelines are found in the Code of Federal Regulations (2019). Other key provisions of the federal mandate required each state to:

- only allow a nursing home to operate if it employed an administrator licensed by the state and in accordance with the federal guidelines for that licensure process (471.03);

- follow composition guidelines that effectively represent stakeholder interests without favoring the overseen profession or presenting material conflicts of interest (431.706);

- develop and enforce standards that licensees are at least "of good moral character, otherwise suitable, and qualified to serve because of training or expertise in institutional administration" (431.707); and

- establish procedures for applying the standards governing the issuance or revocation of a license, disciplinary actions, and ongoing assessment of the program's efficacy (431.08-13).

The impetus for forming in 1971 the National Association of Long-Term Care Administrator Boards (NAB) was the need for NHA licensure boards to share information and best practices. This association has been instrumental in coordinating its member boards' efforts to meet and exceed the federal mandate, encourage standardization and cooperation, and meaningfully respond to the changing complexity of the postacute care field—all with the central purpose of public protection.

There are several different professional preparation paths to earning an NHA's license. Someone might become interested in the field by first having worked in a clinical role or in another administrative or support services capacity. Someone else might consider a career change from another field because they recognize the myriad of challenging opportunities and accompanying rewards this work offers. An increasing number of new licensees are entering the profession right from college, having engaged in a course of study designed to prepare them for it.

Regardless of one's starting point, their unique blend of experience, knowledge, and skills make *tailoring* an optimal entry point and career trajectory feasible, unlike many other health professions. Core leadership competencies are organized by the NAB into five categories, called "domains of practice," and most of the academic preparation, examinations, and continuing education programming in our field utilize this classification system.

Educational Preparation

In most licensing jurisdictions, the formal education minimally required to qualify as an applicant for a NHA's license is a bachelor's degree. Some licensing boards add expectations about—or preferences for—the focus of the degree earned, such as business or healthcare administration, gerontology, or social sciences. Some leave the door open for further evaluation by the board concerning the appropriateness of the applicant's academic preparation, adding a phrase such as "…or other discipline or course of study relevant to the practice of nursing home administration." Only a few boards have a minimum educational requirement of less than a baccalaureate degree, and those all require at least a high school diploma or equivalency credential, such as a general educational development (GED) certificate.

In recent years, interest has begun to heighten among institutions of higher education in offering academic programs of study that focus more intentionally on developing leaders for the postacute care setting, at both the undergraduate and graduate school levels. Such a program may take the form of an academic major, concentration, or minor within a broader context, tied to a degree awarded in health and human services or business administration, public administration, gerontology or aging services, or social and public policy. Some schools encourage blending the major, concentration, or minor with a complementary one in the social sciences (psychology, sociology, family or women's studies, industrial or organizational behavior), communications, or a related business segment (accounting, finance, marketing, entrepreneurship, or analytics).

The host academic units also vary widely, largely because of the interdisciplinary nature of the field. Colleges and universities are organized differently based on their size of enrollment, sponsorship (public or private), history and tradition, and relative emphasis on research, teaching, and service. However, academic programs in long-term care administration are most commonly anchored in a higher education institution's college, school or division of business, health professions or public health, or arts and sciences.

The NAB offers a voluntary accreditation process for an academic program to demonstrate that it meets or exceeds NAB's minimum standards for training students to become successful and effective leaders in our field. Those standards are built around demonstrating one's knowledge and skills concerning each of the five domains of practice introduced in Table 12.1. An objective external assessment of an academic program's curriculum—including an experiential learning component (internship) of at least 1,000 hours—faculty qualifications, staff and other resources, institutional and provider community support, strategic plan, graduation rate and student performance on the licensure exam, and impact by its alumni in the field all contribute to the NAB accreditation process.

According to the NAB's website, "students of NAB-accredited schools score higher than the national average on the NHA Exam and are best-prepared to work as long-term care administrators" (NAB, 2019a). The NAB also encourages its member boards and agencies to include in their respective rules and regulations special recognition of graduates of NAB-accredited academic programs for meeting the required educational and/or experiential learning preparation for becoming a licensed NHA. (For a current list of jurisdictions that do so, visit www.nabweb.org/academic-accreditation.) Finally, graduates of NAB-accredited HSE™ degree programs are eligible to apply for the HSE™ qualification (see later in this chapter).

Two additional nongovernmental organizations (NGOs) offer support and guidelines for academic programs in health services administration. The Association of Undergraduate Programs in Health Administration (AUPHA) has as its members over 200 healthcare management education programs in North America (AUPHA, 2019), which have programs awarding degrees at the bachelor's, master's, and/or doctoral levels. The Commission on Accreditation for Healthcare Management Education (CAHME) accredits graduate programs in healthcare management that meet or exceed its standards. Neither organization has established specific requirements or expectations for training long-term care administrators, so it is not unusual for an academic program with that focus—or academic track—to maintain membership in AUPHA plus accreditation by the NAB, and if it is a graduate program, to maintain CAHME accreditation as well. Their collective goal is to serve the public interest by advancing the quality of healthcare management education in general, and to prepare long-term care leaders of tomorrow, particularly.

Practicum

Regardless of the formal education pathway, most licensing jurisdictions expect an applicant to complete a field learning experience prior to taking the licensure exam, which is often referred to as an "administrator-in-training (AIT)" requirement. This

TABLE 12.1 NAB Domains of Professional Practice

Domain	Knowledge and Skills About
1. Customer care, supports, and service	Planning, developing, implementing, monitoring, and evaluating all services based on care recipient preferences and assessed needs; compliance with applicable federal and state rules and regulations.
2. Human resources	Systems that provide for a consistent, fair, and predictable method of job development, and the recruitment, hiring, training, evaluating and retaining of staff; compliance with applicable federal and state rules and regulations.
3. Finance	Developing, implementing, and evaluating the service provider's budget; financial policies and procedures that comply with GAAP; contractual agreements, insurance, and risk management; systems to optimize financial performance; changes in public policy or reimbursement sources that may affect financial performance; and compliance with applicable federal and state rules and regulations.
4. Environment	Planning, development, implementation, monitoring, and evaluation of a safe, secure, clean and home-like environment; proper use of physical plant, grounds, systems, equipment, and resources; infection control and sanitation; emergency and disaster preparedness; environmental services, housekeeping, laundry and maintenance; HIPAA compliant technology infrastructure; and capital replacement and improvement.
5. Management and leadership	Ensuring compliance with applicable federal and state laws, rules, and regulations; developing, implementing, monitoring, and evaluating policies and procedures that reflect the organization's mission, values, and vision and comply with the directives of the governing body; strategic planning; monitoring internal and external stakeholder satisfaction; risk management; records management and retention; sales, marketing, and public relations; contract management and business affiliation agreements; QAPI; internal and external communication strategies; professional development and training.

GAAP, generally accepted accounting principles; HIPAA, Health Insurance Portability and Accountability Act; QAPI, quality assurance and performance improvement.

Source: National Association of Long-Term Care Administrator Boards. (2019b). *AIT program manual.* Retrieved from https://www.nabweb.org/filebin/images/AIT_Program_Manual_FINAL .pdf

typically involves observing and learning about the roles of people working in each department—their responsibilities and duties, methods and approaches, policies and procedures—and how that all gets coordinated to benefit the residents. It may also include exposure to external stakeholders, such as residents' families, volunteers, regulatory agency representatives, vendors, and community groups. Learning objectives are generally organized to address each of the five NAB domains of professional practice (NAB, 2019d, 2019e).

The licensure applicant completing this process is also often referred to as an "AIT." The host organization's leader who serves as the experienced supervisor during the practicum is frequently called a "preceptor" (NAB, 2019c). Some jurisdictions maintain qualifying standards for prior approval of a preceptor, such as a certain minimum score on their licensure exam or a minimum number of years of experience as a licensed NHA. All boards require a preceptor to at least hold an NHA license "in good standing," meaning that their license is current and that there are no outstanding or recent board disciplinary actions against the licensee.

The preceptor serves as a coach and mentor to the AIT, verifies that the prescribed course of experience gets completed, and attests to the AIT's readiness to take the licensure exam. The NAB and the American College of Health Care Administrators (ACHCA) collaboratively developed and offer an online training program for preceptors and a template framework for designing a comprehensive AIT departmental rotation schedule. Both are voluntary and available without charge at either organization's website (www.nabweb.org or www.achca.org). Many academic programs in long-term care administration and provider organizations utilize this tool kit as an integral part of their practicum requirements (ACHCA, 2019c; NAB, 2019c).

Licensure Examination

The NAB offers a practice entry examination in cooperation with its member licensing boards. Some jurisdictions rely solely on an applicant's performance on the national exam to determine whether to issue a license; others also require successful completion of a supplemental, board-specific test focused on unique requirements of that jurisdiction. Someone applying for an NHA license in a location that requires both must pass both exams to receive a license there.

The entry exams are designed to allow an applicant to demonstrate that they have acquired sufficient knowledge and skills across the five NAB domains to apply them effectively in real, everyday situations (NAB, 2019d). A significant part of the NAB's ongoing work is to exercise due diligence in maintaining examinations that reflect current practice—relevant changes in applicable laws, regulations, and standards—and to assist its member boards in doing likewise.

Licensure by Reciprocity, Endorsement, or Equivalency

An NHA license provides permission to practice only in the jurisdiction for which it is issued. However, most boards have provisions in their rules or regulations that make it possible for a licensee to move from one jurisdiction to another with minimal disruption. Licensure by…

- "Reciprocity" is bidirectional acceptance of a licensee from another jurisdiction; one board accepts licensees from another state if the recognition is mutual.

- "Endorsement" occurs when a licensure board reviews an application submitted by a person who holds a license in good standing from another jurisdiction's board and determines that they meet all the expected requirements for a license—and the board waives any additional demonstration of skills or knowledge to issue an additional license. Many states recognize, for endorsement purposes, an applicant's qualification by having an advanced professional credential, such as certified nursing home administrator (CNHA) or certified assisted living administrator, both issued by the ACHCA.

■   "Equivalency" happens when a board accepts the NAB's HSE™ qualification as fulfilling its licensure requirements for any postacute service line (see later in this chapter).

Residential Care/Assisted Living

The administrative leaders in facility-based communities that are not licensed as either a nursing facility or skilled nursing facility (SNF) typically are not required to become licensed health professionals. There is not yet a comparable federal mandate compelling states to establish and enforce practice standards for administrators working in these settings. However, the public protection motive for moving in that direction in a field that serves frail elders and their families appears to be gaining steam. Although only a few states have yet expanded the purview of their licensing boards for NHAs to include the managers of additional postacute care settings, several are at least exploring the merits of the following suit. In the meantime, Argentum, a national association representing the interests of assisted living communities, offers training about effectively leading an organization engaged in that service line (see Certified Director of Assisted Living under Professional Continuing Education).

Residential care and assisted living (RC/AL) facilities are defined with great variation from state to state, but they consistently fall somewhere between SNF and independent living along the postacute continuum of care. The complexity of resident care needs and services offered is generally limited to intensity levels beneath those of an SNF. Other terms that are used either synonymously or to further segment the range of services include personal care home, home for the aged, and congregate living. "Affordable Senior Housing with Services and Supports" describes publicly funded (most commonly the Department of Housing and Urban Development [HUD] or the U.S. Department of Agriculture [USDA]) dwellings for low-income, frail elders that have expanded to include coordination of services to help residents successfully age in place.

Educational Preparation

Virginia began licensing assisted living administrators in 2008, and its initial requirements have served as a model template for other licensing boards pursuing a similar path. Table 12.2 provides a summary of the educational expectations Virginia has for someone to become a licensed assisted living administrator (Virginia DHP, 2020b).

Most states do not have formal education requirements beyond a high school diploma or general education diploma (GED) for a person to serve as the lead administrative agent of an operation considered part of the RC/AL category of postacute services.

Practicum

Except where licensure for the administrator has become the law, completing a practicum or apprenticeship before assuming a key leadership position in an organization that provides RC/AL services is certainly beneficial and advisable but still voluntary. Many long-term care academic programs encourage students to become familiar with this setting through structured field learning experiences, community service projects, or volunteering.

TABLE 12.2 Licensed Assisted Living Administrator Qualifications— Commonwealth of Virginia

Education *and* one of the following	High school diploma or GED
a. AIT program	Complete an educational program: a. of at least 30 semester hours at an accredited college or university (any subject) plus 640 hours in an approved ALF-AIT program; or b. as a licensed practical nurse and hold a current, unrestricted license or multistate licensure privilege plus 640 hours in an approved ALF-AIT program; or c. as a registered nurse and hold a current, unrestricted license or multistate licensure privilege plus 480 hours in an approved ALF-AIT program; or d. at least 30 semester hours at an accredited college or university with courses in the content areas (NAB domains of practice of client/resident care, human resources management, financial management, physical environment and leadership and governance), plus 480 hours in an approved ALF-AIT program; or e. awarding a master's or a baccalaureate degree in a healthcare-related field (or a comparable field) without an internship or practicum, plus 320 hours in an approved ALF-AIT program. *Or* Hold a master's or baccalaureate degree in an unrelated field plus complete 480 hours in an approved ALF-AIT program.
b. Certificate program	Hold a baccalaureate or higher degree in a field unrelated to healthcare from an accredited college or university. *And* Complete a certificate program (21 credit hours or greater) at an accredited college or university in a healthcare-related field. *And* Complete an internship or practicum of at least 320 hours that addresses the (NAB domains of practice) content areas, conducted in a licensed assisted living facility as part of the certificate program and under the supervision of a preceptor.
c. Degree and practical experience	Hold a baccalaureate or higher degree in a healthcare-related field, from an accredited college or university that addresses the (NAB domains of practice) content areas. *And* Complete an internship or practicum of at least 320 hours that addresses the (NAB domains of practice) content areas, conducted in a licensed assisted living facility as part of the certificate program and under the supervision of a preceptor.

AIT, administrator-in-training; ALF, assisted living facility; GED, general equivalency diploma; NAB, National Association of Long-Term Care Administrator Boards.

Source: Data from Virginia Department of Health Professions, Board of Long-Term Care Administrators. (2020a). *Law*. Retrieved from https://law.lis.virginia.gov/vacode/title54 .1/chapter31/; Virginia Department of Health Professions, Board of Long-Term Care Administrators. (2020b). *Laws and regulations*. Retrieved from https://www.dhp.virginia.gov/ nha/nha_laws_regs.htm#reg (Under Final Regulations, click on ALF Regulations)

Examination

There is not yet a national examination *required* for RC/AL administrators because not all states license them. In jurisdictions that do license RC/AL administrators, there is generally a qualifying examination that is built around the NAB's domains of practice. Although they have the same five headings as the NHA domains of practice, the practical application of them in the RC/AL setting differs, reflecting a contrasting set of needs among those residents. Many of the certificate programs designed to enhance an RC/AL administrator's knowledge and skills also include a minimum proficiency examination component.

Home- and Community-Based Services

Typically included in a discussion of organizations providing home- and community-based services (HCBS) are home health agencies (medical or personal care), hospices (inpatient and outpatient), and adult day care programs. The NAB completed in 2015 a professional practice analysis that found that the core competencies required to serve as an HCBS administrator aligned closely with its five domains of professional practice for both NHA and RC/AL administrators (Lindner, 2015). In fact, over 82% of the knowledge and skills needed were the same across this continuum of postacute care. The most variance was shown in the knowledge and skills related to reimbursement and regulatory compliance.

There are additional supports and services that can also be characterized as belonging in the HCBS realm because of their nonresidential nature and shared goal of fostering a person's probability of successfully aging in place, preventing—or at least delaying—a person's institutionalization. This includes services such as transportation, emergency security alert systems, home modification and installing "smart home" devices, and professional geriatric care management.

Educational Preparation, Practicum, and Examination

The realm of HCBS includes a broader scope of services than either the NHA or RC/AL setting. Consequently, the qualifications required or expected of the person charged with leading each type of enterprise vary greatly. This is the segment of postacute care that is anticipated to grow the most profoundly, so it is reasonable to predict that professional standards for those in leadership will continue to emerge (Consumer Direct Care Network, 2020; Mullaney, 2018).

For a person to serve as the lead administrative agent of an operation considered part of the RC/AL category of postacute services, most states do not currently have formal education requirements beyond a high school diploma or GED. In the absence of widespread adoption of uniform professional practice standards for HCBS administrators, a few states and associations have led the way in developing and championing the value of having them—for both public protection and enhancing quality of care. Table 12.3 provides some illustrative examples of such initiatives.

CAREER LATTICE

Professional advancement in many fields is referred to as "climbing the career ladder"—a metaphor for rising through the ranks of an organization in almost linear fashion. In our discipline, a more suitable image is a "career lattice," depicting the many intersecting lines of service and a broad range of options for professional

TABLE 12.3 Sample HCBS Administrator Qualifications

HCBS Service Line	Licensure	Voluntary
Home health agency or hospice	**Ohio** (like most states) does not license the individual HCBS administrator, but it does license the agency. However, the administrator must meet the same minimum hiring standards as other employees: Background check (criminal record, abuse, and sex offender registries). (Ohio, 2019)	Relevant continuing education to enhance one's knowledge and skills regarding home health and hospice leadership is available from the following associations: • NAHC • NHPCO Depending on the size of the organization, employers generally *prefer* at least a bachelor's degree in a healthcare-related field or in business administration with experience in a health or human services setting.
Adult day program/center	**Oklahoma** requires one of the following combinations of education and experience: • 5 consecutive years of supervisory experience in a long-term care or geriatric setting *and* a HS/GED diploma; *or* • 1-year supervisory experience (preferably in a social or health services setting *and* a bachelor's degree); *or* • 2 years of nursing experience *and* an active Oklahoma nursing license (either RN or LPN). *Plus* a. Completion of state-approved 1-day training course b. Passing the state ADC exam c. 12 CEUs/year for renewal (Oklahoma, 2019)	The NADSA offers guidelines and tools for administrators, as well as an Internet portal to the relevant facility licensing standards in each state (which include minimum requirements for the administrator and other personnel). Commonly expected to provide a physician's statement of good health, TB and hepatitis immunizations, basic first aid, and CPR training. Depending on the size of the organization, employers generally *prefer* at least a bachelor's degree in a healthcare-related field or in business administration with experience in a health or human services setting. (NADSA, 2019)
Geriatric care managers	Some jurisdictions require a business license and registration with the Secretary of State, but not a license specifically for this service.	Relevant continuing education to enhance one's knowledge and skills regarding leadership of an organization providing this service is available from the Aging Life Care Association (2019).

(continued)

TABLE 12.3 *(continued)*

HCBS Service Line	Licensure	Voluntary
Home modification	Some jurisdictions require a business license and registration with the Secretary of State; not a license specifically for this service, but for certain trades (i.e., electrician or plumber).	The NAHB offers training and a proficiency-based credential known as the "Certified Aging-in-Place Specialist," as well as continuing education concerning the business aspects of this service. (NAHB, 2019)

HCBS, home- and community-based services; HS/GED, high school/general equivalency diploma; NADSA, National Adult Day Services Association; NAHB, National Association of Home Builders; NAHC, National Association of Home Care and Hospice; NHPCO, National Hospice and Palliative Care Association Organization; TB, tuberculosis.

Source: Aging Life Care Association. (2019). *Formerly: National Association of Professional Geriatric Care Managers.* Retrieved from https://www.aginglifecare.org/; National Adult Day Services Association. (2019). *About NADSA.* Retrieved from https://www.nadsa.org/; National Association of Home Builders. (2019). *Certified aging-in-place specialist.* Retrieved from https://www.nahb.org/learn/designations/certified-aging-in-place-specialist/how-to-earn -caps.aspx; Ohio Administrative Code. (2019). *3701-60-home health agencies.* Retrieved from http://codes.ohio.gov/oac/3701-60; Oklahoma State Board of Examiners for Long Term Care Administrators. (2019). *Adult day care administrator qualifications.* Retrieved from https:// www.ok.gov/osbeltca/documents/ADC%20FAQs.pdf

development and career trajectory. Moving across the lattice's various combinations of care needs, qualifications required, and recommended knowledge and skills, the relevance and applicability of the NAB's five domains of professional practice remain throughout one's career as a postacute care leader.

Health Services Executive

This evolution opened the door for the NAB to launch an initiative intended to reflect the changing nature of the postacute care environment—to replace career ladders leaning against adjacent silos of care with a career *lattice* that touches each of them. The NAB introduced a new credential, the HSE™ qualification. It has served as a catalyst for the profession to move toward recognizing the value and utility of broadening an administrator's scope of practice.

This new approach reimagined how long-term care leaders are educated, trained, and licensed to practice along the continuum of postacute care. In tandem with this initiative, the NAB committed to addressing the challenges of bolstering the profession's image, minimizing inconsistent practice standards, improving licensure portability, meeting the needs of employers and regulators, and supporting the NAB's member regulatory boards and agencies in their role of public protection.

According to Randy Lindner, the NAB's president and CEO, the first step was to validate the role of the contemporary long-term care leader to practice along the continuum of care and within lines of specialized service. This was accomplished through conducting a professional practice analysis (PPA) that examined both common and specialized tasks, knowledge, and skills required along multiple lines of service. The results of the PPA validated the hypothesis that a significant common core of tasks, knowledge, and skills (over 82%) cross multiple lines of service, supporting the establishment of a broad-based approach to how LTC leaders are trained, educated, and licensed (Lindner, 2015).

Additional support for this direction came from the 2015 White House report, "Occupational Licensing: A Framework for Policy Makers" (U.S. Department of the Treasury, 2015). Its authors emphasized the need for health professions licensure to become both more uniform and portable. Not officially endorsing, but strongly encouraging the success of this model, was the Centers for Medicaid & Medicare Services (CMS). Major associations, including LeadingAge, the American Health Care Association (AHCA), and the ACHCA, supported this approach, recognizing that it could expand career opportunities, as well as enhance recruitment and retention of a talented, highly qualified leadership workforce.

The HSE™ qualification recognizes one's command of knowledge, skills, and tasks within a common core across the NAB's five domains of practice *plus* entry-level competencies unique to each postacute care line of service—NHA, RC/AL, and HCBS (Figure 12.1). Successful demonstration of this combination of competencies—measured by one's education, experience, and examination—meets or exceeds the current requirements for licensure in most jurisdictions to practice as an NHA, as an RC/AL administrator, and as an HCBS administrator. Thus, the NAB describes and positions this approach as "Licensure by Equivalency."

This approach offers an additional option for licensure portability, providing an acceptable and practical pathway for entry-level and experienced practitioners to demonstrate qualification for licensure in more than one jurisdiction. Licensure portability models that are based on common competency standards have been successful in other health professions, such as for nurses, occupational therapists, and pharmacists (Lindner, 2015).

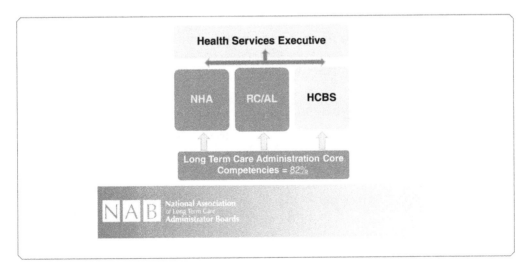

Figure 12.1 Exploring a New Vision for the Profession

HCBS, home- and community-based services; NHA, nursing home administrator; RC/AL, residential care and assisted living.

Source: Reproduced with permission from the National Association of Long-Term Care Administrator Boards.

Licensure by Equivalency allows a long-term care administrator board to consider any person qualified as an HSE™ by the NAB as meeting the minimum qualifications for licensure of an NHA, RC/AL, or HCBS administrator (as applicable to state licensure requirements). A board may additionally require a state jurisprudence examination, and it continues to make all final decisions about licensure. This does not replace any board's individual existing pathway to licensure for an NHA, RC/AL, or HCBS administrator, it merely enhances license portability and supports professional leadership standards for practice in multiple lines of postacute care services.

INVOLVEMENT BEYOND THE WORKPLACE

Network Cultivation

An important element of effective leadership in long-term care is developing a network of colleagues and associates who can serve as helpful resources—and for whom you might serve as one. That requires getting away from your workplace and getting involved in outside organizations associated with the profession, the field, or the community-at-large. Regularly engaging in their activities not only advances those organizations' respective missions but adds positively to the reputation of an administrator's employer, further develops an administrator's leadership skills, and establishes relationships that can prove beneficial—personally and professionally.

Senior living leaders must look beyond their own communities to consistently seek new ideas and validation of current practices, and one of the best places to do this is through involvement in professional societies or trade associations. Involvement in one's own professional society can serve to help keep our saw sharpened through formal educational offerings and informal networking; to challenge our paradigms. It can afford opportunities to give back to the profession through our experiences, contributions and time. It often results in being more fully engaged, energized and professionally enriched. Most importantly, in addition to our own growth, our organizations— staff, residents, and their families—reap the positive outcomes that can result.

Robert Lane, MA, CNHA, FACHCA
Director, BKD, and Past Chair, ACHCA

Professional Societies

American College of Health Care Administrators   The ACHCA is the professional society that specifically represents the interests of long-term care administrators throughout North America. Founded in 1962, the ACHCA is a nonprofit professional membership association, which provides advocacy, continuing education, peer support and recognition, networking, and career development opportunities for its members. Its mission is to serve as the catalyst for excellence in postacute and aging services leadership (ACHCA, 2019a).

"Fellowship" is an honor bestowed by the ACHCA to recognize leaders who are deemed by their peers as the best of our profession. Receiving the "FACHCA" designation reflects a senior living leader's "distinguished contributions to the field of long-term care administration through such avenues as education, publications, teaching, contributing to the public awareness of long-term care, leadership of professional organizations, involvement in civic and community organizations, serving as a board member or officer of an ACHCA chapter, and attending the national ACHCA Convocation" (ACHCA, 2019b). Fellow status indicates to consumers, community, and peers alike one's professional achievement and ongoing adherence to the ethical and professional standards of the ACHCA.

The ACHCA's professional code of ethics is either incorporated or referenced in many jurisdictions' licensing regulations. The designation "Fellow" is a peer recognition designation given to members who demonstrate extraordinary commitment to their residents and families, profession, and communities. Its professional certification program for either NHA or AL administrators is designed to demonstrate advanced proficiency in applying each of the NAB's five domains of practice, and it is recognized by nearly one half of state licensure boards for determining either reciprocity or endorsement.

The ACHCA's membership is organized geographically into regional districts and state or local chapters. There are also "student societies" as recognized student organizations at postsecondary educational institutions with academic programs in long-term care administration. Continuing education programs and networking opportunities occur at each organizational level and sometimes interface with conferences sponsored by one of the trade associations. (Visit www.achca.org for more information about ACHCA.)

American College of Healthcare Executives   The ACHE is the professional society for healthcare executives who lead healthcare organizations, predominantly in acute care settings. Founded in 1933, the ACHE is known for its credentialing and educational programs, its annual Congress on Healthcare Management, and its career development and public policy programs. The ACHE's publishing division, Health Administration Press, is one of the largest publishers of books and journals on all aspects of health services management. The ACHE's professional code of ethics serves as a model for other health and human services disciplines, as well.

With healthcare systems broadening their scope of services, either formally or informally, administrators who frequently operate across the acute/postacute divide typically find value in ACHE membership. The ACHE's membership is organized geographically into 78 local chapters. There are also "student associates" who are currently enrolled in a health administration academic program at a college or university (ACHE, 2019).

Related Disciplines   While the two professional societies described earlier are the premier ones for administrators, there are similar organizations for other postacute care leaders in which a progressive HSE™ should encourage appropriate team members to participate. Table 12.4 introduces some of the more influential ones in postacute care.

TABLE 12.4 Professional Societies in Postacute Care

Position or Profession	Professional Society	Website
Director of nursing or chief clinical officer	National Association of Directors of Nursing in Long-Term Care (NADONA) American Association of Directors of Nursing Services (AADNS)	www.nadona.org www.aadns-ltc.org
Medical director	American Medical Directors Association (AMDA) American Geriatrics Society (AGS)	www.paltc.org www.americangeriatrics.org
Chief financial officer	Healthcare Financial Management Association (HFMA) Long Term Care Finance Association (LTCFA)	www.hfma.org www.ltcfa.org
Information/technology	National Association for the Support of Long-Term Care (NASL)	www.nasl.org
Human resources	American Society for Healthcare Human Resources Administration (ASHHRA) Society for Human Resource Management (SHRM)	www.ashhra.org www.shrm.org
Dining services	Association of Nutrition and Foodservice Professionals (ANFP)	www.anfponline.org
Facilities maintenance	American Society for Healthcare Engineering (ASHE)	www.ashe.org
Environmental services and infection control	Association for the Health Care Environment (AHCE) Association for Professionals in Infection Control and Epidemiology (APIC)	www.ahce.org www.apic.org
Activities	National Association of Activities Professionals (NAAP)	www.naap.org
Medical records	American Health Information Management Association (AHIMA)	www.ahima.org
CNA/SRNA	National Association of Health Care Assistants (NAHCA)	www.nahcacna.org
Senior housing manager	National Center for Housing Management (NCHM)	www.nchm.org

CNA, certified nursing assistant/aide; SRNA, state-registered nursing assistant/aide.

Trade Associations

A trade association differs from a professional society in that it represents the interests of member *organizations*, not those of individuals. A trade association forms to address the collective needs of provider organizations in similar lines of service. It typically advocates on behalf of the association's members regarding public policies that would affect them, provides relevant continuing education for its members' employees, and offers other benefits, such as group purchasing, pooled risk management, or access to training scholarships. Leadership development opportunities through committee involvement and special programs are readily available from trade associations.

American Health Care Association   The ACHA is the nation's largest association of postacute care providers. The AHCA advocates for quality care and services for frail, elderly, and disabled Americans by representing the long-term care community to government, business leaders, and the public. Directly and through its state affiliates, it provides its members information, education, and administrative tools that enhance quality care. (Visit www.ahca.org for further information about the AHCA.)

Argentum   Formed in 1990 as the Assisted Living Federation of America, this association's member organizations operate senior living communities offering primarily assisted living, but also independent living, continuing care, and memory care services. Directly and through its state affiliates, Argentum (which means "silver" in Latin) provides its members information, education, and administrative tools that foster quality services and consumer choice. (Visit www.argentum.org for further information about the Argentum.)

LeadingAge   Not-for-profit and faith-based providers of long-term care and senior housing from around the nation came together in 1961 to establish the American Association of Homes for the Aging, now known as LeadingAge. According to the association's website, their initial goals were to learn from each other, advocate together, and inspire the nation to view aging differently. Two audiences it uniquely includes are its members' governing boards and customers. LeadingAge is also part of the "Global Ageing Network," an international collection of leaders in aging services, housing, research, technology, and design with the shared goal of developing and implementing innovative ideas in senior care. Directly and through its state affiliates, LeadingAge provides its members information, education, and administrative tools to improve the quality of life experienced by those served by its members. (Visit www.leadingage.org for further information about LeadingAge and www.globalageing.org/ to learn more about the Global Ageing Network.)

National Adult Day Services Association   The National Adult Day Services Association's (NADSA's) members include adult day center providers, associations of providers, corporations, educators, students, retired workers, and others interested in working to build better lives for adults in adult day programs. The NADSA developed national recommended operating standards and guidelines for providing adult day services, initiated national accreditation standards, and designed professional development curriculum for adult day services managers and direct care workers. (Visit www.nadsa.org for further information about the NADSA.)

National Affordable Housing Management Association   The National Affordable Housing Management Association (NAHMA) is the leading voice for affordable housing management, advocating on behalf of multifamily property managers and owners with the common interest of providing quality affordable housing. According to its website, the NAHMA "supports legislative and regulatory policy that promotes the development and preservation of decent and safe affordable housing, is a vital resource for technical education and information, and fosters strategic relations between government and industry." The NAHMA's membership represents 75% of affordable housing providers, including 19 regional, state, and local affordable housing management associations nationwide. (Visit www.nahma.org for more information about the NAHMA.)

National Association of Home Care and Hospice   The National Association of Home Care and Hospice (NAHC) is the largest association representing the interests of chronically ill, disabled, and dying Americans of all ages, as well as the caregivers who provide them with in-home health and hospice services. The NAHC is a unique trade association because its membership includes both care providers and recipients. Through its organizational affiliates and directly, the NAHC provides its members information to improve the quality of life for those receiving home health and hospice services (NAHC, 2019).

National Hospice and Palliative Care Organization   The National Hospice and Palliative Care Organization's (NHPCO's) mission is "to lead and mobilize social change for improved care at the end of life" (NHPCO, 2019). It was founded in 1978 as the National Hospice Organization and has grown to become the nation's largest nonprofit membership organization representing hospice and palliative care programs and professionals. The NHPCO is committed to improving end-of-life care and expanding access to hospice and palliative care by advocating for the terminally ill and their families. It also develops public and professional educational programs and materials to enhance understanding and availability of hospice and palliative care, provides technical informational resources to its membership, conducts research, monitors regulatory activities, and collaborates with other organizations interested in improving end-of-life care. (Visit www.nhpco.org for further information about the NHPCO.)

Duty: Advocacy and Public Policy

The postacute care lines of service operate amid an extremely dynamic political environment. With the anticipated rise in the number of Americans who will reach advanced ages comes the likelihood that the demand for more supports and services will also increase. In addition to the challenges surrounding both public and private financing, there will be ongoing concerns about ensuring service quality and public protection, provider accountability and transparency, workforce development and the contributions of technology, and preserving an individual's privacy, dignity, and self-determination. The HSE™ simply *must* remain informed about the pertinent issues under consideration at the local, state, and federal levels and proactively engage in the legislative process as both a concerned citizen and content expert for others. This is a foundational responsibility; it is not optional. There is simply too much at stake to leave it to others to manage and then live with the results.

Public Service

Licensure boards for long-term care administrators determine the qualifications for serving as—and enforce the regulations governing—administrators of nursing homes, RC/AL facilities, HCBS organizations, or some combination of two or more of these lines of service. The governor (or chief executive branch officer for Washington, DC and U.S. territories) typically appoints a licensure board's members from a list of nominees, and the enabling legislation specifies the professional composition of the board. Common professional categories of board members include representatives of consumers or the public-at-large, higher education, relevant trade associations, or professional societies. The board members' terms of office are generally staggered so that continuity and institutional memory are preserved. Serving on a licensure board is a rewarding experience and an opportunity to advance the standards of the profession. Some boards periodically recruit nonboard members to participate in a task force with a time-limited, focused charge concerning a licensure-related issue.

National Association of Long-Term Care Administrator Boards   Although its voting delegates are selected by each member licensing board, the NAB invites others to participate as volunteers in its ongoing efforts to preserve the relevance and quality of its programs: examinations, continuing education approval and recordkeeping, and academic accreditation. Extensive training and support are provided by the NAB for its delegates and volunteers. The NAB convenes semiannually in various locations around the country, and its various committees and work groups connect between those meetings either electronically or in person. (Visit www.nabweb.org for information about engaging with the NAB.)

Public Advisory Bodies   Many state governments form advisory boards or councils to assist their executive and legislative branches as technical resources concerning specific public policy interests or topics, such as Alzheimer's disease and related disorders, Medicaid, health technology, or workforce development. For the executive branch, members are generally appointed by the state's lead elected officer, its governor, or by an agency's director. For the legislative branch, the appointment might be made directly by the legislative body or recommended through nomination by the legislative body for appointment by the executive branch. This process varies greatly by location. Some communities utilize a similar approach for informing public discourse about similar issues on a more local scale.

Although offering your professional expertise and insight to public officials can sometimes result in an acceptance, it is generally a better strategy to first develop positive relationships with policy makers and regulators in advance. Do not wait until a crisis or threat presents itself. Here are a few approaches for becoming regarded as a valuable resource by those who develop and/or enforce the rules governing our scope of practice.

1. **Site Visits:** Elected officials are drawn to public service for a wide variety of reasons, but one common denominator among them tends to be the desire for reelection. Fact: Old people vote! (In many instances, this includes the spouses and adult children of residents and clients.) Regardless of the underlying motive for public service, an elected official at *any* level of government is generally receptive to an invitation to visit with their constituents. Suggest that they participate in planned patriotic events (i.e., Memorial Day,

Flag Day, Independence Day, or Veterans Day) or other special celebrations (from a mortgage burning to a resident's 100th birthday). Do this with some regularity—when there is *not* a pressing need for action by them—to build awareness and the **relationship**. When a need for their engagement arises, such as requesting support of or opposition to specific legislation, it will not be the first interaction.

2. **Technical Resource:** Proactively offering to serve as a subject matter expert can prove beneficial, even if it is not accepted each time. It is impossible for public officials to be knowledgeable about the broad array of issues with which they are presented. Becoming known as a reliable and objective resource on topics affecting senior living helps build a reciprocal relationship. (This may include consulting about resolving elder care challenges in their personal life concerning a family member, friend, or neighbor.)

3. **Support Staff Connections:** An elected official often has support staff members who are responsible for granting access to them, following up on constituent requests, and completing assignments tied to commitments made by the official. Depending on the scope of the office, this could be one person or many. Proactively cultivating a positive relationship with support staffers can be as important as doing so with their boss.

4. **Embrace Regulators:** Each of the first three concepts also applies to public employees whose roles center on enforcing pertinent regulations, from planning and zoning proceedings to an agency's on-site inspections. Some administrators stubbornly search for ways to challenge a regulator's judgment or interpretation of the rules; others accept deficiency citations and related penalties wholesale. There is wisdom somewhere between those extremes, with plenty of room for capitalizing on each regulator's expertise as a publicly funded consultation on QAPI.

5. **Alignment With Allies:** There is often strength in numbers. This is one of the greatest values derived from active membership in one's professional society and trade association—the ability to join forces with similarly situated stakeholders. Whether it takes human or financial resources (often it takes both), professional networks that are built prior to a common outside threat or opportunity are generally much more effective in influencing public policy and regulatory enforcement.

Corporate Citizen

A postacute care organization serves as a catalyst for preserving a community's intergenerational continuity. In many suburban and rural communities, it may also be one of the larger employers. The HSE™ is often the face of the organization externally, so its engagement in community groups and activities conveys a commitment to good corporate citizenship. It is virtually impossible to actively participate in *every* civic, fraternal, or charitable organization, no matter how worthwhile the mission. However, one can judiciously apply a combination of filters to arrive at a balanced mix of such memberships: the most impactful for the operation (potential referral source for residents, staff, volunteers, board members, donors, lenders, or other business relationships), the greatest personal interest or under-met community need, or the best opportunity for gaining positive visibility for one's employer.

CHAPTER 12 : PERSONAL DEVELOPMENT: INVESTING IN YOURSELF **301**

Civic and Service Organizations   Civic and service organizations comprise people who come together to provide a service to their community intended to address a public or mutual benefit *other than* the pursuit of profits for owners or investors (BlurtIt.com, 2019). They are typically organized as tax-exempt entities, and there are several categories of them described in Table 12.5.

TABLE 12.5 Overview of Civic and Service Organizations

Organization Type	Primary Purpose	Examples
Civic and social	Promoting the civic and social interests of members; assisting those identified with needs associated with its mission.	• Service club (Rotary International, Kiwanis, Lions, Optimists, or Civitan) • Fraternal lodge (Masons, Knights of Columbus, Elks, Moose) • Ethnic association (League of United Latin American Citizens or Ancient Order of Hibernians) • Veterans' membership organization (VFW or American Legion) • Alumni association and booster club • Parent–teacher organization • Youth organizations (Junior Achievement, Scouting, Boys/Girls Club, or Youth Sports Teams)
Advocacy	Heightening public awareness about issues and fostering the development of policies to effectively address them.	Organizations promoting peace, community action, or taxpayers' rights
Voluntary health	Raise funds for health-related issues, such as disease prevention and treatment, health education, and patient services.	• Disease awareness and research (American Heart Association, Alzheimer's Association) Or • Voluntary health providers (free clinics)
Grantmaking foundation and charitable trust	Support through grants for causes in alignment with the preferences of the grantors or managers or funding a single entity (e.g., museum or zoo).	• Community foundation • Private foundation or philanthropic trust • Corporate foundation • Scholarship trust

(continued)

TABLE 12.5 (continued)

Organization Type	Primary Purpose	Examples
Other grantmaking and giving services	Attract and distribute—through grants—funds for a wide range of social welfare activities, such as educational, scientific, cultural, and health.	• Community Chest • United Way • Fund for the arts
Human rights	Promoting causes associated with human rights, either for a broad or specific constituency.	• Civil liberties and human rights (ACLU) • Nondiscrimination (Anti-Defamation League, NAACP) • Veterans' rights (Disabled American Veterans)
Religious institutions	Administering an organized religion or promoting religious activities.	Churches, mosques, synagogues, and temples Monasteries and seminaries
Environment conservation and wildlife	Promoting the preservation and protection of the environment and wildlife.	• Environmental conservation (Environmental Defense Fund, Sierra Club, Nature Conservancy) • Animal rights (Humane Societies, World Wildlife Fund, PETA)

Source: Modified from MyPlan.com. (2019, March). *Civic organizations.* Retrieved from https://www.myplan.com/careers/industries/religious-charitable-civic-and-professional-organizations/subsectors-02.02.html

Educational Organizations   Local schools at every level—preschool, primary, secondary, and postsecondary—are thirsting for community engagement opportunities for their students, and they typically welcome community subject matter experts to enhance their curricula and learning activities. We work in a field rich in relevant and interesting events, trends, challenges, rewards, and, most of all, people. Think of the many ways in which to capitalize on the wealth of knowledge and experience that lives among our residents. Community service, in this instance, may take the form of facilitating new connections between those we serve and the next generation. It might mean directly teaching students about aging, health and human services, volunteering, or why we find this work so rewarding.

Corporate citizenship can also be exhibited by providing direct sponsorships of school teams, extracurricular activities, publications, or programs or by volunteering as an assistant coach, mentor, or tutor, or fulfilling some other purpose. The main goal is to develop a positive reputation as someone who is keenly interested in the success of the students, and that positive reputation is likely to extend to the organization.

Commitment to "Lifelong Learning" and "Being the Best"

Building and fostering a *corporate* culture of lifelong learning starts with the person in leadership … the one in the mirror. Its foundation is having the desire to outperform the competition and to continuously improve one's knowledge, skills, and effectiveness as an HSE™. As mentioned at the opening to this chapter, Dr. Steven Covey referred to this as "sharpening the saw" (1989a). He explained that the best investment a leader can make in their future is to develop and embrace a balanced program for self-renewal in the four areas of life: physical, social/emotional, mental, and spiritual. Examples from his writing include the following:

- Physical   Beneficial diet, exercise, and rest
- Social/emotional   Meaningful connections with others
- Mental   Learning, reading, writing, and teaching
- Spiritual   Expanding spiritual self through meditation, music, art, prayer, service, and nature

Professional Development

While all four aspects of life described by Covey are important, let us focus here on sharpening one's *mental* saw. Ours is a rapidly changing field, with a steady stream of new regulations (or varying interpretations of the same ones by different officials), tightening reimbursement levels, innovative techniques, treatments, and approaches to delivering services, designing facilities and programs, and greater consumer and employee expectations. It is not an environment for either the faint of heart or someone who thrives on predictability and stability!

However, one strategy that the HSE™ can employ to enhance their probability of successfully meeting the demands accompanying so many changes is to plan for and engage in ongoing professional development activities. In fact, it is beneficial to create and follow a professional development plan (PDP), strategically planning one's continuing education journey with an eye toward enhancing existing skills and expertise, as well as building new ones. The PDP might include formal or informal educational endeavors, or some blend of both, depending on the learning objectives selected. Employers increasingly place a premium on the following capabilities, traits, and trends, which should be given consideration as key factors in framing a PDP:

- **Flexibility and Relevance:** Leave the door open to become an early adapter of new technology, approaches, and techniques; welcome disruption in the marketplace; and prepare to capitalize on it by staying ahead of the curve. Constantly prowl trade and professional journals for industry news and applicable research findings.
- **Leadership Versus Technocrat:** While it is important to understand rules, regulations, standards of practice, and corporate compliance, progressive provider organizations place a premium on *leaders* with the capacity for envisioning a better future and inspiring others to join them in pursuit of it. Learn about the theoretical bases for various leadership styles and experiment with applying them.
- **Advocacy:** Compassion and passion are not enough to trigger meaningful change; there is an art to effective advocacy. It starts with developing effective

written and verbal communication skills. Learn more about business or creative writing, history, and civics.

- **Transparency:** It is not necessarily synonymous with truth telling. Exercising wisdom about how much to say when is essential. An old saying advises, "When someone asks you for the time, you don't also need to report where you bought the watch." Ethics, philosophy, and logic are often overlooked as core disciplines, but they inform all five of the NAB domains of practice.

- **Informatics and Predictive Analytics:** They are emerging as key tools in our field, starting with the mantra, "measure what matters" (not just whatever is measurable). While it may not become necessary to know how to write computer code, functional mastery of spreadsheets, statistics, and probability will soon become considered a survival skill.

- **Emotional Intelligence (EI) and Emotional Quotient (EQ):** These are terms coined by two researchers, Peter Salavoy and John Mayer, and later popularized by Daniel Goleman (2012). He emphasizes the importance of developing awareness that emotions can drive our behavior and impact people (positively and negatively) and learning how to manage those emotions—our own and others—especially when we are under pressure. EQ can count for twice as much as IQ and technical skills *combined* in determining who will be successful.

Committing to lifelong learning as standard operating procedure is simply a must in today's dynamic, challenging world of senior living, regardless of service line. Developing and following a professional development plan, mentoring and being mentored are essential. They are like care planning for the professional and personal growth of the person in the mirror.

Liz Fowler
President and CEO, Bluegrass Care Navigators,
and Board of Directors, National Hospice and
Palliative Care Organization

One's PDP provides a road map for professional growth. In addition to identifying learning objectives, it is often helpful to establish a destination and milestones for the journey, to estimate a timeline for reaching them, and to update the PDP periodically. Another habit described by Steven Covey, the second of his seven, is "to begin with the end in mind." Perhaps that is an advanced degree or professional certification, or a position in the company that requires additional credentialing. Completing each class in a course of study required to earn that degree or credential represents a milestone marker. The pace of completion may be set by the academic program (although asynchronous online and hybrid courses are becoming increasingly popular). Finally, temptations sometimes surface to pause, change, or abandon direction ... staying the course can get tough! The very best litmus test is to continuously evaluate how the additional knowledge and skills will improve the lives of those served by the organization.

Formal Education

Pursuing additional formal education is one path that can help achieve those learning objectives, and it often qualifies the degree recipient for career advancement. For someone transitioning from a clinical role, such as a nurse or dietitian, a program of study that strengthens one's proficiency in business-related topics may have the greatest impact, such as accounting and financial management, strategic planning, leadership, governance, and marketing. For someone who is solidly grounded in those disciplines, either by training or experience, it might prove advantageous to emphasize other operational elements in the PDP, such as human resources management, organizational behavior, medical terminology, and customer service. Many organizations offer tuition assistance as an incentive for its promising emerging leaders to add to their knowledge, skills, credentials, and prospects for advancement.

Professional Continuing Education

Relevant and useful training can also be acquired through professional continuing education, the providers of which do not award a formal academic degree but typically offer verification of completion, a certificate, or even professional certification. An important distinction is the difference between licensure, which is only granted by a government agency, and other professional, competency-based credentials.

Various professions apply slightly different standards for recognizing continuing education, but most track the number of contact instruction hours: 1 classroom hour = 1 continuing education unit or "CEU." In most licensure jurisdictions, renewal requires some prescribed number of CEUs, usually in the range of 15 to 20 per year. Some long-term care administrator boards also permit online learning activities to result in awarding CEUs.

The NAB provides two services to its member boards that directly affect continuing education for licensed administrators. First, its National Continuing Education Review Service (NCERS) approves continuing education providers and their seminars as having relevant content delivered by qualified instructors. This relieves state boards from the task of reviewing and approving continuing education programs that are offered across multiple states by national firms or associations. Second is the National Continuing Education Registry, an online repository for CEUs earned by every licensed administrator, made available to licensees and their respective boards for verification at time of renewal. Continuing education providers report attendance and completion of NCERS-approved programs directly to the CE Registry, so licensees no longer need to maintain copies for submission with their renewal applications.

The various lines of service have different entry-level thresholds for administrators—educational preparation, experience, or examination—all of which are intended to verify an administrator's command of *minimum* standards and practices. Licensure is only required uniformly for NHAs, even though some jurisdictions have begun also licensing RC/AL and some HCBS administrators. In the absence of licensure, a few of the trade associations began offering leadership training and proficiency-based certification programs for administrators in other service lines.

■ *Certified Occupancy Specialist (COS)* from the National Housing Management Association (NHMA) for administrators of HUD affordable housing.

- ■ *Certified Director of Assisted Living (CDAL)* from the Senior Living Certification Commission (affiliated with Argentum) for administrators of RC / AL communities.

- ■ *Hospice Management Development Program* (MDP I, II, and III) from the NHPCO for administrators of hospice organizations.

Teaching and Guiding

Teaching others—whether in the classroom, in the workplace, or through a professional network—is also a form of continuing *self*-education and professional development. Serving as a guest lecturer or adjunct faculty member at an area high school, community college, or university and providing information and insights about health services and senior living leadership is not only professionally rewarding, but it can pay dividends along the recruiting trail for both staff and volunteers. Facilitating staff development efforts within the organization can also be an effective way to demonstrate one's expertise in ways that bolster confidence and respect among employees.

"Mentor" is a term often used to describe someone who is a positive, guiding influence in the life of another—usually younger—person's life. We acquired "mentor" from the literature of ancient Greece. In Homer's epic *The Odyssey*, Odysseus was journeying and fighting battles far from home for two decades. During that time, Telemachus, the son he left as a babe in arms, grew up under the supervision of an old and trusted friend named Mentor.

Mentoring is a two-sided coin. First, it is important to identify and associate with a colleague who is more experienced and can offer relevant, insightful advice along one's professional journey. For service lines that require licensure, the first formal mentoring occurs between a preceptor (supervisor) and an AIT. Preceptor qualifications vary somewhat by jurisdiction and only apply when licensure is required. The role is like that of an athletic coach, providing instruction on relevant knowledge, skills, and tasks, plus inspiration, and challenging the AIT to grow.

The NAB and ACHCA collaborated to develop the "National AIT/Preceptor Program Manual," available for no charge as the "AIT/Preceptor Toolkit" at either organization's website (ACHCA, 2019c; NAB, 2019c). The Interactive AIT Program Manual guides both the preceptor and the AIT through the internship experience, with recommended schedules for complementary time commitments in each department. The online training program for preceptors includes four complementary modules of education, and preceptors earn 1.25 NAB-approved CEUs for completing each one.

Module	Focus
1	Structure of the AIT/practicum and the role of the preceptor
2	Fostering a culture of learning
3	Developing the AIT from a novice to an emerging leader
4	Moving beyond the domains of practice; explore other resources and mentoring

Most licensing jurisdictions currently expect an applicant for licensure to secure their preceptor. However, they typically maintain a list of approved preceptors, and the ACHCA provides limited assistance with linking aspiring AITs and prospective preceptors. It is standard practice for the licensing board to expect an approved preceptor to attest to the AIT's program completion and recommend them for taking the licensure exam.

Once a person enters the profession, the need for—and utility of—having a professional mentor continues. This could be someone within the same company or not. It is generally beneficial to have a mentor within the same or related professional field, but not required. (A seasoned executive from another business can often provide sound guidance about a wide range of leadership topics but is likely to have limited input about matters specific to postacute care operations.) This might involve, at least initially, extending the AIT–preceptor partnership.

One can establish such a relationship either informally or formally. The ACHCA has developed a structured mentoring program to "provide a mechanism through which both established and emerging leaders in the field can better prepare themselves for changes in the profession" (ACHCA, 2019d). It is open to emerging leaders in long-term care who are ACHCA (nonstudent) members and employed in a long-term care or aging services setting, and it matches them with seasoned administrators who have earned the rank of Fellow as ACHCA members. In this program, mentors and protégés commit to a minimum of 1 hour per month to the successful development of the relationship.

Taking a less experienced administrator under wing and serving as a mentor to them is both professionally rewarding and a challenging growth opportunity for the mentor. The rewards are experienced through building another leader in our field and from knowing that the protégé's professional growth will likely result in positive outcomes for many—residents and staff, the families of both, and other stakeholders. The challenges presented by mentoring often stretch one's imagination and critical thinking skills to apply one's experience and knowledge to new situations.

To capture the essence of the variety of forms that mentoring can take, we propose a synonym for mentor: *"Yoda-ship,"* invoking the image of the sage character in the Star Wars movies, who guided protégés about harnessing and applying life energy. It is a playful blend of "Yoda" and "Leadership." As Yoda would likely say, "a light saber it comes not with." Serving as a preceptor for an AIT and as a mentor for a less-experienced administrator are two of the most available ways one can proactively exercise good "Yoda-ship."

Personal Development

Covey's other three aspects of sharpening one's saw—for self-renewal aimed at creating a sustainable, long-term, and effective lifestyle—are physical, social/emotional, and spiritual wellness. He writes,

Feeling good doesn't just happen. Living a life in balance means taking the necessary time to renew yourself. It's all up to you. You can renew yourself through relaxation. Or you can totally burn yourself out by overdoing everything. You can pamper yourself mentally and spiritually. Or you can go through life oblivious to your well-being. You can experience vibrant energy. Or you can procrastinate and miss out on the benefits of good health and exercise. You can revitalize yourself and face a new day in peace and harmony. Or you can wake up in the morning full of apathy because your get-up-and-go has got-up-and-gone. Just remember that every day provides a new opportunity for renewal—a new opportunity to recharge yourself instead of hitting the wall. All it takes is the desire, knowledge, and skill. (Covey, 1989a)

Physical Wellness   Wellness is more than good health. It includes ingesting the right things, exercising consistently, and getting an adequate amount of restful sleep. First, it is important to maintain a healthy, balanced diet (including portion control), staying well-hydrated, and going outside for 10 minutes when the sun is shining to enhance one's vitamin D metabolism. Second, there is not a pill that substitutes for movement—for regularly working out, running, bicycling, yoga, walking (maybe with the dog), or swimming.

Third, a recent study found that over one third of Americans aged 18 to 29 years report getting insufficient sleep to function their best and that increases to over 40% for those aged 30 to 59 years (Statista, 2019). According to the Mayo Clinic, an adult needs 7 to 9 hours of uninterrupted sleep every 24 hours, and the quality of sleep is as important as the quantity. Although some people claim to feel rested after just a few hours of sleep a night, the evidence supports that people who sleep so little over many nights do not perform as well on complex mental tasks as people who get closer to 7 hours of sleep a night (Olson, 2019).

Social/Emotional Wellness   This refers to making meaningful social connections with other people. The strength added by forming, growing, and relying on relationships with others should not be overlooked. Humans are a social species. Going it alone may work in a movie or novel, but it rarely does for very long in real life. While there are some notable generational differences in how we remain in touch with one another most comfortably—from meeting in person or by phone, email, or social media—the foundation for social and emotional well-being is interreliance. That often takes exercising some initiative and investment of time; deeper relationships rarely come about through spontaneous generation.

Spiritual Wellness   Not to be confused with religion, spiritual wellness *might* include a religious aspect or participation in a faith tradition. The emphasis here is on being in touch with one's inner self, values, and beliefs. Some people achieve this by making time for stillness, mindful introspection or meditation, or prayer. Others feed this need by connecting with nature—walking in the woods or by the ocean shore, appreciating a colorful sunset, or marveling at the variety of plants and creatures inhabiting a garden or field. Some apply all of these in different combinations over time. The main point is to step back routinely from the hustle and bustle of a busy life, take a deep breath, and experience contentment.

HSEs™ build on the passion for serving others that led them to this profession by committing to become the best version of themselves imaginable—professionally and personally. It is a highly personalized form of QAPI. Partnering with the person in the mirror on this is one of the purest forms of leadership by example, modeling for others in the organization behaviors that together foster a corporate culture of lifelong learning and excellence.

POLICIES AND PROCEDURES

Codify the importance lifelong learning and professional development by including them prominently in the organization's policies and procedures—do not leave them to chance or spontaneous generation. Make it standard procedure for every employee to frame and follow a PDP—expect the best in order to get the best from them. Then lead by example.

SUMMARY

Being competent to be a leader in senior care and services is not only a societal expectation, but it is also an important foundation for an individual to start building confidence. The career of a health services executive in senior care and services is a marathon, not a sprint. Taking care of yourself and staying current by taking advantage of the plentiful opportunities for lifelong learning is critical. Individuals are wise to take ownership of their own development and growth. People that choose this profession will also find very soon in their career that there are a plethora of incredible people that they can draw upon as both peers and colleagues (and ultimately lifelong friends) for feedback and support.

KEY POINTS

1. HSE™ leadership is not an event, it is an expedition.

2. NHAs are licensed as health professionals due to a federal mandate:

    a. Requirements for educational preparation, field training and experience, demonstrating proficiency of knowledge and skills by examination, and continuing education vary by licensing board and by line of service.

    b. Some jurisdictions have moved toward also licensing administrators of other lines of postacute care services.

3. The NAB's five domains of professional practice—the knowledge, skills, and tasks minimally required of a long-term care administrator—are based on a periodically updated PPA and include the following:

    a. Customer care, supports, and services

    b. Human resources

    c. Finance

    d. Environment

    e. Management and leadership

4. Over 82% of the core competencies for leading organizations across the three major postacute care lines of service—NHA, RC/AL, and HCBS—are common to all three; knowledge, skills, and tasks pertaining to reimbursement models and regulatory compliance comprise the remainder.

5. The HSE™ qualification offered by the NAB is a mechanism to both improve licensure portability and apply evidence-based administrator standards across the postacute care service lines of NHA, RC/AL, and HCBS.

6. External engagement in each of the following is key to an HSE™'s success:

    a. Professional societies and trade associations

    b. Advocacy and public policy

    c. Community-at-large as a good "corporate citizen"

    d. Educational institutions

7. Commitment to lifelong learning and self-improvement—professionally and personally; take the time necessary to "sharpen your saw."

    a.　Create and adhere to a PDP

        i.　Include purposeful and focused elements of formal and continuing education

        ii.　Seek and acquire credentials that are relevant to career interests and enhance professional value

    b.　Strive for personal balance and growth in mental, physical, social/emotional, and spiritual wellness.

LEADERSHIP ROLES

1. Regardless of one's entry line of service—NHA, RC/AL, or HCBS—seek and acquire the NAB's "HSE™ qualification" to optimize career opportunities and effectiveness.

2. Actively and purposefully engage in external activities that foster professional and personal growth, enhance the image and probability of success of the organization, and provide value for those that the organization serves—and encourage others to do likewise.

3. Model the value of lifelong learning and individual QAPI; others are more likely to embrace this philosophy when their leader is "all in."

4. Find and connect with a mentor, someone with greater experience and solid executive judgment who can be a resource, sounding board, and coach. Serve as a mentor, either as a preceptor for someone about to enter the profession or as a trusted guide—"Yoda"—for an administrator with less experience.

HIGH-IMPACT PRACTICES

1. *The 7 Habits of Highly Effective People* (Covey, 1989b) belongs in the personal library of every HSE™, and it should bear plenty of highlighting and underlining, Post-it notes, and turned-down corners. It is widely viewed as one of the most useful and influential frameworks for understanding and achieving personal effectiveness. Covey presents an "inside-out" approach to effectiveness centered on principles and character, suggesting that meaningful change starts within oneself. He maintains that character is a collection of one's habits

Habit	Example
1. Be proactive	Achieve extraordinary results by consistently executing resourcefulness and initiative to break through barriers.
2. Begin with the end in mind	Develop an outcome-oriented mind-set in every activity— projects, meetings, presentations, contributions, etc.
3. Put first things first	Eliminate energy and time-wasting tendencies by focusing and executing on the team's wildly important goals with a weekly planning cadence.
4. Think "win-win"	Lead teams that are motivated to perform superbly through a shared expectation and accountability process.

(continued)

Habit	Example
5. Seek *first* to understand, and *then* to be understood	Create an atmosphere of helpful give-and-take by taking the time to fully understand issues and by providing candid and accurate feedback.
6. Synergize	Demonstrate innovative problem-solving skills by seeking out differences and new and better alternatives.
7. Sharpen the saw	Tap into the highest and best contribution of everyone on a team by unlocking the total strength, passion, capability, and spirit of each.

and that habits consist of knowledge, skills, and desire. Knowledge allows one to understand what to do, skill represents the ability to know how to do it, and desire is the motivation for doing it. This work and other related information are available from Franklin-Covey, Inc. (www.franklincovey.com).

2. **AIT Outside the Box:** Beyond the minimum standards for departmental rotations recommended jointly by the NAB and ACHCA for becoming licensed as an NHA, some progressive postacute provider organizations have found it beneficial to include in an AIT's schedule an experience meeting with or observing any of the following:

a. **Inspectors and Regulatory Compliance:** Office of Inspector General/state survey team; health department; OSHA; U.S. Department of Labor (Wage and Hour Division's local office); or elevator inspector.

b. **Other relevant government entities:**
   i. Federal—U.S. Representative and U.S. Senators (or staff); Social Security Administration (local office); Veterans Affairs (local office).
   ii. State—State Representative and Senator (or staff); state or area agency on aging; Adult Protective Services; Certificate of Need staff (if applicable).
   iii. Local—City/County legislative representative; executive branch department for aging services; police department division for elder crimes.

c. *Business Stakeholders:* Operational sites of high-volume purveyors (i.e., food, paper goods, chemicals, medical supplies, linens, pharmacy) or key services (i.e., clinical laboratory, payroll processing, financial auditor, electronic medical record and other technology assistance, or employee assistance program).

d. **Related Service Providers:**
   i. RC/AL: Communities providing RC, AL, personal care, independent senior living (market rate and affordable/subsidized housing); continuing care retirement community (aka life plan community).
   ii. Facilities/services for other constituents: Pediatrics, intellectual and developmentally disabled, long-term acute care hospital, or corrections infirmary (hospital-based or on prison campus).
   iii. HCBS: Home health (medical and nonmedical), hospice (inpatient and nonresidential), adult day center (medical and social models), PACE

(Program of All-Inclusive Care for the Elderly), emergency and none-mergency transportation provider, home modification contractor.

iv. Other consultants (shadow): Medical director / geriatrician, dentist, optometrist, podiatrist, pharmacist, dietitian, hospital discharge planner, geriatric care manager, elder law attorney, or bank trust officer.

3. **Comprehensive PDP:** Must understand to begin by assessing one's own strengths—knowledge, skills, emotional intelligence, credentials, and other assets—and comparing them to those needed to advance in the profession, as well as to develop short-term (this year), medium-term (1–3 years), and longer-term (3–5 years) PDP goals and action steps. Two critical success factors that are often overlooked, inadequately researched, or simply underestimated are the time and money required to achieve those goals. An effective PDP includes a calendar with milestones, the frequency of checkpoints, and a method for proactively performing a real-time analysis of work–life balance (perhaps involving others, and not just in times of crisis). It also should have a budget and a cash flow projection (sources and uses of funds), as well as metrics for calculating the PDP's return on investment.

QUESTIONS FOR DISCUSSION

1. Discuss the central purpose of licensing a health profession and the key differences among licensure, certification, and other credentials aimed at establishing standards of professional practice.

2. What are the determinants of licensure by reciprocity, endorsement, and equivalency?

3. Should a participant in a continuing education seminar be expected to pass a postprogram test that demonstrates key learning objectives were met? Why or why not?

4. Select a community civic organization—visit the website to learn about its mission and service activities, membership requirements, estimated time commitment, and leaders.

5. What would you likely include in your PDP?

6. Which one of Covey's four life balance elements offer you the most opportunity for improvement, and what are three things you are willing to *try* that might produce the desired result?

CASE PROBLEMS

1. Molly was an RN with several years of experience in palliative care both in a hospital setting and through a home health agency. The local hospice organization hired her to manage its newly opened office in a nearby community, to which Molly decided to move. Her realtor advised that the civic organization in town with the highest community profile was the Rotary Club. She requested financial support for the dues and release time for participation in the group's weekly meetings and outreach activities, which was authorized

by the organization's CEO. **Results:** Molly's active participation as a Rotarian shortened her tenure as a newcomer to town. It accelerated the speed with which she became a trusted subject matter expert on aging and associated family dynamics, advance directives, death and dying, and the region's healthcare network. In turn, this led to several direct and indirect referrals—for both patients and staff members. The hospice even received a charitable grant to fund a community education outreach program that trained family caregivers.

Questions:

a. In addition to the patient and employee recruitment referrals, as well as the grant awarded, what other beneficial outcomes might Molly expect her new civic organization relationships to foster?

b. How would you justify civic organization involvement and balance that with work-related duties and demands?

2. **Residential Care/Assisted Living (RC/AL) Administrators:** An organization operating AL communities in a state that does not issue professional practice licenses to RC/AL administrators had plans for expansion. The CEO wanted to establish criteria for hiring new administrators, either promoting internally or recruiting new talent. The human resources director gathered information available from the Commonwealth of Virginia's licensure regulations for AL administrators, Argentum's CDAL program, and the NAB's Study Guide for the Residential Care and Assisted Living portion of the HSE™ exam. **Results:** The company's administrator position description and performance evaluation tool were refined with greater focus on relevant knowledge and skills; the CEO decided that the organization should become a member of the Argentum; and when the state began exploring the possibility of licensing AL administrators, the CEO advocated for following the Virginia regulations as a possible template.

Questions:

a. What other resources might the organization have included in its research about effective standards and relevant, evidence-based practices for an AL executive?

b. How could the company best prepare to promote from within the ranks of its current employees?

3. **Nursing Home Administrator (NHA):** Tom had been licensed as an NHA for 10 years. He had been approached in recent years by multiple people who were seeking a preceptor, so they could complete AIT requirements to become licensed as NHAs. The timing just never seemed to suit, and he did not feel prepared to serve in that role. At the suggestion of a colleague who was a member of the ACHCA, he decided to complete the online training available for preceptors. **Results:** Tom learned what is expected of a preceptor when supervising an AIT and what learning objectives and experiences should ideally be emphasized in an AIT's program, and he earned 6.0 CEUs. Since trying it for the first time, he has not gone longer than 3 months without serving as an AIT's preceptor. Furthermore, he has the satisfaction of knowing that each one passed the NAB exam on the first try and is now capably leading a long-term care facility of their own. (Now he wonders why he did not do this sooner.)

Questions:

a. What do you see as the most difficult obstacles to overcome in matching an aspiring future administrator with a seasoned senior living executive?

b. Propose a solution for each issue identified in question (a).

NAB DOMAINS OF PRACTICE

10 CUSTOMER CARE, SUPPORTS, AND SERVICES

10.19 Ensure the provision of a customer service culture that leads to a quality experience for care recipients.

20 HUMAN RESOURCES

20.03 Establish the planning, development, implementation, monitoring, and evaluation of employee training and development programs.

20.10 Establish the planning, development, implementation, monitoring, and evaluation of leadership development programs.

20.13 Facilitate effective written, oral, and electronic communication among management and employees.

30 FINANCE

30.05 Develop, implement, monitor, and evaluate financial policies and procedures that comply with Generally Accepted Accounting Principles (GAAP).

30.10 Monitor and address changes in the industry that may affect financial viability.

40 ENVIRONMENT

40.09 Identify opportunities to enhance the physical environment to meet changing market demands.

40.10 Establish, maintain, and monitor an environment that promotes choice, comfort, and dignity for care recipients.

50 MANAGEMENT AND LEADERSHIP

50.01 Ensure compliance with applicable federal, state, and local laws, rules, and regulations.

50.19 Promote professional development of all team members.

A summary of the related knowledge, skills, and core expectations across service lines, and unique features of each service line are available at www.nabweb.org/filebin/pdf/Annotation_of_Tasks_Performed_Across _LOS_in_LTC.pdf.

Source: Reproduced with permission from the National Association of Long-Term Care Administrator Boards. (2016). *Annotation of tasks performed and knowledge and skills used across lines of service in long term care.* Retrieved from https://www.nabweb.org/filebin/ pdf/Annotation_of_Tasks_Performed_Across_LOS_in_LTC.pdf

REFERENCES

Aging Life Care Association. (2019). *Formerly: National Association of Professional Geriatric Care Managers*. Retrieved from https://www.aginglifecare.org/

American College of Health Care Administrators. (2019a). *About ACHCA*. Retrieved from https://www.achca.org

American College of Health Care Administrators. (2019b). *Advancement to fellow*. Retrieved from https://www.achca.org/advancement-to-fellow

American College of Health Care Administrators. (2019c). *AIT/preceptor toolkit*. Retrieved from https://www.achca.org/index.php?option=com_content&view=article&id=115:AIT-Preceptor-Program&catid=20:site-content&Itemid=208

American College of Health Care Administrators. (2019d). *Guiding to greatness—Mentoring tomorrow's leaders*. Retrieved from https://www.achca.org/mentoring-program

American College of Healthcare Executives. (2019). *About ACHE*. Retrieved from https://www.ache.org/

Association of University Programs in Health Administration. (2019). *Explore AUPHA*. Retrieved from https://www.aupha.org/membership/explore

BlurtIt.com. (2019). *What is a civic organization?* Retrieved from https://business-finance.blurtit.com/70259/what-is-a-civic-organization-

Consumer Direct Care Network. (2020). *Role of home and community based services* (White Paper). Retrieved from https://2evjda20n77c34y15z2q1eoh-wpengine.netdna-ssl.com/wp-content/uploads/2018/01/Trends-in-HCBS_White-Paper-FINAL.pdf

Covey, S. (1989a). *Habit 7: Sharpen the saw*. Retrieved from https://www.franklincovey.com/the-7-habits/habit-7.html

Covey, S. (1989b). *The 7 habits of highly effective people*. New York, NY: Free Press and Simon & Schuster.

Goleman, D. (2012). *Emotional intelligence: Why it can matter more than I.Q.* New York, NY: Random House Publishing Group.

Lindner, R. (2015). *NAB's professional practice analysis aligns leadership core competencies across expanding continuum of care* (White Paper). Washington, DC: National Association of Long-Term Care Administrator Boards.

Mullaney, T. (2018, February 14). Home health spending projected to outpace all other types of care. *Home Health Care News*. Retrieved from https://homehealthcarenews.com/2018/02/home-health-spending-projected-to-outpace-all-other-types-of-care/

MyPlan.com. (2019, March). *Civic organizations*. Retrieved from https://www.myplan.com/careers/industries/religious-charitable-civic-and-professional-organizations/subsectors-02.02.html

National Adult Day Services Association. (2019). *About NADSA*. Retrieved from https://www.nadsa.org/

National Association of Home Builders. (2019). *Certified aging-in-place specialist*. Retrieved from https://www.nahb.org/learn/designations/certified-aging-in-place-specialist/how-to-earn-caps.aspx

National Association for Home Care and Hospice. (2019). *About NAHC*. Retrieved from https://www.nahc.org/

National Association of Long-Term Care Administrator Boards. (2019a). *Academic accreditation*. Retrieved from https://www.nabweb.org/academic-accreditation

National Association of Long-Term Care Administrator Boards. (2019b). *AIT program manual*. Retrieved from https://www.nabweb.org/filebin/images/AIT_Program_Manual_FINAL.pdf

National Association of Long-Term Care Administrator Boards. (2019c). *NAB—AIT/preceptor toolkit*. Retrieved from https://www.nabweb.org/nationalaittoolkit

National Association of Long-Term Care Administrator Boards. (2019d). *NAB candidate handbook*. Retrieved from https://www.nabweb.org/filebin/pdf/NAB_Handbook_July_2017_CM5.pdf

National Association of Long-Term Care Administrator Boards. (2019e). *NAB study guide*. Retrieved from https://www.nabweb.org/studyguide

National Hospice and Palliative Care Organization. (2019). *About NHPCO*. Retrieved from https://www.nhpco.org/

Ohio Administrative Code. (2019). *3701-60-home health agencies*. Retrieved from http://codes.ohio.gov/oac/3701-60

Oklahoma State Board of Examiners for Long Term Care Administrators. (2019). *Adult day care administrator qualifications*. Retrieved from https://www.ok.gov/osbeltca/documents/ADC%20FAQs.pdf

Olson, E. (2019). *How many hours of sleep are enough?* Retrieved from https://www.mayoclinic.org/healthy-lifestyle/adult-health/expert-answers/how-many-hours-of-sleep-are-enough/faq-20057898

Statista. (2019). *Percentage of adults in the U.S. who reported they get enough sleep as of January 2017, by age*. Retrieved from https://www.statista.com/statistics/668092/sleep-sufficiency-among-us-adults-age/

U.S. Code of Federal Regulations. (2019). *CFR 431.700–431.715, Licensed nursing home administrators*. Retrieved from https://www.govinfo.gov/app/details/CFR-1999-title42-vol3/CFR-1999-title42-vol3-sec431-700

U.S. Department of the Treasury, Office of Economic Policy, Council of Economic Advisers, and the U.S. Department of Labor for the White House. (2015). *Occupational licensing: A framework for policymakers*. Retrieved from https://obamawhitehouse.archives.gov/sites/default/files/docs/licensing_report_final_nonembargo.pdf

Virginia Department of Health Professions, Board of Long-Term Care Administrators. (2020a). *Law*. Retrieved from https://law.lis.virginia.gov/vacode/title54.1/chapter31/

Virginia Department of Health Professions, Board of Long-Term Care Administrators. (2020b). *Laws and regulations*. Retrieved from https://www.dhp.virginia.gov/nha/nha_laws_regs.htm#reg (Under Final Regulations, click on ALF Regulations)

ADDITIONAL RESOURCES

Civic and Service Organizations

AmeriCorps and Senior Corps: Volunteering in America: https://www.nationalservice.gov/serve/via

Public Service and Volunteer Opportunities: https://www.usa.gov/volunteer

Service Clubs: https://blogs.voanews.com/tedlandphairsamerica/2012/08/30/join-the-club-please/

Professional Development Plans

The Balance Careers: https://www.thebalancecareers.com/how-to-create-a-professional-development-plan-2059790

Career Development International: https://careerdirectionsllc.com/develop-management-development-plan/

Other

Professional Examination Service, Department of Research and Advisory Services. (2014). *Final report: Practice analysis of long-term care administrators across multiple lines of service*. Washington, DC: National Association of Long-Term Care Administrator Boards.

CHAPTER 13

Conclusion

There is a growing demand for talented individuals to lead senior living organizations. It is our societal responsibility to make sure that we develop a solid foundation and platform for preparing leaders with a head for business, hands for working with people, and a heart for caring for the deserving elders of our country. The importance of trained professionals to manage and lead skilled care facilities, assisted living residences, senior housing properties, and managing home- and community-based services is paramount for the services offered and provided today and tomorrow. Quality leadership makes a tremendous difference to the residents, caregivers, and other customers who rely on the services we provide.

In a recent talk, Robert Kramer, a longtime advocate for considering the exciting possibilities for careers in long-term care and support services discussed a broader view of aging that deserves thoughtful consideration and reflection. He challenged us to rethink our personal and professional views and attitudes toward aging and those we serve.

1. *Changing the paradigm (perspective) on how we view the field and our customers is crucial to success.*

   - **Aging:** *Viewing aging as a stage of life rather than a disease that is terminal. Phrases such as "Silver Tsunami" convey that the growing number of people living longer is an unmitigated disaster versus thinking about the "Silver* **Stimulus**" *and the benefit that the longevity bonus offers not only older adults, but our entire society.*
   - **Age:** *We need to rethink our chronological sense of age and what it means to be growing older. People reaching 65 today have another third of their adult lives ahead of them, and we should be helping them to get the maximum sense of satisfaction and enjoyment from this longevity bonus.*
   - **Retirement:** *Rather than viewing retirement as a time of disconnecting, disengaging, and decline, until the ultimate form of disappearance—death—we need to rethink retirement as a time to "**refire**" our sense of purpose, meaning, and engagement.*
   - **Health:** *We need to rethink our understanding of what produces health. Health is not primarily determined by the amount or quality of healthcare, but rather by the setting or environment in which we live and the behaviors that we follow.*

2. *"Broaden our focus in what we do from one of just providing care for people with physical or cognitive limitations." That leads to many people, including potential future customers, viewing senior living primarily as places where people go to die. Instead, we must demonstrate that our primary role is to reconnect individuals with what gives them a sense of purpose, connection, and engagement. We must reimagine the role of our activities directors as purpose matchmakers for our residents.*

3. *"See the future in terms of who our customers are going to be and what they will expect, and train leaders for a longevity economy." The phrase "senior living" will be an anachronism in 5 to 10 years, as it represents for boomers their parents' notion of retirement and aging—not theirs. The boomer customer will be more racially and ethnically diverse and will seek settings that offer a sense of connection and engagement, not just care. To recruit future leaders to our industry, we must develop winning cultures in our companies that attract individuals who want to make a difference. Success over the next decade will not be primarily due to access to capital or a great product strategy. Rather, the key to success will be a company culture that attracts and retains talent.*

4. *The new bottom line, "We need to invest time, talent, and resources to move the needle and solve this problem."*

Robert Kramer, Senior Advisor at the National Investment Center

The future of this profession is bright and ever changing, with lots of possibilities for reimagining and reshaping the culture of what we do and how we do it. For individuals, especially this next generation of leaders that want to make a difference for people, this vocation is an excellent choice with lots of benefits and rewards.

Serving as a Health Services Executive is a dynamic career choice and profession. The world of senior care is constantly changing and without ongoing professional development an individual runs the risk of falling behind. A person has to stay both current and fresh especially at this time. Professional development is what helps you recharge your batteries, so you are open to try new things, and to be at the top of your game.

Bill McGinley, President and CEO, American College of Health Care Administrators

This text has covered a lot of landscape when it comes to knowledge, technical competencies, leadership, and management skills required to be successful in leading an organization committed to serving the needs and wants of the future elder consumer group. A high-impact practice of leadership in senior care by exceptional individuals is that they understand the need to stay focused on their core product of excellent care and customer service, knowing that a good work environment and positive financial performance will be an expected part of their results. These leaders understand and embrace that they are part of a noble profession that this country needs now more than ever. They accept the humanistic call to action for being professionals who practice with integrity and have a spirit of lifelong engagement in this vocation. The opportunity to be a health service executive in the broader continuum of aging services is an excellent choice with plentiful benefits and rewards.

One must also accept the responsibility of "paying it forward" by taking the next natural step of giving back to the professional community. We challenge you to take that role seriously yet also have fun and enjoy the journey as a member of a wonderful community of senior living leaders across the country!

Afterword: COVID-19 and Senior Care and Services

INTRODUCTION

The COVID-19 global pandemic has had a major impact on the world, and the United States has been struck particularly hard with the first wave of reports starting in February and community spread continuing well into the summer and early fall. Senior living has been hit by a perfect storm with the virus being both contagious and spread by asymptomatic and symptomatic staff or visitors to these congregate settings serving a frail and vulnerable population.

As would be expected with the introduction of a new and fast communicable virus, many of the cases and deaths are occurring in skilled nursing facilities, with significant outbreaks and deaths also being reported in both assisted living facilities and senior housing. The special needs of residents also present significant challenges in managing this population's complexities of care and service needs. Compounding these factors has been the substantial shortage of personal protective equipment (PPE) made available for senior care communities. The focus on hospitals has certainly been highlighted by federal and state leadership priorities, yet the PPE needs of senior care providers have been underemphasized in the public dialogue. The elders that we serve deserve the focus and attention that this pandemic demands. Senior care communities already had faced staffing challenges prior to the pandemic, and this disease has only amplified the pressing needs in these facilities. Staff need to feel respected, safe, and valued by both their own organizations and society as a whole. We have let them down. Administrative leaders have worked tirelessly to support these often-unsung heroes. Misconceptions compounded by poor communication coming from a variety of sources, such as governmental leaders and news outlets and social media, have further added fuel to a fire that has required caring, proactive messages of hope and support to staff. Further, there is mixed evidence about whether the quality of care centers is correlated with infiltration or spread of COVID-19 (Abrams, Loomer, Gandhi, & Grabowski, 2020; Li, Temkin-Greener, Gao, & Cai, 2020). The appropriate role of the government should be one of assistance and support, not one of overly aggressive scrutiny and levying of fines (Centers for Medicare and Medicaid Services [CMS], 2020a). There has been some evidence that CMS and state health departments have been attempting to move in this direction (CMS, 2020b).

The senior living provider community must reconsider inconsistent admission and discharge policies and approaches that have not always served the best interests of their residents and patients. Treatment protocols have been advanced with only modest scientific support, which has further added to a confusing environment. There have also been some providers that have not advanced or maintained the proper infection control processes nor have monitored adherence to the proper use of PPE. Overall, there are many who should be held accountable for not providing adequate support for direct care staff who have served—or are now serving—patients on the frontlines of the fight.

There are some things we learned quickly that helped the senior care community weather the storm. First and foremost, access to adequate PPE is a necessary factor for success. Second, the importance of having a strong infection control training program for all staff in place cannot be underestimated. One of the key related success factors has been to have adequate testing available for both consumers and staff. Another necessary condition has been a strong leadership presence, including the administrator, medical director, and clinical leadership. There has also been some success with using COVID-19 designated facilities across the country, especially among multisite organizations. For many providers, using isolation strategies has been an internal approach that has yielded positive results in controlling the spread of this virus. An example of a related practice effort has been to make sure that advance directives are in place and updated using a frailty assessment, especially with patients who are potentially at higher risk. (Buslovich, Nazir, & Wasserman, 2020).

There are several lessons that have been relearned by organizations. These areas have been amplified during this pandemic and, although covered in the text, deserve additional emphasis related to the situation the senior living field finds itself in for the foreseeable future.

■ Infection control and prevention is a critical practice that has been highlighted and will need to be solidly in place going forward. Protocols as simple as promoting good handwashing techniques and following appropriate precautions are essential going forward. These approaches also send a positive signal to your staff that you are committed to taking care of them as caregivers.

■ One of the bigger lessons has been the practice of effective and efficient operational communications. The variety of stakeholders and the limitations on in-person interaction because of the pandemic have required different communication approaches. Due to the ever-changing nature of this situation, the senior living field finds itself needing to provide regular, weekly, or even daily informational messages to residents, tenants, clients, and staff to ease apprehensions and provide clarity for the road ahead. The importance of communicating with families of all of these groups has also been amplified, answering questions and boosting confidence that the leadership is doing everything possible to ensure a safe environment and remain as attentive and accessible as possible. Leaders must also communicate appropriately to their governing boards and corporate ownership—garnering their support during this unprecedented event yet avoiding the unintentional inclination to overcommunicate and for them to get immersed into the tall weeds. Leadership needs to balance what constitutes enough and too much information. When communicating to the broader community, the specific content of the information being communicated should determine the approach. Pausing to evaluate what you are trying to accomplish or convey is a first step with all of these messages.

■   Paying attention to the broader wellness factors of your audiences has taken on a whole new meaning during this pandemic. The most obvious is their physical well-being, which has had to be front and center, especially for residents and clients, along with employees and volunteers. The mental and emotional toll this has taken on everyone requires both thought and action, in the form of resources made available to help individuals cope and survive this challenging time. The changes to the conventional religious gathering and methods for providing spiritual support have added challenges for many already facing hardships. Lastly, the economic struggles go well beyond just one's own organization, as just about every family circle has felt some of the financial stresses of this period.

Successful leaders must be tuned into many of these reemphasized facets of organizational life when running their healthcare businesses. It has taken extra energy and insight to navigate these uncharted waters.

Lessons revealed during this pandemic have touched a wide array of issues, and many have had a significant impact on the senior care services field. They include the broad categories of infection control, coordination, operations, staffing, and holistic wellness.

INFECTION CONTROL AND PREVENTION

Beyond the health precautions required of everyone, the importance of paying attention to community spread factors is critical. The world also understands better the many ways in which we are interdependent when it comes to travel and shipping. Social distancing, often now called "physical distancing," is a new construct that we have all gotten to know. This has had a major impact on senior care services, especially concerning visitors and memory care venues. Quarantining for 10 to 14 days after coming into contact with an individual with COVID-19 or even visiting a community that has confirmed cases is a new expectation for any person entering the building who does not reside there. Another new concept has been the policies required to limit group assembly, which has been viewed in some settings as one that has competing rights: one's civil liberties versus another's right to remain healthy. For purposes of senior care, the public health field has weighed in heavily with the limitations of these gatherings or visits to help protect the vulnerable population of senior care communities. This has been a challenge for both providers and families. Lastly, we have learned that senior living belongs on the list of businesses considered "essential" during a pandemic.

There have also been clinical protocols that have been important to practice after using them only infrequently and to learn because they were unfamiliar in senior living settings. Two of the most obvious examples have been proactive diagnostic testing and widespread use of PPE (e.g., particularly masks and eyewear). Testing for the presence of the virus provides an opportunity for early detection, but it is only a snapshot in time. Testing survivors for the antibody gives some assurances that they are unlikely to remain contagious—even if still symptomatic—but we do not have enough evidence accumulated yet about how long they will remain so. How do you ensure that you have an adequate supply? How do you administer or encourage tests? What do you do when a staff member or resident (or his/her guardian) refuses to test? How do you use the information provided by the results?

There is also a matter of priority-setting for the use of tests, depending on the supply. The "when" and "frequency" of testing are also important considerations. An organization must have a contingency plan for responding if it receives positive results. Federal and state agencies issued inconsistent—sometimes conflicting—guidance about whether to rely on a symptom-based or test-based strategy for resident admissions, discharge, or transfer, as well as for personnel returning to work.

Given COVID-19's multiple avenues of transmission, PPE has been crucial (Centers for Disease Control and Prevention, 2020). The availability and distribution of these supplies have been an issue, and the supply chain has been tested on multiple levels. A few of the issues have been:

- appropriate supply levels on hand,
- setting priorities and tiers for distribution,
- the competition among states for access to the federal stockpile, and
- fluctuations in actual market prices.

At the provider level, inventory management has been tested, including how to:

- initiate real-time inventory tracking,
- calculate the right "burn-rate," and
- manage all the logistics so customers and staff are safe and have the appropriate PPE.

COORDINATION

This is a tale of success (and the lack thereof) with both the public and private sectors. Starting with government agencies, there have been new kinds of challenges for the coordination of support among federal, state, and local levels. Emergency manufacturing and distribution of desperately needed ventilators and PPE, as well as providing some shared staffing support, were accomplished with remarkable speed, but with significant disparities among regions and levels of care. Members of the healthcare provider continuum have also been tasked with working better within their ranks to communicate and manage COVID-19 patients. The role of suppliers that provide vital goods, from pharmaceuticals and medical equipment to food and cleaning products, has brought tremendous value to organizations. Even the ancillary services, such as utilities, trash collection, communications, education, and electronic health technology, have all adjusted to support people and organizations. The communication and coordination of all these resources and services have been magnified. The Trump Administration even directed the CMS to create an Independent Coronavirus Commission on Safety and Quality in Nursing Homes (CMS, 2020c).

OPERATIONAL COMMUNICATION

Communication has been front and center for senior care leaders with this pandemic, with lots of stakeholders. Staff need to be assured that you are doing everything you can to keep them safe. They also need to know that you appreciate their efforts. Residents, tenants, clients, and their families need many of the same messages of assurance of their safety. They also need to know that you care and understand their anxieties and fears. The more formal communications with agencies and the public media are largely focused on specific requests and reactions. One of the frustrations is that the general media continues to play the blame card more often than not, and of course negative news attracts more attention (in most cases). The role of an effective leader is to wade through some of this news and create some calm by not yelling "Fire" in a crowded theater. It is also clear that greater transparency helps to squelch the fear of the unknown that was very present in the early stages of the pandemic. Lastly, being proactive with communication and transparent with all efforts has been critically important.

STAFFING

The real heroes of this pandemic have been the frontline staff. They have accepted the risk and cared for the elders that deserve our very best. A number of proactive management decisions have helped, including implementation of dedicated assignments, tracking of multisite workers (within the same organization or among multiple employers), provider-issued transportation (rather than reliance on public transportation or rideshare), and even creation of temporary staff housing to protect staff families from COVID-19 transmission. The communities we serve have also responded with tremendous support of our staff. There have been many stories of communities and families reaching out to help support staff with meals and childcare assistance.

This environment has also required the mobilization of human resources from a variety of sources to help fill the staffing needs caused by vacant positions or staff illness. The National Guard, unemployment insurance enrollees, furloughed health professionals (especially from acute care), and college students have all represented emergency sources of labor. One of the by-products of using temporary staff has been modest relaxation of some licensure standards, which has relied on the flexibility and sound judgment of state licensing boards and the related health professions. As an example, there has temporarily been a reduction of the training requirements for certified nursing assistants. This has long-term implications, depending on when and how the normal standards are reinstated, for the public protection afforded by licensure concerning qualifications, credentials, and regulatory oversight.

The governing boards and owners of these care and service organizations are also facing a new fiscal climate, and their budgets have had to both evolve and be refined. This has also required a new engagement with public officials to ensure the most appropriate support during such an unanticipated world event. The guidance and support for executive leadership have had to be at the forefront of these boards and corporate owners as they weather the storm of COVID-19.

HOLISTIC WELLNESS

A new essential perspective required of leadership—to take care of the caregivers, care recipients, and families of both—is a broader view of the individual and the organization's role in their lives. This includes considering their physical, mental, emotional, spiritual, and economic health. In some cases, it means considering how to support them to meet their basic security needs. What happens to the lifelong nursing assistant who exhausts all sources of supplemental income, such as paid-time-off and unemployment benefits, because he or she contracts COVID-19 while working for a senior living organization? These are difficult choices for an organization, but ones that can readily emerge. This has been a difficult time for our country, with many false choices, such as pitting the reopening of the economy against people surviving and living. Our field has risen to the challenge and has nobly responded with compassion and common sense.

LESSONS TO APPLY GOING FORWARD

As a country, we have certainly been reminded of the need to invest in our public health infrastructure. There will be much work ahead to revise public health protocols, policies, and procedures. We must blend these efforts with the healthcare system's emergency disaster planning infrastructure. We must also invest in preparation for similar events in the future. This should include contingency planning, supply chain management and inventory control for supplies and equipment, a training and distribution strategy for people, supplies and equipment, and a better, more seamless and technology-assisted approach for contact tracing. People are also taking a step back to reconsider our reliance on foreign resources and reevaluating the necessary funding level needed for truly fostering public health.

Regarding our senior living field, we have made great strides with a number of new or renewed practice efforts. The use of designated COVID-19 facilities or units, often described as Centers of Excellence, has been a shared healthcare system accomplishment. The use of remote patient monitoring, novel data-driven testing, and the development of frailty-driven care pathways for COVID-19 patients are all examples of strides forward. There is a renewed emphasis on training for infection control and a broader perspective on disaster preparedness, as various systems have embraced the value of proactively addressing these new threats for the benefit of our customers, staff, and organizations.

Although it may be a reach to identify any positives while facing this pandemic, several good things have emerged as we reexamine how we do things. The following list captures a few of these approaches or practices that we can possibly reimagine in the future.

- The need for reconsidering congregate living may leave us in place where semi-private rooms in skilled nursing facilities may not be an acceptable practice or policy. This change will have both quality and price considerations, but the time for the discussion is now.

- Relationships among the acute care system, senior care providers, and public health agencies will need to continue to develop and evolve, especially after great progress has been made.

- Communication modes for all stakeholders will get better. The use of telemedicine will not only be maintained but will be expected to improve as we press forward. Families will communicate with loved ones more frequently, with access to and use of technology becoming even more prevalent.

- A new, broader look at crisis-related staff assistance and trauma-informed supports provided by both employers and the broader society will emerge.

The value of senior care as an "essential" service will continue to be more widely understood, although there is no question that we need to continue to press forward with building the respect this field deserves.

There will be many more new and reimagined opportunities that present themselves in the next few years, and there is still a lot of hard work ahead of us.

In closing, we can only scratch the surface in our expression of all the amazing efforts and stories of this often-unsung field of senior care and services during the pandemic. We appreciate the many people across the country doing this work every day. We are hopeful that America will make the choice that the elders of today and tomorrow—and all of their caregivers across the country—deserve the very best support. This is a time in our country where actions speak louder than words.

REFERENCES

Abrams, H., Loomer, L., Gandhi, A., & Grabowski, D. (2020). Characteristics of U.S. nursing homes with COVID -19 cases. *Journal of the American Geriatrics Society, 68*(8). doi:10 .1111/jgs.16661

Buslovich, S., Nazir, A., & Wasserman, M. (2020, June 30). *COVID-19 learnings and strategies from medical directors on the front lines.* Pathway Health and Patient Patterns webinar.

Centers for Disease Control and Prevention. (2020). *How COVID-19 spreads.* Atlanta, GA: Author. [Google Scholar]

Centers for Medicare and Medicaid Services. (2020a). *Trump Administration unveils enhanced enforcement actions based on nursing home COVID-19 data and inspection results.* https:// www.cms.gov/newsroom/press-releases/trump-administration-unveils-enhanced -enforcement-actions-based-nursing-home-covid-19-data-and

Centers for Medicare and Medicaid Services. (2020b). *Trump Administration announces new resources to protect nursing home residents against COVID-19.* https://www.cms.gov/ newsroom/press-releases/trump-administration-announces-new-resources-protect -nursing-home-residents-against-covid-19

Centers for Medicare and Medicaid Services. (2020c). *CMS announces membership of Independent Coronavirus Commission on Safety and Quality in Nursing Homes.* https://www.cms.gov/ newsroom/press-releases/cms-announces-membership-independent-coronavirus -commission-safety-and-quality-nursing-homes

Li, Y., Temkin-Greener, H., Gao, S., & Cai, S. (2020). COVID-19 infections and deaths among Connecticut nursing home residents: Facility correlates. *Journal of the American Geriatrics Society.* doi:10.1111/jgs.16689

ADDITIONAL RESOURCES

There is a vast array of association-related resources available for providers.

Centers for Disease Control and Prevention: Coronavirus Disease 2019 (COVID-19): Retirement Communities: https://www.cdc.gov/coronavirus/2019-ncov/community/retirement/ index.html

Centers for Medicare & Medicaid Services: Toolkit on State Actions to Mitigate COVID-19 Prevalence in Nursing Homes: https://www.cms.gov/files/document/covid-toolkit -states-mitigate-covid-19-nursing-homes.pdf

AARP: Family Caregiving: Protect Nursing Home Residents: https://www.aarp.org/caregiving/ nursing-homes/

Glossary of Senior Living Acronyms and Selected Terms

One constant challenge in senior living leadership is keeping up with the seemingly ever-evolving list of relevant acronyms, abbreviations, and terms of art—the "jargon" frequently used across the senior living continuum. The following compilation includes many of the most commonly used ones, most of which appear in this text at some point. Some might be rather unfamiliar or surface only periodically. Acronyms and abbreviations may have more than one meaning—inside the profession and externally; only the definitions applying to senior living leadership are included here. This glossary is not an exhaustive list of the terms encountered in aging services and long-term care administration, but it can serve as a handy desk reference for the health services executive in deciphering the "alphabet soup" of senior living terminology.

A

AA   Alzheimer's Association: Nonprofit NGO with the mission "to eliminate Alzheimer's disease and all other dementia through the advancement of research; to provide and enhance care and support for all affected; and to reduce the risk of dementia through the promotion of brain health." https://www.alz.org

AAA   Area Agency on Aging: Designated planning and service areas to provide specific programming funded by the state and Administration on Aging to meet the needs of older adults and disabled persons, as well as evaluate program effectiveness. (See also N4A.)

AADNS   American Association of Directors of Nursing Services: Nonprofit professional society advocating for and addressing the interests of its member senior living directors of nursing departments. https://www.aadns-ltc.org

AAH   American Association of Homecare: Nonprofit trade association advocating for and addressing the interests of its member home healthcare provider organizations. https://www.aahomecare.org

AAIDD   American Association on Intellectual and Developmental Disabilities: Nonprofit NGO with the mission of promoting "progressive policies, sound research, effective practices, and universal human rights for people with intellectual and developmental disabilities. https://www.aaidd.org/

AALTCI   American Association for Long-Term Care Insurance: Nonprofit professional association advocating for and addressing the interests of its member providers of long-term care insurance and life planning solutions. https://www.aaltci.org

AAO   American Association of Ophthalmology: Nonprofit professional society advocating for and addressing the interests of its member ophthalmologists, with the mission "to protect sight and empower lives by serving as an advocate for patients and the public, leading ophthalmic education, and advancing the profession of ophthalmology." https://www.aao.org

AAPC   American Academy of Professional Coders: Nonprofit professional society advocating for and addressing the interests of its members, with the mission of providing "education and professional certification to physician-based medical coders and to elevate the standards of medical coding by providing training, certification, networking, and job opportunities." https://www.aapc.com

AARP   American Association of Retired Persons: Nonprofit, nonpartisan membership organization for people age 50 years and over advocating for and addressing the interests of its members, with the mission "to empower people to choose how they live as they age." The organization is dedicated to enhancing quality of life for all seniors. https://www.aarp.org

AASA   Aging and Adult Services Administration: The principal agency of the U.S. Department of Health and Human Services designated to carry out the provisions of the Older Americans Act of 1965. (See also OAA.) https://acl.gov/about-acl/administration-aging

AAUAP   American Association of University Affiliated Programs for Persons with Developmental Disabilities: Nonprofit trade association advocating for and addressing the interests of its member university-affiliated programs (UAPs), with a shared vision that foresees a nation in which all Americans, including Americans with disabilities, participate fully in their communities. (See also UAP.) http://aauap.org

ABA   American Barbers Association: Nonprofit professional society advocating for and addressing the interests of its member barbers, with the mission of giving its members the resources they need to be a "cut above the rest." https://americanbarber.org

or

American Board of Audiology: Nonprofit professional society advocating for and addressing the interests of its member audiologists, with the mission of creating, administering, and promoting "rigorous credentialing programs that elevate professional practice and advance patient care." https://www.boardofaudiology.org

or

Board Certified in Audiology: Credential awarded by the American Board of Audiology for demonstrating advanced proficiency in relevant knowledge and skills for serving as an audiologist. (See also CCC-A.)

ABI Waiver Acquired Brain Injury Waiver Program/Services: Federal Medicaid waiver that permits approved states to provide rehabilitative home- and community-based services to individuals with brain injuries as an alternative to nursing home facility services and to support individuals' efforts to return to a community setting with existing resources.

ABN Advance Beneficiary Notice (of Noncoverage)—Medicare Form CMS-R-131: Issued by Medicare-certified providers to Original Medicare (fee for service—FFS) beneficiaries in situations where Medicare payment is expected to be denied in order to transfer potential financial liability to the Medicare beneficiary in certain instances. https://www.cms.gov/Medicare/Medicare-General-Information/BNI/ABN

ACA Affordable Care Act: Shortened name for the Patient Protection and Affordable Care Act of 2010; comprehensive healthcare reform law and its amendments addressing health insurance coverage, healthcare costs, and preventive care. (See also PPACA.)

ACHCA American College of Health Care Administrators: Nonprofit professional society advocating for and addressing the interests of its members and dedicated to administrative leadership and excellence in postacute care and aging services across the spectrum of healthcare services. https://achca.memberclicks.net

ACHE American College of Health Care Executives: *Nonprofit professional society advocating for and addressing the interests of its members— people who* lead hospitals, healthcare systems, and other healthcare organizations— with the mission of advancing "healthcare management excellence." https://www.ache.org

ACL Administration for Community Living: Federal agency in the U.S. Department of Health and Human Services that combines the interests of the Administration on Aging and other agencies representing the needs of individuals with both intellectual and physical disabilities.

ACO Accountable care organization: Group of doctors, hospitals, and other healthcare providers who voluntarily affiliate to deliver coordinated high-quality care to Medicare patients, aiming to ensure that patients get the right care at the right time, while avoiding unnecessary duplication of services and preventing medical errors. When successful in both delivering high-quality care and cost containment, the ACO can share in the savings it achieves. https://innovation.cms.gov

ACP Advance care planning: Process that supports a person's understanding of—and expressly sharing—their personal values, life goals, and preferences regarding future medical care, with the goal of ensuring that they receive medical care that is consistent with those values, goals, and preferences.

AD   Advance directive: Legal document that takes effect if one cannot make decisions due to illness or incapacity, such as a living will (instructions on which measures can be used to prolong life) or medical power of attorney (appointment of a surrogate decision-maker for medical questions).

or

Alzheimer's disease (also DAT—dementia of the Alzheimer's type): A degenerative and progressive brain disease with varying combinations of symptoms, from memory loss, confusion, and cognitive decline to irritability, paranoia, and behavior changes.

ADA   American Dental Association: Nonprofit professional society advocating for and addressing the interests of its member dentists, with the mission of "promoting good dental health." https://www.ada.org

or

Americans with Disabilities Act: Federal civil rights law that prohibits discrimination against individuals with disabilities, guaranteeing them equity in public accommodations, employment, transportation, state and local government services, and telecommunications.

ADC   Average daily census: Average number of service recipients (residents, patients, participants, clients or customers) per day over a specific period (week, month, quarter of year).

or

Adult day care: Services provided during the day at a community-based center with programs that are designed to meet the needs of functionally and/or cognitively impaired adults through an individual plan of care. The structured programs provide a variety of social and support services in a protective setting during any part of a day, but less than 24-hour care. Many adult day service programs include health-related services. (See also ADHC.)

ADEA   Age Discrimination in Employment Act: Federal law that protects certain applicants and employees 40-and-older from discrimination on the basis of age in hiring, promotion, discharge, compensation, or terms, conditions, or privileges of employment.

ADHC   Adult Day Health Care: An adult day care program that is also licensed to provide continuous supervision of a participant's medical and health needs, such as administering medications and providing therapeutic services. (See also ADC.)

ADL   Activities of daily living: Blended metric for determining whether a person requires assistance in performing common functions: bathing, dressing, eating, continence and toileting, transferring; maintaining personal hygiene or walking (ambulating) might also be included to evaluate self-care and mobility.

ADON   Assistant Director of Nursing: Chief lieutenant in nursing administration; duties vary by scope and size of the organization.

ADR   Alternative dispute resolution: Any method of resolving disputes without litigation. Arbitration and mediation are two major forms of ADR.

ADRD   Alzheimer's disease or related disorder: The National Institute on Aging (NIA) includes in this group of dementias Alzheimer's disease, frontotemporal degeneration (FTD), Lewy body dementia (LBD), vascular contributions to cognitive impairment and dementia (VCID), and mixed etiology dementias (MED).

Advancing states   Nonprofit association advocating for and addressing the interests of its member state agencies on aging and disabilities, with the mission of designing, improving, and sustaining state systems delivering long-term services and supports for older adults, people with disabilities, and their caregivers. www.advancingstates.org

AE   Adaptive environment: Home modifications and provision of assistive technologies that support independent living among older adults, such as adaptations to the physical environment, such as eliminating slip and trip hazards, installing grab bars or railings.

AFC   Adult foster care: System in which adults are placed into group or private homes with caregivers. Adult foster care is typically arranged through governmental or private agencies, but it may be arranged by relatives who are unable to care for the adult in question.

Aging in place   Providing a familiar, stable, and supportive environment where an elder can receive needed services as their care needs evolve.

AHA   American Hospital Association: Nonprofit trade association advocating for and addressing the interests of its member hospitals and health systems, with the mission of advancing "the health of individuals and communities; AHA leads, represents, and serves hospitals, health systems, and other related organizations that are accountable to the community and committed to health improvement." https://www.aha.org

AHCA   American Health Care Association: Nonprofit trade association advocating for and addressing the interests of its member senior living provider organizations—the nation's largest association of long-term and postacute care providers—with the mission of "improving lives by delivering solutions for quality care" (affiliated with NCAL). https://www.ahcancal.org

AHIMA   American Health Information Management Association: Nonprofit professional society advocating for and addressing the interests of its members, with the mission of "transforming healthcare by leading HIM, informatics, and information governance." www.ahima.org

AHIP   America's Health Insurance Plans: Nonprofit trade association "whose members provide coverage and health related services that improve and protect the health and financial security of consumers, families, businesses, communities, and the nation." https://www.ahip.org

AHRQ   Agency for Healthcare Research and Quality (previously the Agency for Health Care Policy and Research): Federal agency with the mission of producing evidence to make healthcare safer, higher quality, more accessible, equitable, affordable, understood, and used. https://www.ahrq.gov

AIDS   Acquired immunodeficiency syndrome (also stage 3 HIV): Condition when the HIV (human immunodeficiency virus) has caused serious damage to one's immune system, making one more vulnerable to contracting infections. (See also HIV.)

AIT   Administrator-in-training: A person serving an internship with a qualified preceptor/mentor in order to meet the experiential requirements of a state professional licensing board to practice as a licensed senior living administrator; requirements and applicable service lines vary by state.

AL   Assisted living: Type of housing facility for older or disabled adults who may require assistance with their activities of daily living; licensure requirements vary by state. (See also ACLF.) Related terms:

- AL/RC: Assisted living/residential care facility
- ALC: Assisted living community
- ALF: Assisted living facility
- ALR-RC: Assisted living residence–residential care
- ALR-SRHC: Assisted living residence–supported residential healthcare
- RC/AL: Residential care/assisted living

ALS   Amyotrophic lateral sclerosis: Progressive nervous system disease that affects nerve cells in the brain and spinal cord, causing loss of muscle control; sometimes called "Lou Gehrig's disease" after famous professional baseball player with this diagnosis.

AMA   American Medical Association: Nonprofit professional society advocating for and addressing the interests of its member physicians, with the mission to promote the art and science of medicine and the betterment of public health. https://www.ama-assn.org

AMDA   American Medical Directors Association (now the Society for Post-Acute and Long-Term Care Medicine or SPALTCM)

ANA   American Nurses Association: Nonprofit professional society advocating for and addressing the interests of its member professional nurses, with the mission of leading the profession to shape the future of nursing and healthcare. https://www.nursingworld.org/ana

ANFP   Association of Nutrition and Foodservice Professionals: Nonprofit professional society dedicated to the practice of providing optimum nutritional care through foodservice management. https://www.anfponline.org

AOA   Administration on Aging: Federal agency under the Department of Health and Human Services designated to carry out the provisions of the Older Americans Act. https://acl.gov/about-acl/administration-aging

APC   Association of Professional Chaplains: Nonprofit professional society advocating for and addressing the interests of its member healthcare chaplains, with the mission of promoting "quality chaplaincy care through advocacy, education, professional standards, and service to its members." www.professionalchaplains.org

APHA   American Public Health Association: Nonprofit trade association advocating for and addressing the interests of its member public health agencies and professionals, with the mission to "improve the health of the public and achieve equity in health status." https://apha.org

APMA   American Podiatric Medicine Association: Nonprofit professional society advocating for and addressing the interests of its member podiatrists, with the mission of https://www.apma.org

APS   Adult Protective Services: Social services provided by state and/or local governments serving older adults and adults with disabilities who are in need of assistance; investigates cases of abuse, neglect, or exploitation. (See also NAPSA.)

APTA   American Physical Therapy Association: Nonprofit professional society with the mission of "building a community that advances the profession of physical therapy to improve the health of society." www.apta.org

Arbitration Alternative dispute resolution (ADR) method in which one or more persons review a dispute and render a binding decision.

Arc   "The Arc" (formerly the Association for Retarded Citizens): Largest national community-based organization advocating for and with people with intellectual and developmental disabilities (I/DD) and their families, with the mission of promoting and protecting "the human rights of people with intellectual and developmental disabilities and actively support(ing) their full inclusion and participation in the community throughout their lifetimes." https://thearc.org

ARNP   Advanced registered nurse practitioner: Credential earned by an RN who completes further clinical training reflecting their advanced proficiency in the profession.

ASA   American Society on Aging: Nonprofit membership organization advocating for and addressing the interests of its members, with the shared goal "to support the commitment and enhance the knowledge and skills of those who seek to improve the quality of life of older adults and their families." https://www.asaging.org

ASCP   American Society of Consultant Pharmacists: Nonprofit professional society advocating for and addressing the interests of its member consulting pharmacists who focus on the unique medication needs of older adults, with the mission "to promote healthy aging by empowering pharmacists with education, resources, and innovative opportunities." https://www.ascp.com

Asepsis   The absence of pathogens (harmful microbes); clean and sanitary.

ASHA   American Speech-Language-Hearing Association: Nonprofit professional society advocating for and addressing the interests of its member speech, language, and hearing therapists, with the mission of "empowering and supporting audiologists, speech-language pathologists, and speech, language, and hearing scientists through advancing science, setting standards, fostering excellence in professional practice, and advocating for members and those they serve." https://www.asha.org

ASL   American sign language: Form of sign language developed in the United States and used also in English-speaking parts of Canada.

Assault   Intentionally giving another person reasonable concern about an imminent harmful or offensive contact.

AUPHA   Association of University Programs in Health Administration: Nonprofit association advocating for and addressing the interests of its member undergraduate academic programs in health services administration, with the mission of fostering "excellence and innovation in health management and policy education, and scholarship." https://www.aupha.org/about/visionmissionvalues

Autonomy   Ethical concept focused on the importance of a person's independence, freedom of choice, and self-determination.

AWP   Average wholesale price: The average value at which wholesalers sell prescriptions drugs to pharmacies and other customers, and it is the generally accepted standard measure for calculating the cost of a medication.

B

Bargaining unit   Distinct group of employees whose job responsibilities and/or pay level might justify classifying them together for the purpose of unionization or collective bargaining.

Battery   Intentionally causing harmful or offensive contact with another person without their consent.

BBA   Balanced Budget Act of 1997: Established a Medicare prospective payment system for skilled nursing facility services.

BCBS   Blue Cross and Blue Shield: Federation of 36 insurance companies providing hospital (Blue Cross) and medical (Blue Shield) insurance products and services in both the group and individual markets.

BCC   Board-certified chaplain: Credential awarded by the Association of Professional Chaplains for demonstrating advanced proficiency in relevant knowledge and skills for serving as a healthcare chaplain. (See also APC.)

BENHA   Board of Examiners for Nursing Home Administrators: State government agency overseeing the professional licensing of long-term care administrators.

Best Friends™   Best Friends™ approach to Alzheimer's and dementia care: Program model pioneered by David Troxel and Virginia Bell that recasts the caregiver-recipient relationship from staff-patient to "best friends." http://bestfriendsapproach.com

BHO   Behavioral healthcare organization: Provider focused on coordinating preventive and treatment services concerning behavioral factors in chronic illness care, non–disease-related physical symptoms, and health behaviors.

BHP   Behavioral health plan: Insurance program covering behavioral health conditions and interventions.

BIW	Brain injury waiver: Federal waiver permitting a state Medicaid program to provide home- or community-based services to persons with a brain injury.
BLS	Bureau of Labor Statistics: The U.S. Department of Labor bureau that tracks economic indicators (such as the Consumer Price Index) and employment data (such as the unemployment rate, pay and benefits, workplace safety performance and productivity). https://www.bls.gov
Board and care home	Congregate housing that provides basic shelter, food, nonmedical personal assistance, and safety monitoring.
BRFSS	Behavioral risk factor surveillance system: Collaborative project among all of the states and participating U.S. territories with the Centers for Disease Control and Prevention (CDC) to collect uniform data on adults' health-related risk behaviors, chronic health conditions use of preventive services.
Bundled payment	Combined payment (per the Affordable Care Act) for services that Medicare reimburses separately in a fee-for-service model to each provider for the services it renders.

C

CADE	Commission on Accreditation for Dietetics Education: Governs curriculum and related standards for academic programs preparing dietitians.
CAH	Critical Access Hospital: Centers for Medicare & Medicaid-designated primary healthcare hospital that provides limited outpatient and inpatient hospital services to people in rural areas.
CAHME	Commission on Accreditation of Healthcare Management Education: Private nonprofit NGO that offers objective assessment of graduate academic programs in health services management through its accreditation programs.
CARF	Commission on Accreditation for Rehabilitation Facilities: Independent, nonprofit organization focused on advancing the quality of services delivered by rehabilitation providers through its program accreditation programs.
Case mix	Acuity-based classification system to depict the care need profile of a patient population.
CASPER	Certification and Survey Provider Enhanced Reporting (formerly OSCAR): Centers for Medicare & Medicaid's operational data resource for monitoring the status of a provider's short- and long-term quality measure rates and the effectiveness of applied improvement strategies.
CAST	Center for Aging Services Technologies: LeadingAge's initiative to unleash the potential of technology for innovative development across the continuum of healthcare, housing, and services for the aging. https://www.leadingage.org/leadingage-cast-mission-and-vision
CBO	Community-based organization: Noninstitutional provider of senior living services. or

Congressional budget office: Federal agency charged with producing independent, impartial, and nonpartisan analyses of budgetary and economic issues to inform the Congressional budget process; does not make policy recommendations. https://www.cbo.gov

CCC-A   Certificate of Clinical Competence in Audiology: Credential awarded by the American Speech and Hearing Association for demonstrating advanced proficiency in relevant knowledge and skills for serving as an audiologist. (See also ABA.)

CCC-SLP   Certificate of Clinical Competence in Speech-Language Pathology: Credential awarded by the American Speech and Hearing Association for demonstrating advanced proficiency in relevant knowledge and skills for serving as an speech-language pathologist.

CCGP   Commission on Certification of Geriatric Pharmacy: Coalition of 11 professional organizations focused on creating uniform standards for pharmacy credentials and certifications.

CCO   Chief clinical officer: Lead executive staff member overseeing all clinical aspects of a provider organization's operations especially QAPI and quality of life. (See CMO.)

CCRC   Continuing care retirement community: Senior living option with multiple levels of care co-located, from independent and assisted living to memory care, skilled nursing, and rehab care, as well as home health services, to accommodate changing needs. (See also life plan community.)

CDBG   Community Development Block Grant: The U.S. Department of Housing and Urban Development program that funds local community development activities that provide affordable housing, antipoverty programs, and infrastructure development.

CDC   Centers for Disease Control and Prevention: Federal agency under the Department of Health and Human Services, with the main goal of protecting public health and safety through the control and prevention of disease, injury, and disability.

CDM   Certified dietary manager: Credential awarded by the Association of Nutrition and Food Service Professionals for demonstrating basic proficiency in relevant knowledge and skills for serving as a dietary/dining services manager.

CDO   Consumer-directed options: Medicaid waiver that offers eligible beneficiaries more choices about how and when nonmedical services are provided and by whom. (Varies by state.)

CE/CEU   Continuing education professional learning experiences designed to augment knowledge and skills of healthcare professionals after completing their initial academic preparation; required for relicensure and/or specialty certification in most health professions. (Varies by state and discipline.)

CEO   Chief executive officer: Lead executive staff member overseeing all management and leadership aspects of a provider organization's operations, especially strategic planning, social impact, governing board relations, and resource development.

CFO   Chief financial officer: Lead executive staff member overseeing all financial management aspects of a provider organization's operations, especially budgeting, financial performance, and resource management.

CFR   Code of Federal Regulations: The codification of the general and permanent rules published in the Federal Register by the federal government's departments and agencies.

CHAMPUS   Civilian Health and Medical Program of the Uniformed Services: Supplemental program to the Uniformed Services Direct Medical Care System (USDMCS); similar to private insurance programs; designed to provide financial assistance to CHAMPUS beneficiaries for certain prescribed medical care obtained from civilian sources.

CHAMPVA   Civilian Health and Medical Program of the Department of Veterans Affairs: Comprehensive healthcare program in which the VA shares the cost of covered healthcare services and supplies with eligible beneficiaries. https://www.va.gov/

CHC   Community health center: Community-based health provider organization that delivers comprehensive, culturally competent, high-quality primary healthcare services to the nation's most vulnerable individuals and families, including people experiencing homelessness, agricultural workers, residents of public housing, and the nation's veterans.

CHF   Congestive heart failure: Condition in which the heart muscle is weakened and cannot pump normally, triggering fluid retention, particularly in the lungs, legs, and abdomen; major causes include coronary heart disease (most common), hypertension, idiopathic cardiomyopathy, and other heart diseases.

CHRO   Chief human resources officer: Lead executive staff member overseeing all personnel and human resources management aspects of a provider organization's operations.

CIL   Center for Independent Living: Private non-governmental organization that is consumer-controlled, community-based, cross-disability, and nonresidential, designed and operated within a local community by individuals with disabilities, and provides an array of independent living services.

or

Centers for Independent Living: Federal agency under the Administration for Community Living, U.S. Department of Health and Human Services; focused on supporting community living and independence for people with disabilities. https://acl.gov/programs/aging-and-disability-networks/centers-independent-living

CIO   Chief information officer: Lead executive staff member overseeing all technology, information, and communication aspects of a provider organization's operations, especially protected health information (PHI), cybersecurity, infrastructure, and redundancy. (See also CTO.)

CMA or CMT   Certified medication aide/technician: Nursing assistant with additional pharmacology training in fundamental pharmacology and relevant observation protocols. (Not all states.)

CMD   Certified medical director: Credential awarded by the Society for Post-Acute and Long-Term Care Medicine (formerly American Medical Directors Association) for demonstrating advanced proficiency in relevant knowledge and skills for serving as medical director in the senior living field.

CME   Continuing medical education: Professional learning experiences designed to augment knowledge and skills of physicians after completing their initial academic preparation; required for relicensure and/or specialty certification. (Varies by state and speciality.)

CMHC   Community Mental Health Center: Publicly funded, not-for-profit center that contracts with the government (federal, state, and/or local) to provide mental healthcare through inpatient, outpatient, day treatment, and emergency services.

CMO   Care Management Organization: NGO (for-profit or not-for-profit) that develops, coordinates, and monitors individualized service plans, typically for Medicaid beneficiaries. (See also MCO.)

or

Chief medical officer: Lead executive staff member overseeing all clinical aspects of a provider organization's medical operations, especially quality assurance and performance improvement (QAPI) and quality of life. (See also CCO.)

CMP   Civil monetary penalty: Fine levied by Centers for Medicare & Medicaid Services in response to a Medicare/Medicaid-certified provider's severe or consistent noncompliance with the regulations governing program participation.

CMR   Computerized medical record: Automated record of patient treatment information. (See also EHR or EMR.)

CMS   Centers for Medicare & Medicaid Services (formerly HCFA): Federal agency under the Department of Health and Human Services charged with overseeing program operations of Medicare and Medicaid. www.cms.gov

CNA/ SRNA   Certified nursing assistant/aide or state-registered nursing assistant/aide: Provide direct or care services to residents/patients/clients/participants under the supervision of licensed nursing staff.

COB   Coordination of benefits: Centers for Medicare & Medicaid Services program that allows plans that provide health and/or prescription coverage for a Medicare beneficiary to determine their respective payment responsibilities.

COBRA   Consolidated Omnibus Budget Reconciliation Act of 1985: Federal law that affords qualified workers and their families who lose their health benefits the right to continue group health benefits provided by their group health plan for limited period under certain circumstances (i.e., voluntary or involuntary job loss, reduction in hours worked, transition between jobs, death, divorce, and other life events).

COLA   Cost of living adjustment: Periodic modification to wage rates or retirement payments to reflect inflation, generally based on the Consumer Price Index or some similar measure.

CON	Certificate of Need: Authorization from state health planning for a provider to make a significant capital investment for initiating or expanding a covered service. (Varies by state.)
Conditions of Participation	(Now Requirements of Participation): Centers for Medicare & Medicaid Services rules governing provider qualification for certification by Medicare and Medicaid.
Controlled Substance	Drug that is governed by the Controlled Substances Act, which categorizes drugs into five classifications ("schedules") based on their potential for abuse, status in international treaties, and any medical benefits they may provide; includes hallucinogens, narcotics, depressants, and stimulants.
COO	Chief operating officer: Lead executive staff member overseeing and coordinating all aspects of a provider organization's daily operations, especially regulatory compliance, quality assurance and performance improvement, resource optimization, and quality of life. (See also CCO.)
Cost report	Financial report filed by providers that informs Medicare and Medicaid reimbursement.
COTA	Certified occupational therapist assistant: Works under the direct supervision of an occupational therapist by performing specified treatments, documenting therapeutic interventions, and providing feedback on a patient's progress.
CPC	Certified professional coder: Credential awarded by the American Academy of Professional Coders verifying basic proficiency in medical records coding. (Related: RHIT.)
CPE	Clinical pastoral education: Postgraduate academic program teaching pastoral care techniques and approaches to clergy and others; primary method of training healthcare chaplains and spiritual care providers in the United States, Canada, Australia, and New Zealand.
CPOE	Computerized/computer-based physician/provider order entry: Application that allows healthcare providers to directly enter medical orders electronically in EMR systems in a variety of care settings, replacing the more traditional order methods of paper, verbal, telephone, and fax. (See also CPOM.)
CPT	Current procedural terminology: Medical code set maintained by the American Medical Association (AMA) designed to communicate uniform information about medical services and procedures among physicians, coders, patients, accreditation organizations, and payers for administrative, financial, and analytical purposes; similar to ICD-10 coding, but identifies services rendered rather than diagnoses; revised each October.
CPTAS	Certified physical therapist aide specialist: Credential awarded by the National Career Certification Board for demonstrating basic proficiency in relevant knowledge and skills for serving as a PTA.
CQI	Continuous quality improvement: See QAPI.
CTO	Chief technology officer: Lead executive staff member overseeing all technology, information, and communication aspects of a provider organization's operations, especially PHI, cybersecurity, infrastructure, and redundancy. (See also CIO.)

Cultural competence	Ability of a senior living provider organization to design and deliver services in alignment with the cultural needs and preferences of its customers.
Culture change	Senior living's movement toward person-centered care, where the elder's values, preferences, practices, and personhood are all considered in the planning and delivery of care; emphasis on individual choice, purposeful living, self-determination, and respect.
Custodial care	Nonmedical services, including assistance with performing activities of daily living (ADLs), but not nursing or rehabilitative treatments.
CVA	Cerebral vascular (or cerebrovascular) accident: Stroke; when blood flow to a part of the brain is suddenly stopped, either by a blockage or the rupture of a blood vessel, and preventing oxygen from reaching it.

D

DAT	Dementia—Alzheimer's type: A degenerative and progressive brain disease with varying combinations of symptoms, from memory loss, confusion, and cognitive decline to irritability, paranoia, and behavior changes. (See also AD—Alzheimer's disease.)
DCF	Domiciliary care facility: Designation in some states or insurance policies describing a board-and-care home.
DD	Developmental disability (or developmentally disabled): A chronic condition due to a mental or physical impairment that emerges before adulthood and typically limits a person's ability to learn, communicate, or live independently.
DDA	Developmental Disabilities Administration: State agency that assists individuals with developmental disabilities and their families to obtain services and support based on individual preference, capabilities, and needs. (Varies by state.)
DDS	Doctor of Dental Surgery: Professional degree awarded by accredited academic programs in dentistry for completing the required course of study; dentists diagnose and treat conditions affecting teeth, gums, and the oral cavity. (See also DMD.)
Decision support system	Information technology that provides analytical tools to support effective decision-making, especially for clinical applications, purchasing, and strategic planning.
de minimus **Doctrine**	Legal concept holding that a very small amount of either time or money is so insignificant that it makes accounting for it unreasonable or impractical.
DHHS	U.S. Department of Health and Human Services: Federal cabinet-level agency with the mission of enhancing and protecting the health and well-being of all Americans by providing for effective health and human services and fostering advances in medicine, public health, and social services. The ACL, CDC, CMS, HRSA, and NIH operate as agencies under the DHHS. (See also HHS.) https://www.hhs.gov
DHS	Department of Health Services: State agency responsible for overseeing and coordinating health programs, as well as targeted social programs. Also known as

- DHFS: Department of Health and Family Services
- DHMH: Department of Health and Mental Hygiene
- DHSS: Department of Health and Senior (or Social) Services
- DOH: Department of Health

or

U.S. Department of Homeland Security: Cabinet-level federal agency charged with overseeing the nation's efforts concerning anti-terrorism, border security, immigration and customs, cybersecurity, and disaster prevention and management. https://www.dhs.gov

DI Disability insurance: Type of insurance that provides continuing income if a covered worker is unable to fulfill their job duties due to an acquired disability.

DMAIC Define–measure–analyze–improve–control: Refers to a data-driven improvement cycle used for optimizing and stabilizing an organization's operating processes. Pronounced "də-MAY-ick," it is an integral part of the Six Sigma initiative.

DMD Doctor of Medical Dentistry: Professional degree awarded by accredited academic programs in dentistry for completing the required course of study; dentists diagnose and treat conditions affecting teeth, gums, and the oral cavity. (See also DDS.)

DME Durable medical equipment: Equipment that provides therapeutic benefits to a person in need because of a medical condition, illness, or injury (typically not useful otherwise) and designed to endure repeated use; examples include a wheelchair, walker, or crutches.

DNP Doctor of Nursing Practice: Terminal clinical graduate degree in the profession of nursing.

DNR Do not resuscitate: Medical order written by a physician instructing all members of the healthcare team *not* to initiate cardiopulmonary resuscitation (CPR) if a patient's heartbeat or breathing stops; typically established as an "advance directive" to reflect the patient's preferences.

DNS Director of Nursing Services: Administrative leader of a senior living provider's nursing department. (See also DON.)

DNS-CT Director of Nursing Services—Certified: Credential awarded by the American Association of Directors of Nursing for demonstrating advanced proficiency in managing a senior living nursing department.

DO Doctor of Osteopathy (Physician): Professional degree awarded by accredited academic programs in osteopathic medicine for completing the required course of study; physicians diagnose and treat conditions of the whole body (or specialize in one aspect or body system), and educate patients on medical conditions and preventive care; all states recognize DOs as physicians and license them accordingly.

DoE U.S. Department of Education: Cabinet-level federal agency with the mission "to promote student achievement and preparation for global competitiveness by fostering educational excellence and ensuring equal access." (See also DOE.) https://www.ed.gov

DOJ   U.S. Department of Justice (also Justice Department): Federal agency charged with enforcing national civil and criminal laws, particularly those relating to antitrust, civil justice, civil rights, the environmental protection, and taxes. https://www.justice.gov

DOL   U.S. Department of Labor (also Labor Department): Federal agency administers federal labor laws to protect and guarantee workers' rights to fair, safe, and healthy working conditions, including minimum hourly wages and overtime pay, protection against employment discrimination and provision of unemployment insurance. https://www.dol.gov

DON   Director of Nursing: Administrative leader of a senior living provider's nursing department. (See also DNS.)

DP   Doctor of Pharmacy: Professional degree awarded by accredited academic programs in pharmacy for completing the required course of study. (See also PharmD.)

DPAHC   Durable Power of Attorney for Health Care: Document that designates someone as a person's agent or proxy to make healthcare decisions if the patient is no longer able to make them.

DPH   Department of Public Health: State agency responsible for overseeing and administering programs and services aimed at protecting and fostering public health.

DPM   Doctor of Podiatric Medicine: Professional degree awarded by accredited academic programs in podiatric medicine for completing the required course of study; podiatrists diagnose and treat conditions affecting the foot, ankle, and related structures of the leg.

DPOA   Durable power of attorney: Formal written designation of someone to act as one's agent of proxy in managing legal or financial transactions; "durable" means that if the principal becomes incapacitated, the form would remain valid and in effect.

DPOC   Directed plan of correction: When a Medicare/Medicaid-certified senior living provider receives notice from the Centers for Medicare & Medicaid Services (CMS) that an inspection has identified an Immediate Jeopardy (IJ) situation (alleging that the provider's noncompliance with one or more of the requirements of participation has caused, or is likely to cause, serious injury, harm, impairment, or death to a patient), the CMS may direct the provider to take specific corrective action to achieve specific outcomes within prescribed time frames.

DPT   Doctor of Physical Therapy: Professional degree awarded by accredited academic programs in physical therapy for completing the required course of study; physical therapists treat and guide people to restore movement, relieve pain, improve strength, and/or prevent disability.

DRG   Diagnosis-related group: Cost classification method included in the prospective payment system used by Medicare and other insurers to determine reimbursement rates based on a hospital's mix of diagnoses and related treatments.

DSH	Disproportionate share hospital: Acute care provider that received payments statutorily required payments intended to offset its uncompensated care costs to improve access for Medicaid and uninsured patients, as well as preserve its financial stability as a safety-net hospital.
DSM-5	*Diagnostic and Statistical Manual of Mental Disorders* (Fifth Edition): The standard reference used by healthcare providers to diagnose mental and behavioral conditions, published by the American Psychiatric Association.

E

EAP	Employee assistance plan (or program): Plan or program that provides employees with short-term counseling, referrals to specialized professionals or organizations, and follow-up services to address significant life challenges they may face.
EBM	Evidence-based medicine: Judicious and reasonable application of the most current scientific research evidence in making decisions about the care of individual patients.
ECF	Extended care facility: Medical institution that provides prolonged care; popularly used in the early days of Medicare, but replaced in federal and most state regulations by other terms, such as intermediate care facility, nursing facility, or skilled nursing facility.
ED	Emergency department: Hospital department responsible for the provision of medical and surgical care to patients arriving at the hospital in need of immediate care. (See also ER.)
EEOC	U.S. Equal Employment Opportunity Commission: Agency responsible for enforcing federal laws regarding discrimination or harassment against a job applicant or an employee because of the person's race, color, religion, sex (including pregnancy, gender identity, and sexual orientation), national origin, age (40 or older), disability, or genetic information. https://www.eeoc.gov
e-HIE	Electronic health information exchange: Health information exchange network for securely sharing clinical information over the Internet nationwide; spans all 50 states. (See also HIE.)
EHR	Electronic health record: Automated record of patient treatment information. (See also CHR EMR.)
EJCC	Elder Justice Coordinating Council: Federal entity under the Administration for Community Living charged with identifying and proposing solutions to the problems surrounding elder abuse, neglect, and financial exploitation.
Elimination period	Initial waiting period after admission to qualify for insurance benefits to become active; typically 20–60 days.
Employment-at-will	Doctrine that holds an employer can terminate an employee at any time for any reason (except an illegal one) without incurring legal liability, and an employee can leave a job at any time for any reason with no adverse legal consequences.

EMR Electronic medical record: Automated record of patient treatment information. (See also CHR or EHR.)

EMS Emergency medical services: Network of services providing aid and medical assistance from primary response to definitive care, involving personnel trained in the rescue, stabilization, transportation, and advanced treatment of traumatic medical emergencies.

ENP Elderly Nutrition Program: (See NPE—Nutrition Program for the Elderly)

ER Emergency room: Hospital department responsible for the provision of medical and surgical care to patients arriving at the hospital in need of immediate care. (See also ED.)

ERISA Employee Retirement and Income Security Act of 1974: Federal law that protects Americans' retirement assets by implementing rules that qualified plans must follow to ensure that plan fiduciaries properly manage plan assets.

ESRD End-stage renal (kidney) disease: When gradual loss of kidney function reaches an advanced state, rendering one's kidneys ineffective.

F

FADE Focus–analyze–develop–execute: Quality improvement approach aimed at either strengthening process safety or consumer experience or evaluating changes in efficiency or workflow.

FCA False Claims Act of 1863: Federal law prohibiting knowingly presenting a false or fraudulent claim to the U.S. government for payment; "knowingly" means either having actual knowledge that information is false or acting with reckless disregard of the truth.

FDA U.S. Food and Drug Administration: Federal agency responsible for reviewing, approving, and regulating medical products, including pharmaceutical drugs and medical devices and regulating various other products, including food, cosmetics, veterinary drugs, radiation-emitting products, biological products, and tobacco. https://www.fda.gov

FDAMA Food and Drug Administration Modernization Act of 1997: Federal law that increased patient access to experimental drugs and medical devices, accelerated the review of promising new medications and provided for an expanded database on clinical trials.

Federal Register The daily journal of the federal government; published every business day by the National Archives and Records Administration (NARA)'s Office of the Federal Register (OFR); includes federal agency regulations (proposed rules and notices of interest to the public), executive orders, proclamations, and other presidential documents.

FEHBP Federal Employees Health Benefits Program: System through which health insurance benefits are provided to civilian government employees of the U.S. government and their families.

FEMA U.S. Federal Emergency Management Agency: Federal agency with the purpose of coordinating aid and responding to disasters around the nation when local resources are insufficient. https://www.fema.gov

FFS　Fee-for-service: Health insurance payment system in which a provider is paid a fee for each particular service rendered.

FHA　Fair Housing Act of 1968 (and amendments): Federal law that prohibits discrimination on the basis of disability in all types of housing transactions; disability means mental or physical impairments that substantially limit one or more major life activities, such as blindness, impaired hearing or mobility, HIV infection, intellectual or developmental disability, alcoholism, drug addiction, chronic fatigue, learning disability, head injury, or mental illness.

or

U.S. Federal Housing Administration: Federal agency in the Department of Housing and Urban Development (HUD) that sets standards for construction and underwriting and insures loans made by banks and other private lenders for home building; its central goals are to improve housing standards and conditions, provide an adequate home financing system through insurance of mortgage loans, and stabilize the mortgage market. https://www.hud.gov/federal_housing_administration

FI　Fiscal intermediary: An entity that has a contract with the Centers for Medicare & Medicaid Services to determine and to pay Medicare Part A and some Part B bills submitted by certified providers and to perform other related functions.

FICA　Federal Insurance Contributions Act of 1935 (and amendments): Federal law establishing payroll taxes to fund the Social Security and Medicare programs; composed of the old-age, survivors and disability insurance taxes (Social Security) and the hospital insurance tax (Medicare); different rates apply and are calculated as a percentage of the employee's wages.

FIFO　First-in-first-out: Asset management and valuation method in which assets produced or acquired first are sold, used, or disposed of first; applicable to accounting and inventory control.

Fixed Cost　Operating expense that does not fluctuate with census (i.e., property tax or mortgage).

FLSA　Fair Labor Standards Act of 1938 (and amendments): Federal law that establishes minimum wage, overtime pay, recordkeeping, and youth employment standards.

FMAP　Federal Medical Assistance Percentage: Metric used in determining the amount of federal matching funds to distribute to each state for its expenditures on assistance payments for certain social services and Medicaid program.

FMEA　Failure mode and effects analysis: Proactive and systematic method for evaluating a process, identifying how it might fail, and assessing the relative impact of the failure(s), in order to flesh out which part(s) of the process to consider changing.

FMLA　Family and Medical Leave Act of 1993 (and amendments): Federal law that requires covered employers to provide employees with job-protected and unpaid leave for qualified medical and family events.

FPL	Federal poverty level: Measure of income issued every year by the Department of Health and Human Services used to determine eligibility for certain programs and benefits, from marketplace health insurance to Medicaid and Children's Health Insurance Program (CHIP) coverage. https://www.healthcare.gov
FSBPT	Federation of State Boards of Physical Therapy: Nonprofit professional association of state boards of physical therapy advocating for and addressing the interests of its member professional licensing boards, with the mission of protecting the public by providing service and leadership that promote safe and competent physical therapy practice. https://www.fsbpt.org
FSES	Fire safety evaluation system: Measuring system for ensuring compliance of a provider's blend of safeguards with the standards set forth in NFPA 101—Life Safety Code.
FTD	Frontotemporal degeneration: Clinical syndrome associated with shrinking of the frontal and temporal anterior lobes of the brain; the National Institute of Neurological Disorders and Stroke (NINDS) groups together Pick's disease, primary progressive aphasia, and semantic dementia as FTD. (See also ADRD.)
FTE	Full-time equivalent (or employee): Measure that reflects the number of full-time employees an organization would have during a given period. Example: If 100 employee hours are recorded for the week and assuming a full-time employee works 40 hours per week, the full-time equivalent calculation is 100 hours/40 hours = 2.5 FTEs. (Also known as work-time equivalent or WTE.)
FUTA	Federal Unemployment Tax Act of 1939 (and amendments): Federal law that allows the government to collect a tax on businesses with employees for the purpose distributing funds to state unemployment agencies to provide unemployment benefits to qualified citizens.

G

GA	General assistance (also general relief): Term used in some states to describe social programs intended to benefit adults without dependents.
GAAP	Generally accepted accounting principles: Set of rules recognized by the Financial Accounting Standards Board (FASB) that encompass the details, complexities, legalities, methods, and practices of business and corporate accounting.
GAO	U.S. Government Accountability Office: Federal agency that monitors and audits government spending and operations and provides results directly to Congress. https://www.gao.gov
GDP	Gross domestic product: Total monetary value of all the finished goods and services produced within a country's borders in a specific time period; a comprehensive scorecard of the country's economic health.
Geriatrics	Branch of medicine focused on the health and wellness of older adults.

Gerontol-ogy   Study of aging; area of knowledge concerning the aging process and associated changes.

GHP   Green House® Project: Private non-governmental organization with the mission of partnering with "organizations, advocates, and communities to lead the transformation of institutional long-term and postacute care by creating viable homes that spread the Green House Project vision—demonstrating more powerful, meaningful, and satisfying lives, work, and relationships." https://www.thegreenhouse project.org

GNP   Gerontological (or geriatric) nurse practitioner: Credential earned by an RN who completes further clinical training reflecting their advanced proficiency in gerontological nursing.

GP   General practitioner: Physician who treats acute and chronic illnesses, as well as provides preventive care and health education, to patients of any age and gender.

GPO   Group purchasing organization: Entity that helps service providers realize savings and efficiencies by aggregating their purchasing volume and using that leverage to negotiate discounts with manufacturers, distributors, and other vendors.

GSA   Gerontological Society of America: Nonprofit membership organization addressing the interests of its members, promoting the advancement and dissemination of multi- and interdisciplinary research in aging, and supporting and advocating for aging education and training. https://www.geron.org

G-Tube   Gastrostomy tube: Small tube inserted through the abdomen that delivers nutrition directly to the stomach.

Guardian   A person who has been court-appointed to assume legal responsibility to care for another person (called a "ward"), including their personal and property interests, and to make decisions on the ward's behalf; requires the court to determine the ward as incapable of exercising judgement in their own best interest (incompetent).

H

H&P   History and physical: Documentation of a patient's medical history and assessment of their current condition; typically completed at (or before) admission, and one of the first entries in the medical record.

HAA   Hospice Association of America: Now affiliate of the National Association of Home Care and Hospice (NAHC).

HAB   U.S. HIV/AIDS Bureau: Federal agency under Department of Health and Human Services established to address HIV/AIDS; over one-half of people living with HIV in the United States receive services through its "Ryan White HIV/AIDS Program" annually. https://hab.hrsa.gov

HBPC   Hospital-based primary care: Health professional in an acute care setting serves as the first contact and principal point of continuing care for patients within a healthcare system and coordinates other specialist care that the patient may need.

HCB   Home- and community-based care or services: Formal services provided in home- or community-based settings and covered by either private or public funds (senior living examples: hospice, home health, and adult day care). Related terms:

- HCB-D: Home- and community-based services for the developmentally disabled
- HCB-S: Home- and community-based services
- HCB-W: Home- and community-based care waiver program

HCD   Healthcare directive: Legal document that takes effect if one cannot make decisions due to illness or incapacity, such as a living will (instructions on which measures can be used to prolong life) or medical power of attorney (appointment of a surrogate decision-maker for medical questions). (See also AD—advance directive.)

HCFA   Health Care Financing Administration (now called Centers for Medicare & Medicaid Services)

HCPOA   Health Care Power of Attorney: Legal document that empowers another person to make decisions about one's medical care; term refers to both the document and the specific person appointed with this legal authority.

HFMA   Healthcare Financial Management Association: Nonprofit professional society advocating for and addressing the interests of its members, including helping them achieve optimal performance by providing the practical tools and solutions, education, industry analyses, and strategic guidance needed to address the many challenges surrounding the U.S. healthcare.

HHA   Home Health Agency: Public or private organization that offers skilled nursing care and at least one other therapeutic service in the residence of the client through physicians, nurses, therapists, social workers, and homemakers.

HHS   U.S. Department of Health and Human Services: Federal cabinet-level agency with the mission of enhancing and protecting the health and well-being of all Americans by providing for effective health and human services and fostering advances in medicine, public health, and social services. The ACL, CDC, CMS, HRSA, and NIH operate as agencies under the DHHS. (See also DHHS.) https://www.hhs.gov

HIE   Health information exchange: Electronic transmission of healthcare-related data among medical facilities and providers, health information organizations (companies that facilitate the exchange of these data), and government agencies, according to national standards; with the goal of improving the speed, quality, safety, and cost of patient care. (See also e-HIE.)

HIMSS   Health Information Management and Systems Society: Nonprofit professional society advocating for and addressing the interests of its member health information technology professionals, with the mission of reforming the global health ecosystem through the power of information and technology. https://www.himss.org

HIPAA Health Insurance Portability and Accountability Act of 1996: Federal law ensuring that individual healthcare plans are accessible, portable, and renewable and setting the standards and the methods for how health data are shared across the U.S. health system.

HIT Health information technology: Design, development, creation, use, maintenance, and protection of information systems for the healthcare industry.

HITECH Health Information Technology for Economic and Clinical Health Act of 2009: Federal law that creates incentives related to healthcare information technology and the use of electronic health record (EHR) systems among providers.

HIV Human immunodeficiency virus: A virus that can lead to immune system deterioration in humans, eroding its capacity for working normally; can lead to the development of AIDS (stage 3 HIV). (See also AIDS.)

HL-7 Health level 7: Most widely recognized standards for measuring the degree of meaningful use achieved by interfacing computer software programs come mainly from a not-for-profit organization called Health Level Seven International. www.hl7.org

HMO Health maintenance organization: A network or organization that provides health insurance coverage through doctors and other providers who are under contract to the HMO, typically exchanging increased patient volume from the HMO for lower fees.

HPRD Hours per resident (per) day: Total number of hours worked divided by the total number of residents/patients/clients/participants/customers.

HSA Health savings account: Tax-advantaged personal savings account that enables an employee with an HSA-qualified health plan save money on many out-of-pocket medical expenses, such as co-pays for doctor visits, prescriptions, or vision and dental care.

HSE Health services executive (qualification): Credential awarded by the National Association of Long-Term Care Administrator Boards (NAB) in recognition of demonstrating relevant knowledge and skills to lead senior living organizations across the postacute continuum of care.

HUD U.S. Department of Housing and Urban Development: Cabinet-level federal agency with the charge of providing affordable housing and community development assistance, and to ensure that all citizens have "fair and equal" access to housing. https://www.hud.gov

I

I&R Information and referral: Active process of linking a person with a need or problem with a service, which will meaningfully address the need or satisfactorily solve the problem.

IAA Intra-agency agreement: Written contract in which one federal agency agrees to provide to, purchase from, or exchange with another federal agency services, information, supplies, or equipment.

IADL   Instrumental activities of daily living: Activities or tasks performed by an individual daily that are not essential to basic self-care and independent living but add quality to the way of life, such as operating the telephone, shopping, meal preparation, or light housekeeping.

ICD-10   *International Classification of Diseases and Related Health Problems* (10th Edition): Medical classification list of the World Health Organization (WHO) that assigns codes to diseases, signs and symptoms, abnormal findings, complaints, social circumstances, and external causes of injury or diseases; standard used for justifying billable charges and care planning.

ICDR   Interagency Committee on Disability Research: Federal agency established to promote coordination and collaboration among federal departments and agencies conducting disability, independent living, and rehabilitation research programs, including research related to assistive technology and principles of universal design. https://icdr.acl.gov

ICF   Intermediate care facility: Healthcare facility for individuals who are disabled, elderly, or nonacutely ill, usually providing less intensive care than that offered at a hospital or skilled nursing facility.

ICF/MR   Intermediate care facility for persons with mental retardation or a developmental disability.

ICFDD   Healthcare facility providing residential and rehabilitation services to people with intellectual disabilities or a related condition.

ICU   Intensive care unit: Specialized section of a hospital that provides comprehensive, continuous care for persons who are critically ill.

IDD   Intellectual and developmental disabilities: According to the American Association on Intellectual and Developmental Disabilities, the latter is an umbrella term that includes not only intellectual disability but also other disabilities that are apparent during childhood. **Developmental** disabilities are severe chronic disabilities that can be physical, cognitive, or both. **Intellectual** disability refers to a person's limited ability to learn at an expected level and function in daily life.

IDEA   Individuals with Disabilities Education Act: Federal law that provides rights and protections to people with disabilities and to their parents or legal guardians.

IDR   Informal dispute resolution: Process in which two disagreeing parties can engage to avoid legal proceedings, meeting with a third party who facilitates discussions and negotiations to arrive at a resolution. Many states maintain an IDR process for providers to contest survey findings with which they disagree.

IDT   Interdisciplinary team: Group of healthcare professionals representing different fields who work together to optimally plan, provide, and evaluate care for a person.

ILU   Independent living unit: Housing option for senior living when little or no additional services are routinely required by the tenant; examples: apartment, condominium, or continuing care retirement community (CCRC).

IMPACT	Medicare Post-Acute Care Transformation (IMPACT) Act of 2014: Federal law requiring Medicare- and Medicaid-certified providers (SNFs, IRFs, and HHAs) to submit standardized patient assessment data (i.e., MDS, PAI, and OASIS-D, respectively).
Interoper-able	Electronic medical record data that are compatible across multiple operating systems.
IOM	Institute of Medicine: Nonprofit non-governmental organization established in 1970 as a component of the U.S. National Academy of Sciences that works outside the framework of government to conduct and advance evidence-based research and recommendations concerning public health and science policy.
IQIES	Internet quality improvement and evaluation system: Centers for Medicare & Medicaid Services's online system for SNFs, IRFs, and HHAs to submit their IMPACT data.
IRB	Institutional review board: Administrative body established to protect the rights and welfare of human research subjects recruited to participate in research activities conducted under the auspices of the institution, typically a university, with which it is affiliated.
IRC	Internal Revenue Code: Title 26 of the U.S. Code that covers all relevant rules pertaining to income, gift, estate, sales, payroll, and excise taxes.
IRF	Inpatient rehabilitation facility: Free-standing rehabilitation hospital or rehabilitation unit in an acute care hospital that provides an intensive rehabilitation program of at least 3 hours per day.
ISN	Intensive skilled nursing: High-tech and sophisticated skilled nursing care for people with complex comorbidities.
I-SNP	Institutional special needs plan: Insurance model that allows nursing homes to provide a higher level of care and control the disbursement of funds.
ISP	Individual service plan: Assessment tool for use by residential care/assisted living communities; typically focused on supporting emotional, psychosocial, and spiritual wellness and on addressing cognitive impairment and accessing appropriate community resources.
IT	Information technology: Use of computers, infrastructure, and processes to create, process, store, secure, and exchange all forms of electronic data.

J

JCAHO	The Joint Commission on Accreditation of Healthcare Organizations: (Now The Joint Commission)
Joint Com-mission	Nonprofit non-governmental organization offering unbiased, objective assessment of quality achievement by inpatient care and safety through its accreditation programs for healthcare provider organizations. https://www.jointcommission.org
JV	Joint venture: Separate organization formed by two or more existing organizations with the intent of pursuing a common mission or business purpose.

K

Kickback   Payment or item of value given to someone as compensation or reward for providing favorable treatment. Example: Incentivizing patient referrals by paying or providing in-kind gifts to a physician.

L

LANE   Local area networks for excellence: Coalition of stakeholders at the state level formed for the collective purpose of supporting providers and consumers in achieving the goals of the "National Nursing Home Quality Improvement Campaign" (formerly known as "Advancing Excellence in Nursing Homes Campaign"), a national collaborative effort to transform the quality of care and quality of life for nursing home residents. (See also NNHQI.)

LBD   Lewy body dementia: Disease associated with abnormal deposits of α-synuclein protein in the brain, called Lewy bodies, which can lead to problems with thinking, movement, behavior, and mood. (See also ADRD.)

LCSW   Licensed clinical social worker: Assists care recipients with obtaining needed services, as well as provides counseling for them and their families.

LDS   Limited data set: Collection of identifiable patient information as defined in the Privacy Regulations issued under the Health Insurance Portability and Accountability Act (HIPAA).

Leading Age   Formerly the American Association of Homes and Services for the Aging (AAHSA): Nonprofit age trade association representing faith-based and mission-driven providers of senior housing, postacute, and long-term care services. https://www.leadingage.org/

LHI   Leading health indicator: High-priority health issues and actions that can be taken to address them identified by Department of Health and Human Services' Office of Disease Prevention and Health Promotion in "Healthy People 2020."

Life plan community   Senior living option with multiple levels of care co-located, from independent and assisted living to memory care, skilled nursing, and rehabilitation care, as well as home health services, to accommodate changing needs. (See also CCRC.)

LNHA   Licensed nursing home administrator. (See NHA.)

LOC   Level of care: Classification term used by providers, regulators, and third-party payers to describe the type and amount of care a person requires.

LOI   Letter of intent: Nonbinding document detailing a planned action on the part of an organization or individual.

LOS   Length of stay (or service): Period of time a person remains in a healthcare facility as an inpatient (or receives home- and community-based services (HCBS).

LPN   Licensed practical nurse: Professional nurse who has completed a state-approved academic program and passed the NCLEX-PN[R] exam. (See also LVN.)

LSC	Life Safety Code, NFPA 101: Most widely adopted standards for building design safety, published by the National Fire Protection Association (NFPA) with three central goals—protection of life, protection of property, and restoration and use of a building following a fire or other emergencies, such as earthquakes, floods, blackouts, and terrorism.
LSOA	Longitudinal Study of Aging (I and II): Collaborative effort of the National Center for Health Statistics (NCHS) and the National Institute on Aging (NIA) to perform a prospective study of noninstitutionalized persons 70 years of age and over from 1984—1999.
LTAC	Long-term acute care: Treatment of persons with serious medical conditions requiring ongoing care, but no longer requiring intensive care or extensive diagnostic procedures.
LTACH	Long-term acute care hospital: Facilities that specialize in the treatment of persons with serious medical conditions requiring ongoing care, but no longer requiring intensive care or extensive diagnostic procedures.
LTC	Long-term care: Supports and services that include medical and non-medical care provided to people who are unable to perform basic activities of daily living, whether at home or in a congregate living setting.
LTCF	Long-term care facility: Residential community that provides long-term care services.
LTCI	Long-term care insurance: Insurance policy that provides reimbursement for services performed by a long-term care provider for a person who needs constant supervision due to having a chronic or disabling condition.
LTC Partnership	Joint federal state policy initiative to promote the purchase of private long-term care insurance by shielding contract holders from Medicaid spend-down requirements through innovative coverage design (not available in all states).
LTD	Long-term disability insurance: Private insurance coverage that, following a qualifying period (typically 3–6 months), at least partially replaces a person's income in the event of a medical condition that stops them from working; commonly provided by employers under a group policy.
LVN	Licensed vocational nurse: Professional nurse who has completed a state-approved academic program and passed the NCLEX-PN[R] exam. (See also LPN.)

M

MA	Medical assistance: Synonym for a state's Medicaid program.
	or
	Medical assistant: Person who performs a variety of routine administrative and clinical tasks in a clinical healthcare setting, under the direction of a qualified licensed health professional.

MAC   Medicare administrative contractor: Private health insurer that has been awarded a geographic area or "jurisdiction" to regionally manage the policies and process medical claims for Medicare beneficiaries.

MAR   Medication administration record: Schedule for administering medications to a patient for a defined period of time, including dosing, timing of administration, and details about the physician's orders.

Market segmentation   Process of dividing a large market into smaller units in order to more finitely describe an organization's target market.

MCO   Managed care organization: Non-governmental organization (for-profit or not-for-profit) that develops, coordinates, and monitors individualized service plans, typically for Medicaid beneficiaries. (See also CMO.)

MD   Medical doctor (physician): Professional degree awarded by accredited academic programs in allopathic (traditional) medicine for completing the required course of study; physicians diagnose and treat conditions of the whole body (or specialize in one aspect or body system) and educate patients on medical conditions and preventive care.

MDS   Minimum data set: Tool for implementing standardized assessment and for facilitating care management in Medicare-certified skilled nursing facilities (SNFs) and noncritical access hospital swing beds (SBs).

MED   Mixed etiology dementias: In a person with mixed dementia, it may not be clear exactly how many of a person's symptoms are due to Alzheimer's disease or another type of dementia. (See also ADRD.)

Mediation   Alternative dispute resolution (ADR) method with a neutral person helping the parties find a solution to their dispute.

Medicaid   Title 19 of the Social Security Act; jointly funded federal state health insurance program for medically indigent citizens that is administered by each participating state; largest public pay source for senior living services. (See also Title 19.)

Medically Indigent   Person who does not have—and cannot afford—health insurance.

Medicare   Title 18 of the Social Security Act; federal healthcare entitlement and insurance program for older and certain disabled adults, as well as people with end-stage renal disease (ESRD). (See also Title 18.)

MedPAC   Medicare Payment Advisory Commission: Nonpartisan federal legislative agency established by the Balanced Budget Act of 1997 to provide Congress with analysis and policy advice concerning the Medicare program. http://medpac.gov

MEPS   Medical Expenditure Panel Survey: Set of large-scale surveys of families and individuals, their medical providers, and employers across the United States that provides the most comprehensive source of data available on the cost and use of healthcare and health insurance coverage.

MFCU   Medicaid Fraud Control Unit: State agency that investigates and prosecutes Medicaid provider fraud, as well as patient abuse or neglect, in healthcare facilities and board and care facilities; operates in all states, the District of Columbia, Puerto Rico, and the U.S. Virgin Islands.

MFP	Money follows the person: Federal program designed to move elderly Medicaid recipients out of nursing homes into their own homes (or into their families' homes); the program also includes, in some states, persons considered at risk of nursing home placement.
MGMA	Medical Group Management Association: Nonprofit professional society advocating for and addressing the interests of its member medical group practice managers, with the mission of empowering medical group practices, providers, and patients to create meaningful change in healthcare. https://www.mgma.com
MH/SA (or MHSA)	Mental health and substance abuse. (See SA/MH—Substance Abuse and Mental Health.)
MHA	Master's degree in healthcare administration: Graduate degree awarded by an institution of higher education for completing an academic program in healthcare management and leadership, typically accredited by the Commission on Accreditation of Healthcare Management Education (CAHME).
	or
	Mental Health Authority: Federally recognized state agency with responsibility for overseeing public programs for the benefit of people with mental illness.
MHBG	(Community) Mental Health (Services) Block Grant: Federal grant awarded to states and territories by Substance Abuse and Mental Health Services Administration (SAMHSA) to improve access to community-based healthcare delivery systems for adults with serious mental illnesses and children with serious emotional disturbances.
MHPA	Mental Health Parity Act of 1996: Federal law that prohibits large group health plans from imposing annual or lifetime dollar limits on mental health benefits that are less favorable than those imposed on medical/surgical benefits.
MHSA	Master's degree in health services administration. (See MHA—master's degree in healthcare administration.)
MIG	Medicaid Infrastructure Grant: Competitive federal grant program that has provided funding to states for Medicaid infrastructure development and build supports for people with disabilities who would like to be employed.
MIPPA	Medicare Improvements for Patients and Providers Act of 2008: Multifaceted federal law that introduced new funding for State Health Insurance Assistance Programs (SHIPs), Area Agencies on Aging (AAAs), and Aging and Disability Resource Centers (ADRCs) to help low-income Medicare beneficiaries apply for programs that make Medicare affordable.
MMA	Medicare Prescription Drug Improvement and Modernization Act of 2003: Federal law that among several modifications to Medicare introduced a new voluntary prescription drug benefit program (Part D).
MMIS	Medicaid management information system: Integrated group of procedures and computer processing operations (subsystems) developed at the general design level to meet principal data management objectives for state Medicaid programs.

MMSE   Mini-Mental Status (or Folstein) Examination: Brief, structured test of mental status; the most widely used test to assess problems with memory and other cognitive functions.

MOU   Memorandum of understanding: A nonbinding agreement between at least two parties that outlines the responsibilities of each of the parties to the agreement.

MR/DD   Mental retardation and other developmental disabilities: Mental retardation is a developmental disability that first appears in children under 18 years, which is characterized by an intellectual functioning level that is well below average (as measured by standard tests for intelligence quotient) and significant limitations in performing daily living skills (adaptive functioning). (See also IDD—intellectual and developmental disabilities.)

MRSA   Methicillin-resistant *Staphylococcus aureus*: Bacterium that causes infections and is more difficult to treat than most strains of bacteria because it does not respond to many of the most commonly used antibiotics.

MS   Multiple sclerosis: Chronic, progressive disease involving damage to the sheaths (myelin) of nerve cells in the brain and spinal cord resulting from the immune system abnormally attacking them.

MSD   Musculoskeletal disorder: Injury or illness affecting the connective tissues, such as cartilage, joints, muscles, nerves, tendons, or spinal discs.

MSDS   Material safety data sheet: Documentation concerning potentially hazardous chemicals or components in a particular substance or product.

MSW   Master's degree in social work: Graduate degree awarded by an institution of higher education for completing an academic program in social services, typically accredited by the Council on Social Work Education (CSWE).

N

N4A   National Association of Area Agencies on Aging: Nonprofit association advocating for and addressing the interests of its member Area Agencies on Aging, with the mission of building the capacity of its members so they can help older adults and people with disabilities live with dignity and choices in their homes and communities for as long as possible. https://www.n4a.org

NAAP   National Association of Activities Professionals: Nonprofit professional society advocating for and addressing the interests of its member LTC activity professionals, with the mission of providing excellence in professional support services for activity professionals in the promotion of standards, ethics, competencies, education, and advocacy. https://naap.info

NAB   National Association of Long-Term Care Administrator Boards: Nonprofit association advocating for and supporting the interests of its member professional licensing boards governing the practice of long-term care administration. https://www.nabweb.org

NACA	National Advisory Council on Aging: Advises the Secretary of the Department of Health and Human Services, Director of the National Institutes of Heath, and Director of National Institute on Aging by reviewing and recommending applications for research and training concerning aging services. https://www.nia.nih.gov/about/naca
NADONA/ LTC	National Association of Directors of Nursing Administration/Long-Term Care: Nonprofit professional society advocating for and addressing the interests of its member Directors of Nursing in long-term care settings. https://www.nadona.org
NAHC	National Association for Home Care and Hospice: Nonprofit trade association advocating for and addressing the interests of its member providers of home care and hospice services, with the mission of promoting, protecting, and advancing the highest quality healthcare at home. https://www.nahc.org
NAHMA	National Affordable Housing Management Association: Nonprofit professional society advocating for and addressing the interests of its member managers and sponsors of affordable housing for seniors and families, with the mission of supporting legislative and regulatory policy that promotes the development and preservation of decent and safe affordable housing. https://www.nahma.org
NAMI	National Alliance on Mental Illness: Nonprofit membership association representing the interests of its members, with the mission of providing advocacy, education, support, and public awareness so that all individuals and families affected by mental illness can build better lives. https://www.nami.org
NAPSA	National Adult Protective Services Association: Nonprofit association advocating for and addressing the interests of its member adult protective service agencies, with the mission of strengthening Adult Protective Services programs in order to improve the safety and quality of life of vulnerable adults who are victims of abuse, neglect, self-neglect, or financial exploitation. https://www.napsa-now.org
NASUA	National Association of State Units on Aging. (Now Advancing States.)
NASW	National Association of Social Workers: Nonprofit professional society advocating for and addressing the interests of its member social services professionals, with the mission of promoting the quality and effectiveness of social work practice in the United States through services to individuals, groups, and communities. https://www.socialworkers.org
NBCOT	National Board for Certification in Occupational Therapy: National standards board for the profession of occupational therapy, with the mission of serving the public interest by advancing client care and professional practice through evidence-based certification standards and the validation of knowledge essential for effective practice in occupational therapy. https://www.nbcot.org
NCAL	National Center for Assisted Living: Nonprofit trade association (affiliated with AHCA) representing the interests of its member assisted living and residential care communities, with the mission of leading the assisted living profession through public policy advocacy, knowledge, education, and professional development. https://www.ahcancal.org

NCCAP   National Certification Council for Activities Professionals: Affiliate of the National Association of Activities Professionals; governs practice standards regarding quality of life, activities, and engagement across all senior living care settings.

NCCNHR   National Consumer Voice for Quality Long-Term Care (formerly the National Citizen's Coalition for Nursing Home Reform): Nonprofit consumer advocacy non-governmental organization with the mission of improving the nation's long-term care system and quality of life for consumers of long-term care. http://nursinghomeaction.org

NCCPA   National Council of Certification of Physician Assistants: Standards-setting body governing professional certification for Physician's Assistants. https://www.nccpa.net

NCD   National Council on Disability: Independent federal agency charged with advising the President, Congress, and other federal agencies regarding policies, programs, practices, and procedures that affect people with disabilities. https://ncd.gov

NCEA   National Center on Elder Abuse: Federal agency under the U.S. Administration on Aging charged with serving as a national resource center dedicated to the prevention of elder mistreatment, with the mission of improving the national response to elder abuse, neglect, and exploitation; it aims to gather, house, disseminate, and stimulate innovative, validated methods of practice, education, research, and policy. https://ncea.acl.gov

NCHS   National Center for Health Statistics: Federal agency under the Centers for Disease Control and Prevention (CDC) that compiles statistical information to help guide policies to improve the health of Americans. https://www.cdc.gov/nchs

NCLEX-PN®   National Council Licensure Examination-Practical Nurse: Exam administered by National Council of State Boards of Nursing (NCSBN) to practical nurses (PNs) to measure a person's command of appropriate professional nursing knowledge and skills for state licensure as a practical (or vocational) nurse.

NCLEX-RN®   National Council Licensure Examination-Registered Nurse: Exam administered by National Council of State Boards of Nursing (NCSBN) to RNs to measure a person's command of appropriate professional nursing knowledge and skills for state licensure as a registered nurse.

NCOA   National Council on the Aging: Nonprofit membership association advocating for and addressing the interests of its members, with the mission of improving the lives of older adults, especially those who are struggling. https://www.ncoa.org

NCQA   National Committee for Quality Assurance: Private non-governmental organization dedicated to improving healthcare quality through its evidence-based tools, such as HEDIS (Health Effectiveness Data and Information Set). https://www.ncqa.org

NCSBN   National Council of State Boards of Nursing: Nonprofit professional association that advocates for and represents the interests of its member state boards of nursing, including administration of the national licensing examinations for RNs and LPN/LVNs. https://www.ncsbn.org

NCSL   National Conference of State Legislatures: Nonprofit association representing the interests of legislatures in the states, territories, and commonwealths of the United States with the mission of advancing the effectiveness, independence, and integrity of legislatures, fostering interstate cooperation and facilitating the exchange of information among legislatures. https://www.ncsl.org

NCVHS   National Committee on Vital and Health Statistics: Public advisory body for the Department of Health and Human Services concerning health data, statistics, privacy, national health information policy, and the Health Insurance Portability and Accountability Act (HIPAA). https://ncvhs.hhs.gov

NDC   National Drug Code: Universal product identifier for human medications in the United States that assigns a unique 10-digit or 11-digit, 3-segment number, to each product approved by the FDA (manufacturer + product + commercial packet size).

NDI   National Death Index: National Center for Health Statistics (NCHS)'s centralized database of death record information on file in state vital statistics offices; key resource for epidemiologists and other health and medical investigators with their mortality research activities.

Neglect   Failure to provide nourishment, treatment, care, goods, or services necessary for the health, safety, or welfare of a person receiving care.

Negligence   Failure by an individual to exercise the degree of care or caution that could be reasonably expected.

NF   Nursing facility: Residential healthcare facility licensed by the state to provide room, board, specified nursing care, and therapies, for people with chronic conditions or who need rehabilitation services; sometimes used interchangeably with skilled nursing facility (SNF) or nursing home (NH).

NFCSP   National Family Caregiver Support Program: U.S. Administration on Community Living (ACL)'s assistance program that provides grants to states and territories to fund various supports that help family and informal caregivers care for older adults in their homes for as long as possible.

NFPA   National Fire Protection Association: Nonprofit international non-governmental organization devoted to eliminating death, injury, property, and economic loss due to fire, electrical, and natural hazards through evidence-based building standards. (See also LSC—Life Safety Code.) https://www.nfpa.org

NGO   Non-government organization: Citizen-based group (typically nonprofit) that functions independently of government to serve a specific social or political purpose.

NH   Nursing home. (See NF—nursing facility.)

NHA   Nursing home administrator: Executive leader of a postacute care facility providing skilled nursing care; states are federally mandated to license NHAs as health professionals (this acronym often applies to the licensure credential, as well).

NHIC   National Health Information Center: Federal agency under the Department of Health and Human Services' Office of Disease Prevention and Health Promotion that supports public health education and promotion by raising awareness about National Health Observances year-round and helps connect health professionals and consumers to the organizations that can best answer their questions. https://health.gov/our-work/health-literacy/resources/national-health-information-center

NHPCO   National Hospice and Palliative Care Organization: Nonprofit professional association advocating for and representing the interests of its member providers and professionals who care for people affected by serious and life-limiting illness, with the mission of leading and mobilizing social change for improved care at the end of life. https://www.nhpco.org

NHQI   Nursing Home Quality Initiative: Centers for Medicare & Medicaid Services program that provides consumer and provider information regarding the quality of care in nursing homes. https://www.cms.gov/Medicare/Quality-Initiatives-Patient-Assessment-Instruments/NursingHomeQualityInits

NHRA   Nursing Home Reform Act. (See OBRA—Omnibus Budget Reconciliation Act of 1987.)

NHSC   National Health Services Corps: Federal program administered by the Health Resources and Services Administration (HRSA) that provides scholarships and loan repayment to healthcare professionals practicing at approved sites located in/or serving health professional shortage areas (HPSAs) throughout the United States. https://nhsc.hrsa.gov

NIH   National Institutes of Health: Federal agency under the Department of Health and Human Services that serves as the principal catalyst for health research in the United States through conducting and sponsoring original investigations that support its mission of seeking fundamental knowledge about the nature and behavior of living systems and the application of that knowledge to enhance health, lengthen life, and reduce illness and disability; 27 institutes of health comprise the agency, including the following list of those most closely tied with the senior living field. https://www.nih.gov

- NIA   National Institute on Aging: https://www.nia.nih.gov
- NCI   National Cancer Institute: https://www.cancer.gov
- NEA   National Eye Institute: https://www.nei.nih.gov
- NHLBI   National Heart, Lung and Blood Institute: https://www.nhlbi.nih.gov
- NIAAA   National Institute of Alcohol Abuse and Alcoholism: https://www.niaaa.nih.gov
- NIAID   National Institute of Allergy and Infectious Diseases: https://www.niaid.nih.gov
- NIAMS   National Institute of Arthritis and Musculoskeletal and Skin Diseases: https://www.niams.nih.gov
- NIDCD   National Institute on Deafness and Other Communication Disorders: https://www.nidcd.nih.gov

- ■ NIDDK   National Institute of Diabetes and Digestive and Kidney Diseases: https://www.niddk.nih.gov
- ■ NIDA   National Institute of Drug Abuse: https://www.drugabuse.gov
- ■ NIMH   National Institute of Mental Health: https://www.nimh.nih.gov
- ■ NINDS   National Institute of Neurologic Disorders and Stroke: https://www.ninds.nih.gov

NLC   Nurse Licensure Compact: Agreement among over two thirds of state boards of nursing that enables nurses—RNs and LPN/LVNs—to practice in other NLC states without having to obtain additional licenses. Visit: https://www.ncsbn.org/compacts.htm

NLRA   National Labor Relations Act of 1935 (Wagner Act and subsequent amendments): Federal law that permits employees to organize a collective bargaining unit, typically through joining a union, without fear of retribution from their employer.

NLRB   National Labor Relations Board: Federal agency established by the NLRA to administer the law's provisions, including conducting union recognition elections and investigating allegations of unfair labor practices.

NNHQI   National Nursing Home Quality Improvement Campaign" (formerly "Advancing Excellence in Nursing Homes Campaign"): National collaborative effort to transform the quality of care and quality of life for nursing home residents. https://theconsumervoice.org/issues/recipients/nursing-home-residents/advancing-excellence

NOFA   Notice of Fund Allocation: Announcement notice published each year for the Department of Housing and Urban Development's Discretionary Funding Programs; describes types of funding available on a competitive basis and provides instructions for applying.

NORC   Naturally occurring retirement community: Building or neighborhood that was not originally intended as a senior living environment but has a substantial number or proportion of residents aged 60 years or older, generally because people have moved into a home when they were younger and have aged there.

or

National Long-Term Care Ombudsman Resource Center: Nonprofit NGO funded by the Department of Health and Human Services' Administration for Community Living (ACL) and jointly operated by the National Consumer Voice for Quality Long-Term Care and Advancing States with the objectives of enhancing the skills, knowledge, and management capacity of state long-term care ombudsman programs. https://ltcombudsman.org

NORS   National Ombudsman Reporting System: Federal program of the Administration on Community Living's Administration on Aging (AoA) that collects and analyzes complaints received and investigated by state nursing home ombudsman offices to inform policy decisions. https://acl.gov/programs/long-term-care-ombudsman/ltc-ombudsman-national-and-state-data

Nosocomial Negative health condition caused by a medical or healthcare procedure.

NP Nonprofit: Exempt from taxation, typically under section 501(c)(3) of the U.S. Internal Revenue Code.

or

Nurse practitioner: Advanced nursing professional job title; common for an NP to include MSN or DNP in their professional title in order to disclose level of educational attainment. (See also ARNP—advanced registered nurse practitioner.)

NPA National PACE® Association: Nonprofit professional association advocating for and representing the interests of its member organizations operating a PACE® (Programs of All-Inclusive Care for the Elderly) with the mission of providing leadership and support for the growth, innovation, quality, and success of the PACE® model of care. https://www.npaonline.org

NPE Nutrition Program for the Elderly: Federal program that provides grants to operate nutrition programs for the elderly (i.e., Meals-on-Wheels and congregate dining programs) and additional cash payments or commodity assistance for each meal served; title III of the Older Americans Act.

NPI National provider identifier: Unique 10-digit identification number issued by the Centers for Medicare & Medicaid Services (CMS) to healthcare providers; replaced the unique physician identification number (UPIN) as the required identifier for Medicare services; also used by other payers.

NSCSL National Senior Citizens Law Center: Nonprofit non-governmental organization with the mission of protecting the rights of low-income older adults through its advocacy and education of local advocates, programs, and litigation assistance. http://nsclcarchives.org

O

OAA Older Americans Act of 1965 as amended (42 U.S.C.A. § 3001 et seq.): Federal law that promotes the well-being of older individuals by providing services and programs designed to help them live independently in their homes and communities. The Act also empowers the federal government to distribute funds to the states for supportive services for individuals over the age of 60 years.

OASDI Old-Age, Survivors and Disability Insurance: Official name for Social Security benefits, supported by payroll taxes to provide benefits to retirees and disabled people, as well as their spouses, children, and survivors.

OASIS Outcome and Assessment Information Set: Assessment tool developed by the Centers for Medicare & Medicaid Services for conducting a comprehensive evaluation of an adult home care patient forms the basis for measuring patient outcomes and determines agency reimbursement.

OBRA   Omnibus Budget Reconciliation Act: Although several laws enacted in different years by Congress and signed by the president have this name followed by the year, the one that is often also referred to as the *Nursing Home Reform Act* advanced in 1987, and it is interpreted by 42 CFR 483.

OD   Doctor of Optometry: Degree awarded by accredited academic programs in optometry for completing the required course of study; optometrists diagnose and treat diseases of the eye, perform certain eye surgeries, and prescribe corrective eyeglasses or contact lenses.

OIG   Office of the Inspector General: Many federal and state agencies have a unit charged with combatting fraud, waste, and abuse to improve the efficiency of the agency's programs, commonly titled the Inspector General. The largest OIG at the federal level serves the Department of Health and Human Services, and its major focus is on the Medicare and Medicaid programs; its oversight also extends to the Centers for Disease Control and Prevention (CDC), National Institutes of Health (NIH), and the Food and Drug Administration (FDA). State-level OIG personnel typically perform inspections (surveys) of Medicare-certified provider organizations under contract with the Centers for Medicare & Medicaid Services (CMS).

OIS   U.S. Office of Information Services: Federal agency under the National Archives charged with reviewing compliance of all federal agencies with Freedom of Information Act (FOIA) policies, procedures, identifying, and recommending ways to improve it and resolving FOIA disputes between federal agencies and requesters. https://www.archives.gov/ogis

OMB   U.S. Office of Management and Budget: Federal agency evaluates, formulates, and coordinates management procedures and program objectives among federal agencies, oversees the administration of the federal budget, and advises the President concerning budget proposals and related legislative initiatives. www.whitehouse.gov/omb

OOP   Out-of-pocket: Personal share of expenditures for health and related services.

OSCAR   Online Survey Certification and Reporting: (now CASPER)

OSG   U.S. Office of the Surgeon General: America's lead medical officer, whose mission is to protect, promote, and advance the health and safety the nation. https://www.hhs.gov/surgeongeneral

OSHA   U.S. Occupational Safety and Health Administration: Federal agency under the Department of Labor that ensures safe and healthful workplace conditions by setting and enforcing standards and providing training, outreach, education, and assistance. https://www.osha.gov

OT   Occupational therapy: Healthcare profession that uses purposeful activity or interventions designed to achieve functional outcomes to develop, improve, sustain, or restore the highest possible level of independence.

OT/R Registered occupational therapist: Credential that signifies a person is registered by the National Board for Certification in Occupational Therapy.

OTR/L Occupational therapist registered and licensed: Standard credential that signifies a person is both registered by the National Board for Certification in Occupational Therapy and licensed by at least one state.

P

P&A Protection and Advocacy Systems: Initiative of the U.S. Administration on Community Living, P&As work at the state level to protect individuals with disabilities by empowering them and advocating for their rights to make choices, contribute to society, and live independently.

P&L Profit and loss statement: Financial statement showing performance over a specified period.

P4P Pay for performance: Reimbursement model that offers financial incentives to healthcare providers for meeting certain quality and productivity performance measures. (See also value-based purchasing.)

PA Physician assistant: Must work under the supervision of a licensed physician but generally has a broad spectrum of clinical practice, including authority to diagnose and prescribe medications, approve plans of care and treatment approaches, and document progress.

PAC Postacute care: Chronic, rehabilitation, or palliative services received before, after, or instead of a stay in an acute care hospital, typically in a long-term care facility, at home, or through outpatient therapy.

PACE Program of All-Inclusive Care for the Elderly: Care model that utilizes an adult day program as the hub of the wheel for an HCBS-oriented IDT to coordinate housing, medical, and social supports for people who meet the Medicaid eligibility requirements for nursing home care.

PAH/PPH Potentially avoidable (or preventable) hospitalization: Key metric under the ACA, readmission to an acute care facility within 30 days of discharge for the same primary diagnosis; the diagnoses most commonly associated with PAH/PPH of nursing home residents include pneumonia, urinary tract infection, dehydration, pressure ulcers, cellulitis, heart failure, and chronic obstructive pulmonary disease/asthma.

PAI Patient assessment instrument: Centers for Medicare & Medicaid Services' assessment tool for use in the inpatient rehabilitation facility setting; similar to the minimum data set used in skilled nursing facilities, but geared to patients with higher acuity and/or medical complexity.

Parenteral nutrition Providing nutrients directly into the bloodstream when the gastrointestinal system is not functioning normally.

Parkinson's disease Progressive central nervous system disorder characterized by gait difficulty, postural instability, rigidity, decrease in spontaneous movement, and/or tremors.

Par level   Minimum number of a given supply to maintain in inventory (in use and in storage).

PAS   Preadmission screening: Assessment prior to admission to a facility or HCBS program of care.

PASARR   Preadmission screening and annual resident review: Federal requirement to help ensure that no individual with serious mental illness (SMI) or intellectual and developmental disability (IDD) is inappropriately placed in an skilled nursing facility.

Patient days   Cumulative number of care recipients (patients/residents/clients/participants/customers) over a specified period (census per day × days).

PBM   Pharmacy benefit manager: Company that manages prescription drug benefits on behalf of health insurance carriers, Medicare Part D drug plans, large employers, and other payers, negotiating with drug manufacturers and pharmacies to control drug spending.

PC   Personal care: Nonmedical assistance with activities of daily living (ADL) and instrumental activities of daily living (IADL).

PCA   Personal care aide/assistant/attendant: Unlicensed paraprofessional who provides personal care services.

PCH   Personal care home: Residential, congregate, senior living setting providing room, board, and personal care services; licensed in some states.

PCP   Primary care physician: Specialist in family medicine, internal medicine, geriatrics, or pediatrics who provides comprehensive, point-of-first-contact and continuing medical care, which may include chronic, preventive, and acute care in both inpatient and outpatient settings.

PDCA   Plan–do–check–act (Deming Wheel or Shewhart Cycle): Four-step management cycle that facilitates implementing change, problem-solving, and continuous process improvement.

PDP   Prescription drug plan: Stand-alone health plan covering prescription drugs under Medicare Part C (Advantage) or Part D.

PDPM   Person-driven payment model: Reimbursement system implemented by the Centers for Medicare & Medicaid Services in 2019 for skilled nursing facility care that replaced the prospective payment system (PPS) with case mix classifications based on anticipated resource needs.

PDUFA   Prescription Drug User Fee Act of 1992 (and amendments): Federal law that permits the U.S. Food and Drug Administration (FDA) to collect fees from drug manufacturers to fund the approval process for new drugs.

PEG tube   Percutaneous endoscopic gastrostomy tube: Small tube placed directly into the stomach through an incision in the abdominal wall to provide nutrition to someone unable to ingest food by mouth for an extended period.

Per diem   Per day (i.e., per diem reimbursement = daily revenue rate).

PERS	Personal emergency response system: Aging in place technology that initiates communication with an entity—commercial or private (family or neighbor)—capable of responding directly or indirectly by referral; a wide range of products from the most basic, wearable pendant with a call button to an advanced network of in-home sensors that monitor movement, activity, and/or vital signs and report data in real time to caregivers, family members, and first responders; also referred to as life alerts, medical alerts, fall monitors, electronic home monitoring, or telemonitoring.
Person-centered care	Philosophy of care focused on the care recipient's emotional needs and preferences, emphasizing relationships (social model) rather than a task-centered, institution-driven approach concerned chiefly with physical health (medical model); also referred to as person-centered approach (PCA) or resident-centered care (RCC).
Person-directed care	Philosophy of care that embraces as its foundation person-**centered** care (PCC), adding the expectations that care recipients *direct* their own lives and that staffing and schedules are organized to reflect their preferences.
PHA	Public Housing Authority: Government entity authorized to administer HUD programs. (Varies by state.)
PharmD	Doctor of Pharmacy: Degree awarded by accredited academic programs in pharmacy for completing the required course of study. (See also DP.)
PHI	Protected (or personal) health information: Individually identifiable health data created, received, stored, or transmitted by HIPAA-covered entities and their business associates concerning the provision of healthcare, healthcare operations, and payment for healthcare services.
PHS	U.S. Public Health Service: Federal agency responsible for administering several health agencies critical to the health of Americans, including the Food and Drug Administration (FDA), Centers for Disease Control and Prevention (CDC), and National Institutes of Health (NIH).
PI	Principal investigator: Individual primarily responsible for the preparation, conduct, and administration of a research grant, cooperative agreement, training or public service project, contract, or other sponsored project in compliance with applicable laws, regulations, and institutional policies.
	or
	Performance improvement: Management function of continuous study and improvement of processes with the intent to better services or outcomes, and prevent or decrease the likelihood of problems, by identifying areas of opportunity and testing new approaches to correcting underlying causes of persistent/systemic problems or barriers to improvement (CMS, 2020).
Pioneer network	Nonprofit non-governmental organization advocating for the shared goal of senior living providers interested in moving toward a more person-centered and person-directed approach in their programs and services. https://www.pioneernetwork.net

PIP	Performance improvement project: Key element of quality assurance and performance improvement (QAPI); concentrating on a problem in either one area or organization-wide by systematically gathering information to clarify issues or problems and then intervening to stimulate and foster improvements.
PNA	Personal needs allowance: Monthly amount the state permits a Medicaid-certified senior living beneficiary to keep for noncovered personal expenses as a deduction from what they pay to the provider. (Varies by state, but the Centers for Medicare & Medicaid Services sets minimum and maximum amounts.)
POA	Power of attorney: Legal document designating a person as the agent (attorney-in-fact) for another (principal) to act on their behalf with either limited or broad legal authority concerning the principal's property, finances, and/or medical care; typically used in the event of a principal's illness, disability, incapacity, or unavailability.
POC	Plan of correction: Written document developed by the senior living provider that specifies how each finding of regulatory noncompliance, violation, or deficiency identified by a governmental agency inspection will be abated and how recurrence will be prevented.
	or
	Point of care: Diagnostic testing or documentation completed at or near the time and place of patient care. (See also POS—place or point of service.)
	or
	Political Action Committee: Group organized to engage in political election activities—especially fundraising or campaigning—in support of (or opposition to) a candidate based on their position concerning a social, economic, or political cause viewed as important to the group.
POS	Place (or point) of Service. (See POC—point of care.)
PPA	Preferred provider agreement (arrangement): Third-party payer contract with a group of healthcare providers willing to furnish services at discounted rates in return for increased patient volume and prompt payment. (See also PPO.)
PPACA	Patient Protection and Affordable Care Act of 2010 (and amendments): Comprehensive federal healthcare reform law addressing health insurance coverage, healthcare costs, and preventive care. (See also ACA.)
PPD	Patient per pay: Measure of daily revenues/costs for each resident/patient.
PPO	Preferred provider organization: Group of healthcare providers that agrees to furnish services to customers of a third-party insurer at discounted rates in return for increased patient volume and prompt payment. (See also PPA.)
PPS	Prospective payment system: Reimbursement method by which payment is made based on a predetermined price.
PQ	Partnership qualified: Long-term care insurance policies must include certain features to be eligible for inclusion in the State Long-Term Care Partnership Program, such as designation as federally tax-qualified and inflation protection. (Varies by state.)

PRN	Pro re nata: Latin term that means "as needed"; typically applied to medication administration or scheduling part-time employees.
PRO	Peer (physician) review organization: Independent quality improvement or professional review organization staffed by licensed health professionals who conduct preadmission and service reviews concerning Medicare-certified providers.
ProPAC	Prospective Payment Assessment Commission: Independent advisory body that recommends to Congress and the Department of Health and Human Services Secretary an appropriate percentage change in the payments made by Medicare for inpatient hospital services and adjustments to the diagnosis-related groups (DRGs) classification and weighting factors. (The Balanced Budget Act of 1997 terminated the ProPAC and reassigned its duties to the Medicare Payment Advisory Commission—MedPAC.)
PRTF	Psychiatric residential treatment facility: Nonhospital facility offering intensive inpatient services to persons under 21 years who have various emotional and mental health challenges.
PSDA	Patient Self-Determination Act of 1990 (and amendments): Federal law that requires Medicare- and Medicaid-certified healthcare providers to ask each patient about advance directives and to provide information regarding the applicable state law; does not include physicians.
PSR	Physical status review: Assessment tool for an interdisciplinary team (IDT) to quantify a person's health risk, establish their health care needs, identify related training requirements for direct care staff, and determine the optimal frequency of direct health monitoring; used primarily in MR/IDD service settings.
PT	Physical therapist: Licensed health professional who treats people to restore movement, relieve pain, improve strength, and prevent disability through prescribed exercise, hands-on care, and patient education.
	or
	Physical therapy: Health profession dedicated to the preservation, enhancement or restoration of movement, and physical function diminished or threatened by disease, injury, or disability utilizing therapeutic exercise, physical modalities, assistive devices, and patient education. (Also called physiotherapy.)
PTA	Physical therapy assistant/aide: Direct caregiver who works under the supervision of a PT.
Punitive damages	Monetary award in excess of the actual losses claimed by a plaintiff intended to make an example of a defendant due to extraordinarily egregious conduct.
Q	
QA	Quality assurance: Management process focused on providing confidence that quality requirements and expectations are met or exceeded; specification of standards for quality of service and outcomes; ongoing, both anticipatory and retrospective in its efforts to identify how the organization is performing.

QAA   Quality assessment and assurance: Synonym for quality assurance adding emphasis on initial assessment of quality indicators.

QAPI   Quality assurance and performance improvement: Coordinated application of two mutually reinforcing aspects of a quality management system—quality assurance (QA) and performance improvement (PI). QAPI takes a systematic, comprehensive, and data-driven approach to maintaining and improving safety and quality in nursing homes while involving all nursing home caregivers in practical and creative problem-solving.

QI   Quality improvement. (See QAPI.)

or

Quality indicator: Standardized, evidence-based measures of healthcare quality that can be used to measure and track clinical performance and outcomes.

QIO   Quality improvement organization: One of two CMS-designated groups of health quality experts, clinicians, and consumers organized to improve the quality of care delivered to people with Medicare.

- BFCC-QIO—beneficiary and family-centered QIO: Helps Medicare beneficiaries exercise their right to high-quality healthcare by managing beneficiary complaints, quality of care reviews, and beneficiary appeals of a provider's decision to discharge or discontinue services.
- QIN-QIO—Quality innovation network: Coordinates data-driven initiatives to increase patient safety, improve community health posthospital care, and improve clinical quality.

QM   Quality measures: Tools that help measure healthcare processes, outcomes, patient perceptions, and organizational structure and/or systems associated with either the ability to provide high-quality healthcare or that relate to healthcare quality goals.

QMB   Qualified Medicare beneficiary: Person who is enrolled in both Medicare and Medicaid and has no legal obligation to pay Medicare providers for Part A or B cost sharing (coinsurance, copays, or deductibles); many state Medicaid programs pay for some portion of this cost.

QMHP   Qualified mental health professional: Clinician who is trained and experienced in providing psychiatric or mental health services to persons with a psychiatric diagnosis. (Varies by state.)

QRS   (Hospital inpatient) Quality reporting system: Centers for Medicare & Medicaid Services quality incentive program that rewards hospitals that report designated quality measures with a higher annual update to their reimbursement rates.

Quality Standard of excellence; the World Health Organization (WHO) defines quality care as the extent to which healthcare services provided to individuals and patient populations improve desired health outcomes. In order to achieve this, healthcare must be safe, effective, timely, efficient, equitable, and people-centered.

Quality of life Value of the lived experience; integration of social, emotional, personal, and spiritual wellness with environmental comfort, dignity, autonomy, security, and life fulfillment for a care recipient.

Qui tam relator "Whistleblower" under False Claims Act, who has knowledge of someone or an organization defrauding the government.

R

RAI Resident assessment instrument: Centers for Medicare & Medicaid Services assessment tool designed to collect information for care planning and for monitoring residents in long-term care settings; clinical assessment element for completing the minimum data set (MDS).

RAM Random access memory: Form of computer data storage that can be retrieved randomly and swiftly; referred to as volatile memory (lost when power is discontinued).

or

Reverse annuity mortgage: Loan from a lending institution to someone 62 years or older, which is secured by the borrower's home value in which they receive a lump sum, fixed monthly payments, or line of credit and makes no loan payments; becomes due when the borrower dies, moves away permanently, or sells the home; federal regulations prohibit the loan amount from exceeding the home's value.

RAP Resident assessment protocol: Documents included in CMS resident assessment instrument (RAI) that helps determine which persons are at the risk of specific functional disabilities.

RBRVS Resource-based relative value scale: CMS scale of national uniform relative values for all physicians' services reflecting the sum of relative value units representing a physician's practice expenses net of malpractice and professional liability insurance costs.

RC/AL Residential care/assisted living: Type of housing facility for older or disabled adults who may require assistance with their activities of daily living; licensure requirements vary by state. (See also AL—assisted living.)

RD Registered dietitian: Trained nutrition professional who has met the educational and experiential standards set forth by the Commission on Dietetic Registration (CDR) of the Academy of Nutrition and Dietetics (AND), as well as pass the CDR's Registration Examination for Dietitians; licensure varies by state.

RDT Registered dietetic technician: Credential awarded by the Association of Nutrition and Food Service Professionals for demonstrating basic proficiency in relevant knowledge and skills for serving as a dietetic technician.

Reasonable accommodation Actions to adjust a disabled employee's workspace or restructuring job duties to focus on essential functions so that the employee can be reasonably expected to perform them.

Regulation Administrative interpretation promulgated by an executive branch agency (federal, state, or local) for implementation of a statute enacted by the related legislative body.

Respondeat superior Legal doctrine that holds a corporation responsible for tort law violations of its employees; also known as "vicarious liability."

RFI Request for information: Exploratory process with the purpose of collecting written information about the capabilities of prospective suppliers, service providers, or grant applicants for objective comparison.

RFP Request for proposal: Solicitation of written proposals from prospective suppliers, service providers, or grant applicants on addressing an organization's project.

RHC Rural health clinic: Outpatient clinic engaged in providing primary medical care services to Medicare and Medicaid beneficiaries in underserved, rural areas.

RHIT Registered health information technician: Credential awarded by the American Health Information Management Association verifying basic proficiency in medical records management. (Related: CPC.)

RN Registered nurse: Credential awarded by state boards of nursing for demonstrating basic proficiency to practice as a professional nurse by completing a state-approved academic program and passing the NCLEX-RN[(R)] exam.

ROI Return on investment: A ratio that determines the benefit of doing something. In financial terms, it is often calculated by dividing the net income by the cost of the capital or investment resources.

ROM Read-only memory: Form of computer data storage that cannot be easily altered or reprogrammed; referred to as nonvolatile (contents are retained when power is discontinued).

RoP Requirements of participation: (formerly conditions of participation) Centers for Medicare & Medicaid Services rules governing provider qualification for certification by Medicare and Medicaid.

RPh Registered pharmacist: Credential awarded by state boards of pharmacy for demonstrating basic proficiency to practice as a pharmacist; Pharmacists prepare and dispense prescriptions, ensure medicines and doses are correct, prevent harmful drug interactions, and counsel patients on the safe and appropriate use of their medications.

RPM Remote patient monitoring: Aging in place technology that facilitates observation of a care recipient's movement and behavior in order to inform care planning or initiate an intervention or emergency response; a wide range of products from cameras, motion detectors, and pressure-sensitive mats to personal emergency response systems (PERS).

RPS Representative payee system: Federal program under the Social Security Administration under which an appointed representative (or substitute) payee accepts disability or Social Security payments for someone who is not capable of managing their benefits and assists the beneficiary with money management and protection from financial abuse or victimization.

RUG Resource utilization group: Cost classification CMS applies in grouping a nursing facility's residents according to their clinical and functional status, as identified from data supplied by the facility's minimum data set (MDS).

RVU   Relative value unit: Metric reflecting the dollar value of physician services, determined by applying costs assigned to each current procedural terminology (CPT) code based on the respective time, skill, training, and intensity that was necessary to perform the procedure; key component of the Centers for Medicare & Medicaid Services' resource-based relative value scale (RBRVS) program.

S

SA/MH   Substance abuse and mental health: Disorders such as depression and anxiety are closely linked to substance abuse, and some substance abuse can cause prolonged psychotic reactions; one does not directly cause the other; alcohol and drugs are often used to self-medicate to battle the symptoms of mental health problems. (See also MH/SA.)

SAMHSA   Substance Abuse and Mental Health Services Administration: Federal agency under the Department of Health and Human Services charged with improving the quality and availability of treatment and rehabilitative services for reducing illness, death, disability, and the cost to society resulting from substance abuse and mental illness. https://www.samhsa.gov

Scope and severity   Centers for Medicare & Medicaid Services measures of the prevalence (scope) and seriousness (severity) of the risk posed or actual harm caused by a Medicare/Medicaid-certified long-term care provider's noncompliant practice.

SCSEP   Senior Community Service Employment Program: Federal part-time employment program for low-income persons aged 55 years or over authorized by the Older Americans Act and administered by the U.S. Department of Labor. Participants work at community or government agencies, receive the higher of the federal or state minimum wage, and may receive training that enables them to transition to other employment.

SDP   Structured day program: Individually designed services that are provided either in an outpatient, congregate setting or in the community with goal of improving or maintaining the participant's skills and ability to live as independently as possible in the community; benefits older and/or disabled adults. (Varies by state.)

SE   Supported employment: State or local government programs that provide supports and services to persons with intellectual and developmental disabilities (IDD) or serious mental illness, facilitating their employment among a variety of community-integrated work environments; designed to foster regular interaction with persons without disabilities who are not paid caregivers or service providers.

SEP   Service entry point: Location or name of the first contact made by a person seeking health or human services; also referred to as "service portal."

SFF   Special focus facility: Nursing facilities with a persistent pattern of low performance on its most three recent Centers for Medicare & Medicaid Services standard surveys and complaint surveys; subject to enhanced regulatory agency oversight until compliance is satisfactorily restored.

SFY   State fiscal year: Operating period for a state government; typically, July 1 through June 30 of the subsequent calendar year.

SGA   Southern Gerontological Association: Nonprofit professional association advocating for and representing the interests of its member health and human service professionals, educators and students, re searchers, regulators, and policy makers in 13 southern states and Washington, DC, with the shared purpose of providing the bridge between research and practice by translating and applying knowledge in the field of aging. https://southerngerontologicalsociety.org

SHIP   State Health Insurance Assistance Programs: Federally funded programs in each state (and some territories) that provide free counseling and assistance to Medicare enrollees and their families about benefits, premiums, cost sharing, enrollment windows, and appeals.

SLMB   Specified Low-Income Medicaid Beneficiary Program: Federal subsidies to state Medicaid programs to pay Medicare-B premiums for low-income Medicare beneficiaries.

SLP   Speech-language pathologist (also speech therapist): Licensed health professional who evaluates and treats treatment of speech, language, communication, voice, and swallowing disorders and related cognitive impairments.

or

Speech language pathology: Health profession specializing in the evaluation and treatment of speech, language, communication, voice, and swallowing disorders and related cognitive impairments.

SME   Subject matter expert: Person who has specific and relevant knowledge about a skill, technology, procedure, policy, or field.

SMI   Serious mental illness: Mental, behavioral, or emotional disorder resulting in serious functional impairment and substantially interfering with or limiting one or more major life activities.

SN   Skilled nursing: Services performed most safely and effectively by or under the direct supervision of a registered nurse, such as assessment and observation, medication administration, tube feeding, and wound treatments.

SNF   Skilled nursing facility: Licensed inpatient healthcare facility staffed and equipped to provide skilled nursing care and related services.

SNU   Skilled nursing unit: Distinct part of an acute care hospital licensed to provide skilled nursing care and related services.

Social Security Act   Federal law passed initially in 1935 (and amendments): Federal law that established a system of social programs to aid older adults, blind persons, dependent and disabled children, and unemployed people and to advance public health; amendments added Medicare (title XVIII) and Medicaid (title XIX).

SOD   Statement of deficiency: Report by the state's licensure and certification survey team describing any findings that allege a provider's noncompliance with applicable state regulations or Centers for Medicare & Medicaid Services requirements of participation in Medicare or Medicaid.

SPA   State plan amendment: Contractual change to a state Medicaid plan's policies, included programs or operational approach, which require approval by the Centers for Medicare & Medicaid Services.

SPALTCM   Society for Post-Acute and Long-Term Care Medicine (formerly the American Medical Directors Association): Professional society representing the interests of physicians serving as the medical director for any senior living provider, with the mission of promoting and enhancing the development of competent, compassionate, and committed medical practitioners and leaders to provide goal-centered care across all postacute and long-term care settings. https://paltc.org

SPED   Service Payments for Elderly and Disabled Program: State program that provides services for older or physically disabled adults and those who have difficulty completing tasks that enable them to live independently at home. (Varies by state.)

Spend Down   When a Medicaid applicant's assets exceed the strict financial limits set for eligibility, they can reduce their "countable resources" to the amount required to qualify by purchasing certain allowable personal items or services.

SPIA   Single-premium immediate annuity: Contract between an individual and an insurance company that pays the owner (annuitant) a guaranteed income starting almost immediately; also known as an immediate payment annuity.

SPO   Structure–processes–outcomes: Widely recognized and applied framework for evaluating health service quality introduced by Dr. Avedis Donabedian; structure provides context for care delivery, process influences interactions between care providers and recipients, and outcomes reflect the effects of services provided on the health status of patients and populations.

SSA   U.S. Social Security Administration: Federal agency that administers the Social Security retirement, survivors, and disability insurance programs, as well as the Supplemental Security Income (SSI) program for the aged, blind, and disabled.

SSBG   Social Services Block Grant: Department of Health and Human Services program that provides support to states and territories for social services directed toward achieving economic self-sufficiency; preventing or remedying neglect, abuse, or the exploitation of children and adults; preventing or reducing inappropriate institutionalization; and securing appropriate referrals for institutional care.

SSDI   Social Security Disability Insurance: Federal program administered by the Social Security Administration (SSA) that pays monthly benefits to eligible citizens who are unable to work due to a significant illness or impairment that is expected to last at least a year or to result in death within a year; eligibility and benefit levels are based on a person's accumulated Social Security credits from having worked.

SSI   Supplemental Security Income: Federal program administered by the Social Security Administration (SSA) that pays a monthly stipend to persons 65 or older, blind or disabled who are unable to work for at least 12 continuous months and who meet very specific income and resource limitations; unlike SSDI benefits, claimants do not have to work or earn credits to qualify for SSI benefits, and payments are funded through general tax revenues, not the Social Security Trust Fund.

SSN	Social Security Number: Unique numerical identifier assigned by the Social Security Administration (SSA) to U.S. citizens (and some noncitizen residents) to track their income and determine benefits; also used now for a wide range of purposes, such as to identify individuals for tax purposes, track credit record, or perform a criminal record check.
SSP	State supplemental payment: In most states, SSI recipients can also receive a supplementary payment from their state; some states only provide SSP to persons with a disability living in specified supportive settings, such as an adult care home or nursing home.
ST	Speech therapist: See SLP—speech and language therapist.
	or
	Speech therapy: See SLP—speech and language therapy.
Statute	Law enacted by the legislative branch of government; federal (Congress), state (Legislature), or local (city of county legislative body).
Statute of limitations	Period prescribed by law in which a legal action must be initiated.
STD	Short-term disability insurance: Private insurance coverage that at least partially replaces a person's income for a short period (typically 3–6 months) in the event of a medical condition that stops them from working; often provided by employers as a group policy.
Subroga-tion:	Legal right held by an insurance carrier to legally pursue a third party that caused a loss to one of its insured customers in order to recover the amount of the claim it paid. Example: If a health insurance policyholder who was injured in a traffic accident receives from their carrier $10,000 for medical treatments related to the event, that company may collect up to the same amount from the at-fault party.
T	
TANF	Temporary assistance for needy families: Federal program that provides grants to states and territories to provide families in poverty with financial assistance and related support services, such as childcare assistance, job preparation, and work assistance; replaced Aide to Families with Dependent Children (AFDC).
TB	Tuberculosis: Bacterial, infectious disease that usually affects the respiratory system and is particularly dangerous for persons with compromised immune systems.
TBI	Traumatic brain injury: Brain injury caused by an external force resulting in loss of consciousness, memory loss, dizziness, and/or confusion; can lead to long-term impairments, such as motor and sensory problems, cognitive and behavioral dysfunction, and dementia.
TCM	Targeted case management: Direct assistance provided to person's with behavioral health challenges, including problem resolution, advocacy, and referral to appropriate services.
TCU	Transitional care unit: Distinct part of a healthcare facility that provides care and services following hospitalization and before a patient is ready to return home; typically provided in rehabilitation units, long-term care hospitals, subacute or skilled nursing care facilities, or inpatient hospices.

TEFRA	Tax Equity and Fiscal Responsibility Act of 1982 (and amendments): Federal law that, in addition to providing significant changes to the tax code, mandated the development of a prospective payment methodology for Medicare reimbursement to hospitals.
TIA	Transient ischemic attack: Mild stroke that typically lasts only a few minutes; often a warning sign for a future stroke.
Title 18 (XVIII)	Medicare Law (18th amendment to Social Security Act): Federal healthcare entitlement and insurance program for older and certain disabled adults, as well as people with end-stage renal disease (ESRD). (See also Medicare.)
Title 19 (XIX)	Medicaid Law (19th amendment to Social Security Act): Jointly funded federal state health insurance program for medically indigent citizens that is administered by each participating state; largest public pay source for senior living services. (See also Medicaid.)
Tort	Intentional or unintentional civil wrong, not including a breach of contract, that causes injury to a person, their property, or reputation.
TPN	Total parenteral nutrition: Method of feeding that bypasses the gastrointestinal tract by giving a special formula through a vein when a person cannot receive nutrition by mouth.
TQM	Total quality management: See QAPI—quality assurance and performance improvement.
TRH	Transitional rehab to home: Short-term postacute stay in a health facility with the goal of a person completing rehabilitation treatment that restores enough strength and stamina for them to return home.
TSP	Thrift savings plan: Defined contribution retirement plan for federal employees, including members of the military and Congress, as well as civilian employees participating in the Federal Employees Retirement System or Civil Service Retirement System; works similarly to a private sector 401k retirement savings plan.
TTH	Transition to home: See TRH—transitional rehab to home.
TTW	Ticket to work: Federal program that offers Social Security beneficiaries with disabilities opportunities and supports needed to find and keep employment, increase their earnings through work, and reduce their reliance on cash benefits.
TTWWIA	Ticket to Work and Work Incentives Act of 1999: Federal law that provides SSI and SSDI beneficiaries work incentives and employment-related services to support their movement to financial independence.

U

UAP	University-affiliated program: Authorized by the Developmental Disabilities Assistance and Bill of Rights Act (PL 104-183), there is a UAP in every state and U.S. territory affiliated with a major research university. http://aauap.org

Unfair Labor Practice	Act of an employer or union that violates an employee's right to improve their work conditions, such as prohibiting employees to organize or join a union, retaliation toward an employee for filing a grievance, or conspiring with an employer or union to discriminate against an employee; rules are set by the National Labor Relations Board (NLRB).
Unit dose system	Packaging system utilized by an institutional pharmacy that individually encases each dose of a medication.
Upcoding	Fraudulent clinical documentation or billing codes in order to receive inflated reimbursements.
UPIN	Unique physician identification number: See NPI—national provider identifier.
UR	Utilization review: Objective, retrospective evaluation of the necessity or appropriateness, quality, effectiveness, or efficiency of medical procedures and services.
USDA	U.S. Department of Agriculture: Federal agency that provides leadership on food, agriculture, natural resources, and related issues; Rural development program offers grants and loans to senior living providers in underserved, rural communities. https://www.usda.gov and https://www.rd.usda.gov
USERRA	Uniform Services Employment and Reemployment Rights Act: Federal law that entitles a military service member to return to their civilian employment following completion of military service with the seniority, status, and pay rate that would have applied had they remained continuously working for the employer; prohibits discrimination based on present, past, or future military service.
UTI	Urinary tract infection: Infection of the kidney, ureter, bladder, or urethra.

V

VA	U.S. Department of Veterans Affairs: (Previously U.S. Veterans Administration) Federal agency that administers programs benefiting veterans and their families, offering educational opportunities and rehabilitation services, as well as providing compensation payments for disabilities or death related to military service, home loan guaranties, pensions, burials, and healthcare. https://www.va.gov
VAMC	Veterans Affairs Medical Center: One of over 150 acute care hospitals in the Veterans Health Administration's network of healthcare facilities.
Variable cost	Operating expense that fluctuates with census (i.e., food, medical supplies, and staffing).
VBP	Value-based purchasing/payment: Reimbursement model that offers financial incentives to healthcare providers for meeting certain quality and productivity performance measures. (See also pay-for-performance.)
VCID	Vascular contributions to cognitive impairment and dementia: Encompasses all types of cerebrovascular cardiovascular disease–related cognitive decline. (See also ADRD.)

VHA	Veterans Health Administration: Federal agency that operates America's largest integrated healthcare system, serving military veterans and their dependents at 1,255 healthcare facilities. https://www.va.gov/health
VISN	Veterans Integrated Service Network: System of 19 geographic service regions of the Veterans Health Administration's hospitals and healthcare facilities.
VistA	Veterans Health Information System and Technology Architecture: Electronic medical record (EMR) system designed and developed to support a high-quality medical care environment for the Veterans Health Administration (VHA).
Vital Signs	Clinical metrics that serve as a health status dashboard, typically pulse rate, blood pressure, and respiration rate; abnormalities warrant further investigation.
VNA or VNS	Visiting Nurse Association/Service: Home health agency that provides skilled nursing care and related services in a person's home.
VR	Vocational rehabilitation: Therapeutic regimen that enables a person to overcome functional, psychological, developmental, cognitive, emotional, or health disabilities or impairments to gain or regain employment.

W

Waiver	Exception to a program policy granted by a government agency to foster innovation, such as CMS approving a waiver to a state that proposes a modification to services included in or the eligibility requirements for its Medicaid program.
WC	Workers' compensation: Public insurance program that pays monetary benefits to workers who are injured or become disabled in the course of their employment.
WHO	World Health Organization: United Nations agency charged with improving the health of the world's people and preventing or controlling communicable diseases worldwide. https://www.who.int
WIA	Workforce Investment Act of 1998: Federal law that established a national employment and training program to assist eligible participants with managing their career choices through universal access to information and career-oriented services; replaced in 2014 by the Workforce Investment and Opportunity Act.
WIC	Special Supplemental Food Program for Women, Infants, and Children
WIOA	Workforce Investment and Opportunity Act of 2014: Federal law that establishes the Department of Labor programs to provide and coordinate job search, education, and training for eligible participants seeking to gain or improve their employment prospects.
WtW or W2W	Welfare-to-work: Public policy of encouraging or requiring unemployed people and those receiving state financial support to seek and secure employment, often providing job training or incentivizing employers through subsidies or favorable tax treatment.

ADDITIONAL RESOURCES

Centers for Medicare & Medicaid Services. Retrieved from https://www.cms.gov

Cornell University Legal Information Institute. Retrieved from https://www.law.cornell.edu/wex

Diffen. Retrieved from https://www.diffen.com

Invetopedia. Retrieved from https://www.investopedia.com

Kentucky Institute on Aging. (2016). *Terms and acronyms in aging services.*

Law Insider. Retrieved from https://www.lawinsider.com

McSweeney-Feld, M. H., Molinari, C., & Oetjen, R. (Eds.) (2017). *Dimensions of long-term care management: An introduction* (2nd ed.). Chicago, IL: Health Administration Press.

National Institute on Aging. Retrieved from https://www.nia.nih.gov

National Institutes of Health. Retrieved from https://www.nih.gov

Pratt, J. R. (2016). *Long-term care: Managing across the continuum* (4th ed.) Burlington, MA: Jones and Bartlett Learning.

Singh, D. (2016). *Effective management of long-term care facilities* (3rd ed.). Burlington, MA: Jones and Bartlett Learning.

University of Wisconsin – Eau Claire, Center for Health and Aging Services Excellence. (2019). *Medical terminology e-handbook.*

World Health Organization. Retrieved from https://www.who.int

+

Websites (URL links) cited in descriptions of associations and government agencies.

Index

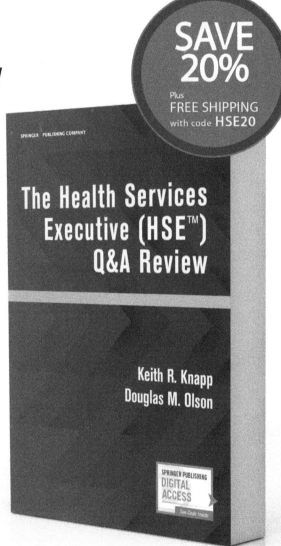
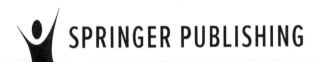